HERBAL TONIC
Therapies

HERBAL TONIC
Therapies

Daniel B. Mowrey, Ph.D.

WINGS BOOKS
New York · Avenel, New Jersey

Herbal Tonic Therapies is not intended as medical advice. Its intent is solely informational and educational. Please consult a health professional should the need for one be indicated.

This 1996 edition is published by Wings Books, a division of Random House Value Publishing, Inc., 40 Engelhard Avenue, Avenel, New Jersey 07001, by arrangement with Keats Publishing, Inc.

Wings Books and colophon are trademarks of Random House Value Publishing, Inc.

Random House
New York • Toronto • London • Sydney • Auckland

Printed and bound in the United States of America

Library of Congress Cataloging–in–Publication Data

Mowrey, Daniel B., 1944–
Herbal tonic therapies / Daniel B. Mowrey.
p. cm.
Originally published: New Canaan, Conn. : Keats Pub., c1993.
ISBN 0–517–18241–6
1. Herbs–Therapeutic use. 2. Tonics (Medicinal preparations) I. Title.
[RM666.H33M675   1996]
615'.321–dc20   96–14551
                                                          CIP

1 2 3 4 5 6 7 8

ACKNOWLEDGMENTS

Thanks to my colleagues at APRL: Evan Bybee and Dennis Gay, who supported me with great patience during the writing of this book. Special gratitude to my wife, Vickie, for her untiring emotional support and patience and for assuming many of the parenting tasks that rightfully should have been mine. Thank you, children, for not complaining too loudly at the frequent absences of your father while laboring over this manuscript.

Finally, thanks to Nathan Keats and Don Bensen and the diligent and meticulous staff at Keat Publishing for laboring to make this book presentable.

A Note on Latin Designations

Botanical names are most often given in Latin, and are commonly followed by a designation denoting the taxonomic system used in naming the plant. These designations are usually presented in the form of the initials or some abbreviation of the name of the system originator. Some of the more common designations are L., Gaert. and Roscoe (e.g., *Zingiber officinale Roscoe*). In this book, these designations are only given when necessary to clearly identify the plant in question.

In addition, the term *spp.* is occasionally used in place of the second term of the botanical name (e.g. *Smilax spp.*); this term is an abbreviation for "species," and means that several members of that particular plant family (e.g. *Smilax*) may be used in common and/or official preparations. The implication is that the different common species would generally be similar in action.

Other Latin terms that occur frequently in the book are:

in vivo = in live organisms

in vitro = in Petri dishes, test tubes, isolated tissue, etc.

in situ = on specific, exposed tissue in live organisms

A Note on APRL Certification

During the last two years, much of the activity at American Phytotherapy Research Laboratory (APRL) has been directed toward reviewing herbal products currently on the shelves of health food stores and circulating across the country on the wings of a multiplicity of multilevel network marketing companies. This review has been geared toward first establishing an array of categories for herbal materials: laxatives, colon cleansers, blood purifiers, PMS-related products, sedatives, energizers, thermogenesis agents, and so forth; then toward determining what characteristics products must have to belong to any given category, and finally toward reviewing individual products to determine whether or not they qualify for inclusion in any given category. Criteria include safety standards and compliance with known and accepted efficacy indications.

The criteria for establishing a product as a tonic are set forth in this book. Any product submitted to APRL that meets these criteria is eligible to receive APRL certification. The same can be said of products that qualify in any other category, although these formulas need not be limited to the tonics discussed in this book. No drug claims are made in the certification, but the APRL seal of certification may appear on the label of the product. These confidential analyses are performed in the hope of raising the quality control standards of the industry. We expect that products failing to comply with APRL standards will be reformulated by the manufacturer to come into compliance. This is, admittedly, a small effort to rectify a huge problem. It is surprising how many herbal products for sale today have been thrown together by marketing managers, advertising types, entrepreneurs with no background in herbal medicine, and others with little or no experience in combining plant materials for impact on health and nutrition.

Look for this seal on herbal products to make sure you are getting what you pay for:

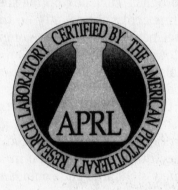

Contents

HERBAL TONIC
Therapies

Introduction: Herbal Tonic Therapies

🌿 What do you think of when someone uses the term "spring tonic"? For most people that term conjures up images of folk remedies, intended for heaven only knows what. For most of us, the tonic is a quaint and outmoded concept that has no place in modern orthodox medicine. Yet, the tonic concept has a firm historical and scientific foundation and represents an approach to health that even moderns would do well to follow. How many of us can say that modern medicine has fulfilled all of our needs for health, vigor and vitality? Or do we sense some gaping holes in the medical model, missing data concerning how to stay well and healthy? Within the vacuum of orthodox ignorance about what makes a person well and whole, it may just be that the concept of the herbal tonic, seemingly beyond the grasp of the modern approach, holds some keys to good health.

The main purpose of this book is to introduce, or reintroduce, to the American public the concept of a "tonic." I believe that very few Americans really know what a tonic is, and even fewer understand what role tonics can play in health. Should the book fail to convert a great number of people to the ranks of dedicated tonic users, it should at least increase the relative level of awareness about these valuable herbs, and may even spark some controversy among practicing herbalists.

Herbal tonics were a major part of earlier schools of medicine. I contend that they are equally useful today. They are appropriate for consumption by everyone, everywhere; furthermore, they embody a medical concept that is actually more advanced than the one from which current drugs are derived. Viewed properly, the tonic is really a space-age concept, one that has yet to be discovered by the developers of orthodox medicines. Perhaps tonics will always be exclusively associated with herbal medicine; it is plain fact that only whole plant materials have been empirically endowed with tonic properties; no synthetic drugs, and not even isolated plant constituents, can lay claim to being tonics.

Definition: A tonic is any substance that balances the biochemical and physiological events that comprise body systems. Instead of "balance," we could use words like "homeostasis" or "equilibrium" or even "normality." The events of any given body system have an optimum operating range that is regulated through dozens of feedback loops to help keep various push-pull tendencies of the events in balance. Balance means health or wellness, so illness may be viewed as a lack in balance, a departure from the optimum state in any given body system. A substance that tends to maintain the optimum state or that moves a system back toward the optimum state is a tonic. An example of a tonic herb for the vascular system is ginseng (*Panax ginseng* or *Eleutherococcus senticosis*), which can either raise or lower blood pressure, depending on the circumstances. The behavior of the whole plant is a composite of these opposing forces, with the force most needed by the body at the time of consumption predominating.

Very few people, including herbalists, understand what a tonic is. Very little attention is paid to the subject. Some herbalists believe that a tonic is anything that strengthens the body, yet they don't have a clear idea as to what "strengthen" means. It could mean "make stronger," or "make healthier," or "make more stable," or "optimize." In practice, herbalists tend to use the word "strengthen" to denote any of those concepts, yet they are by no means identical.

The ambiguity of the term "strengthen" has led to some fuzziness in our attempts to conceptualize the notion of balance. It is like the difference between a body-builder (the weight lifter type) and a gymnast. Outwardly, the body-builder appears to be stronger than the gymnast, and in some ways he is. Yet the gymnast usually has greater agility, and possesses overall a more balanced physique. The body-builder has pushed his body to the limits of human endurance. It is a unidirectional effort. Everything the body builder does has the aim of increasing bulk and muscle. The gymnast has other worries. If he lets the bulk get too large, it interferes with his motion. He must keep the muscles strong, but long. That requires a more balanced approach: if any muscle group gets too large or dominant, he must reverse the process that created that condition until balance is restored, a balance between stretching and bulking. The *optimal* state is one of balance of all processes underlying a body system or function.

BIDIRECTIONALITY

This definition of a tonic clearly excludes the notion of "making stronger" by pushing the body in one direction only. A particular nontonic drug or herb, designed to enhance the function of the immune system for example, might stimulate the production of white blood cells. Goldenseal is an example of this kind of action. Administered to an ailing patient, it would increase T-cell activity and enhance other immunological functions. That's all it would "know" how to do. It would not be able to recognize the difference between a body deficient in white blood cells and one that had too many white blood cells. Its action is *uni*directional. It carries but one signal to the body system: in this example, to produce more white blood cells. This overstimulation could lead to severe imbalances. And it is unlikely that such an agent would be able to address the problem of an over-reactive immune system, as, for example, in a person with an allergy.

In contrast, an immunotonic is an herb that restores balance to immune system function no matter which way it departs from normal. It is *bi*directional. Echinacea is such an herb. It is capable of sending either of two possibly contradictory signals to the body. Thus, in a person with depressed white blood cell counts, echinacea sends a signal to the body to begin producing more white blood cells, and in a person with too many white blood cells, it decelerates the production of white blood cells. It stabilizes the histamine-containing mast cell membrane in persons with hay fever rather than sensitizing it, as do many immune-enhancers.

The concept of a tonic sounds strange to modern ears. We simply have not made room in our medical or nutritional agendas for a concept of a substance that restores balance. This will change as the medical community begins to realize that many modern plagues may be prevented, and even treated, by maintaining optimum health in all body systems. Such a reorientation of thought demands that much less emphasis be placed on finding and killing "germs," and much more on increasing the body systems' natural defense and restorative powers. The concept of the herbal tonic will be a signpost for the new research.

In summary, tonics do not overstimulate the body. They are bidirectional, capable of both increasing and decreasing the activity of body processes. Herbs whose action is bidirectional (or, sometimes, multidirectional) are called tonics. As far as I know, there are no bidirectional drugs, nor is any effort currently under way to invent any. In order to conceptualize drugs as materials for restoring balance, the scientific world will have to undergo a total paradigm shift; and it is not ready to do that.

Conditions of bidirectionality

A legitimate question is: By what virtue do tonic herbs acquire bidirectionality? Bidirectionality presupposes at least two conditions. One, bidirectional agents, or tonics, must contain *op-*

posing groups of constituents, each group capable of sending a different signal, of facilitating reactions in the body opposite (or complementary) to those promoted by the other group. For example, group A would increase white blood cell proliferation, and group B would depress white blood cell production.

Two, the body must be capable of *recognizing and utilizing the correct group of constituents* required to restore and/or maintain functional balance or homeostasis. That is, if the tonic is sending multiple signals, the body must correctly choose the "right" signal.

The first condition, that of opposing groups of constituents, has been the subject of validation ever since science first began to investigate medicinal plants. In the case of ginseng, two fractions, Rb ginsenosides and Rg ginsenosides, have been isolated that possess opposing actions on blood pressure. Similarly, ginseng contains components that raise blood sugar level and substances that lower blood sugar level. Notice that an extract of ginseng that contained only one set of constituents would not behave like a tonic, since the ability to restore balance would be missing. Yet the main goal of medical science, even of some herbalists, is to remove certain constituents from tonic plants in order to create a more powerful drug. The tonic action is thereby lost.

Another example is licorice root. The medical literature is replete with cases of so-called licorice toxicity. Almost all of these cases, however, involve licorice *extract*, as would be found in licorice candy. Some people experience an inexplicable craving for licorice candy (a phenomenon which itself warrants investigation); but, after consuming large amounts over a period of several days or weeks, some of these individuals develop an imbalance in blood chemistry that leads to excessive sodium retention and potassium excretion. Serious, though totally reversible, hypertension may result. The ingestion of whole licorice *root* does not produce this syndrome. The extract, retaining the principle glycyrrhizin but lacking other important substances, becomes incapable of tonic action. As a whole plant, licorice is one of the best tonic plants in the world.

One of the best researched tonic plants is echinacea. This

plant has remarkable actions on the immune system, bringing virtually every aspect of immune function under tonic control. Echinacea *extracts*, however, have been found to have a unidirectional effect on autoimmune and immunosuppressive activity.

As mentioned previously, medical science has not considered developing drugs with tonic actions like these. Drugs tend to be simple agents, unidirectional but powerful, with multiple side effects. But even nontonic medicinal herbs tend to be complex multifaceted substances with dozens of actions, usually mild in nature, with few if any side effects. At the risk of redundancy, I repeat that the concept of a tonic, though of ancient origin, is very advanced relative to current medical orthodoxy; and whole herb materials, due to their complexity, are presently the only agents capable of being tonics.

The second condition demanded by bidirectionality, that the body be able to exclude all signals but the one it needs, or to be able to recognize and utilize only those components it currently requires, is admittedly a more troublesome idea. Yet, the concept is not without precedent; it is related to the idea of *specific hunger*, a valid nutritional notion. Specific hunger refers to the well-established propensity of animals and humans to select from a menu foods containing nutrients the body is lacking at the time. Some sort of interaction between body and mind causes, for example, a selection of fruits instead of candy when a vitamin C deficiency has been created. In a related manner, the metabolic processes of people who ingest nutritional supplements will normally retain those individual vitamins and minerals the body needs at the time and evacuate the rest.

Thus there is some basis for our second condition. In ways not understood at present, the body does utilize needed nutrients while rejecting others. Let's say a person with low blood pressure (hypotension) ingests some high-quality ginseng containing components involved in raising his blood pressure and other components associated with lowering it. Apparently, the feedback mechanisms that tend to raise or restore blood pressure to normal limits when it gets too low have become sensitized and therefore react quickly to hypertensive substances in ginseng, while the feedback mechanisms that tend to lower blood pressure have become unreactive or inhibited by some complementary aspect of the feedback process and react slowly if at all to the hypotensive components in the ginseng.

More on homeostasis

The body contains thousands of metabolic and functional systems that are controlled homeostatically. The body recognizes a range of values that are within normal limits; when values exceed those limits, mechanisms come into play that help restore normality—balance—homeostasis. Usually this takes the form of negative feedback, just like the thermostat in your home. As the furnace responds to the thermostat, these biological processes turn on and turn off in response to changing cellular circumstances. The whole purpose is to maintain things within critical limits. Examples of such processes include: Blood pH, extra-and intra-cellular levels of electrolytes, buffers, blood pressure, heart rate, blood sugar levels, white blood cell/red blood cell ratios, platelet counts, insulin secretion, corticosteroid regulation, neurotransmitter levels, gastric pH, and liver enzymes. There are thousands of others.

STRESS: THE LOSS OF BALANCE

There are probably as many causes of imbalance as there are physiological processes. But in the modern world (and probably the ancient) there is one major factor at the bottom of almost all departures from homeostasis: *stress.* A stressor, according to this view, can be defined as anything that tends to push the body processes away from balance.

All illness is precipitated by stress. Stress comes in many guises: physical, chemical, emotional, mental, even spiritual. What's more, the body's ability to handle stress can be stressed. Much of the junk food we eat, the drugs we take, our chronic lack of exercise, and poor sleeping habits lower the body's ability

to deal effectively with stress. On top of this are the predispositions we are born with, i.e., genetic factors. These tend to dictate
which of our body systems will be most susceptible to disease,
that is, which systems can or cannot handle stress. It may be one
person's heart, another's immune system, yet another's digestive
system or nervous system.

In the final analysis we are all susceptible, to one degree
or another, to the effects of stress. We all get sick, some of us
more often and more seriously than others. One of the main
functions of a tonic is to increase the body's resistance to stress.
My observation is that it takes a lot more stress to move a person
off center who is using tonics on a daily basis.

FUNCTIONAL BODY SYSTEMS:
AN ORGANIZATIONAL NECESSITY

To understand and predict how tonic herbs affect the body,
it is practical to treat the body as a group of systems. The remaining chapters of this book are organized around a series of
body systems, by which are meant groups of organs and tissues
that all serve the purpose of fulfilling the different life-sustaining
functions of the body. Dividing the body into systems is done for
practical purposes, and not as an exercise in explicating absolute
truth. There are no hard and fast rules for combining organs and
tissues into a system, though one would certainly always include
the heart in the cardiovascular system and the sexual organs in
the reproductive system.

In other instances, the situation is not as clear-cut. To what
system(s), for example, does the liver belong? It could belong to
the excretory system, together with the bladder, kidneys, and
skin. Or it could be part of the immune system, since a great
deal of immunity depends upon a properly functioning liver. Or
it could be part of the digestive system, along with the gallbladder
and small intestine (plus others), since it is the source of digestive
bile. Most of the endocrine glands play distinct roles in several
systems; therefore, to speak of an endocrine system makes little

functional sense. And certain functional groups do not seem like systems at all. The excretory system, for example, is apparently designed to rid the body of wastes, but what do exhaling and producing sweat, urine and feces have in common? Also, parts of some systems are not obviously associated with those systems. For instance, the adrenal glands play a major role in nervous system function, but the relationship is not immediately obvious. Finally, some systems seem to be parts of other systems. The immune system, for example, is actually a part of every other system.

Defining systems is, therefore, a rather complex undertaking involving very few absolutes and lots of maybes; it is an enterprise one should not engage in without a great deal of flexible thinking and a bit of a sense of humor.

At times of *general* malaise it may seem proper to treat the body as a whole; usually, however, we can match a particular set of symptoms with one, two or more systems that are out of balance and require restoration. A good deal of research has demonstrated that certain herbs are better suited than others for restoring balance in any given system.

Treating illness, preventing imbalances and maintaining wellness, then, becomes a matter of matching herbs to systems to symptoms. Like this:

Symptom A is a manifestation of an imbalance
in system D and E,
for which herbs Z, O, and M
are normally used to restore balance.

OTHER QUALIFICATIONS

To be regarded as true tonics, herbs must meet requirements additional to those already mentioned, which very few of the world's plants do. Tonic herbs must be free of side effects, and generally free of all contraindications. In addition, tonics should be consumable in small amounts on a daily basis without demonstrating habituation or tolerance. Herbs usually acquire the status of tonic only after centuries of empirical use by people all over the world. There are major tonics and minor tonics, i.e., herbs that affect several systems and broad functional areas, and herbs whose action is limited to a narrow range of physiological processes. The discussion in this book will be focused mainly on the major tonic herbs, though a few minor types have been included.

Finally, some tonic herbs may not be tonic if ingested in large amounts over a period of several days. Echinacea, or purple coneflower, a native herb of North America, is a major immuno-tonic when used in small doses over extended periods of time. But it may also be used in large doses to treat acute infections, particularly those of the throat. For reasons unknown at this time, echinacea in high doses tends to promote continued immune system stimulation rather than balanced immune function. This is not true of most tonics. Most behave like yerba maté, a more or less whole body tonic; yerba maté, even in large amounts, continues to promote balance in many body systems without overstimulating any system.

COMBINATIONS OF TONICS

Without a clear understanding of what a tonic herb is and what it does and doesn't do, it is very difficult to assemble effective tonic combinations. One who believes that tonic herbs exert a simple, unidirectional influence on some physiological processes will not think twice about combining them with herbs whose action is truly unidirectional. This results in a combination skewed in its effects away from normalizing to the extent to which the bidirectional action of the tonic components is overcome by the unidirectional action of the nontonic herbs. Tonic herbs are, as a rule, somewhat milder and more delicate in action than nontonic herbs (hence their low degree of side effects and high degree of tolerance); it is natural, then, that the presence of nontonic herbs in a combination could result in the complete suppression of the action of any tonic herbs present.

It has been the experience of this author that pure tonic combinations of herbs are extremely hard to find. Furthermore, very few people know enough about herbs to identify tonic blends with any degree of confidence or accuracy. One purpose of this book is to put a knowledge of several herbal tonics within the reader's grasp—once a person has a knowledge of tonics, he will find it very easy to combine them freely, and use them with confidence.

SUMMARY

Tonics are substances provided by nature for the repair and maintenance of normal physiology. They restore balance to body systems that are under stress. They do not stress the body themselves, but are suitable for long-term use in small doses. Tonics differ from most medicinal substances in being bidirectional in action, i.e., in correcting illness-promoting imbalances independent of the particular nature of the causes. To meet this demand, tonics contain a wide variety of active principles, many of which may possess opposing actions on a particular body system. Yet, rather than cancel each other out, these actions are brought into play only where and when needed, now one, then the other, responding to the changing state of the organism. A system in balance is a healthy system. A system under stress, from environmental, psychological, microbial, or other sources, is teetering toward an imbalance one way or another. The consumption of tonics is a fail-safe approach to restoring balance and promoting the overall health of the body.

In conclusion, since nobody manages to go through this life in a perfect state of balance, everyone can benefit from the use of the right choice of herbal tonic. It is a worry-free method for handling life's daily challenges to health and happiness. Then, while you experience the rejuvenation of body systems through the action of tonic herbs, you will be in a good position to expand your understanding and knowledge of herbal medicine in general. The study of tonics is a good starting point for the novice herbalist. Herbs are, in general, safer than multivitamins and perhaps more beneficial, and tonic herbs are the safest and most beneficial of all.

Here is a list of the body systems and the herbs discussed in this book.

IMMUNE SYSTEM

Echinacea
Ginseng (American, Asian, Siberian)
Gotu kola
Astragalus
Schizandra
Licorice root
Lapacho

CARDIOVASCULAR SYSTEM

Hawthorn berry
Butcher's broom
Cayenne
Kelp
Turmeric
Rosemary
Motherwort
Valerian root
Centella
Bilberry

NERVOUS SYSTEM

Valerian root
Ginkgo biloba
Hops
Peppermint
Chamomile
Lime blossoms
Passion flower
Balm

DIGESTIVE SYSTEM

Milk thistle
Artichoke
Dandelion root
Gentian root
Ginger root
Turmeric
Schizandra

MUSCULOSKELETAL SYSTEM

Horsetail grass
Alfalfa
Devil's claw
Yarrow
Saw palmetto
Wild yam
Sarsaparilla
Echinacea
Licorice root

FEMALE SYSTEM

Ginger
Dong quai

Black haw
Cramp bark
Valerian root
Fenugreek
Red raspberry
Licorice root
Black cohosh
Vitex agnus castus

MALE SYSTEM

Pygeum
Saw palmetto
Sarsaparilla
Damiana
Muira puama
Siberian ginseng

WHOLE BODY SYSTEM

Yerba maté
Echinacea
Astragalus
Licorice root
Stillingia
Korean ginseng
Siberian ginseng
Chaparral
Hawthorn
Sarsaparilla
Aloe vera
Ginger root
Lapacho

A NOTE ON STANDARDIZATION

Over the years it has become necessary to standardize several herbs in order to insure that they contain enough active material to be biologically active. The technology for standardizing has become very complex and sometimes subject to the whims of the technocrats with nothing better to do than mess around with Mother Nature. Standardization has thus become a double-edged sword; on the one hand it results in the maintenance of high standards of purity and excellence of research, but, it can also be misused to create extracts that do not reflect the true nature of the original plant materials.

Modern medicine has, of course, raised the art of isolating and synthesizing plant constituents to a level at which the new substances bear no relationship to the original plant material, and usually produce severely greater risks of overdose, toxicity, and dangerous interactions. But one gets the impression from some of today's research literature on plants that supposedly enlightened herbal researchers, armed with million-dollar labs, are trying to duplicate the efforts of the medical establishment as fast as possible.

It is the position of this author that standardized plant materials are good, but only when kept within the context of whole plant preparations. The balance in tonic herbs, especially, can be destroyed by improper manufacturing and standardization practices. Many of the plants recommended in this book are most active if obtained as standardized, or Guaranteed Potency, herbs. But only if care has been taken to place the extract back into whole herb material. Guaranteed Potency Herbs are not only standardized, they are subjected to extensive safety and efficacy tests to make sure the delicate balances are not disturbed (for more on Guaranteed Potency Herbs, see my book on the subject*).

One hopes that the standardization process insures the presence of all constituents, or at least those responsible for the bidirectional action of the plant. However, the extract should always be placed in a base of whole herbs to increase the probability that other important constituents are present to at least some small degree. In that way, should the body not need the primary constituents, it can still choose some of the minor, non-standardized, constituents to help maintain its health.

HOW TO USE HERBAL TONICS

Very few tonic herbs are used directly from the field. Typically, as with most herbs, some processing is necessary to get them into a form the body can utilize quickly, easily and effectively. All of the tonic herbs discussed in this book can be found in a powdered form in capsules. One to three capsules per day

---

Next Generation Herbal Medicine, Keats Publishing, Inc., 1990.

is an average number to consume, but at times, several more than that may be indicated. Generally, the more severe the symptoms, the more capsules can be consumed. This rule does not apply to those tonic herbs that are found as Guaranteed Potency Herbs: bilberry, centella, butcher's broom, echinacea, ginseng, pygeum, turmeric and valerian root. These preparations are specifically designed to be used at the rate of 1-2 capsules per day; consuming more is generally of little benefit. The same herbs in non-guaranteed potency form can be used in greater quantities, even if they are found as standardized extracts in the range of 4:1 or lower.

Some herbal tonics, such as licorice root, can be chewed after simply cleansing and drying, but might be more satisfying and effective if ground and encapsulated. Others, such as ginger root and turmeric, may be eaten on some occasions in form of culinary herbs or spices, but taken in capsule form on other occasions. Ginger root should be encapsulated if used to treat nausea.

Tinctures and liquid extracts are alternative forms and work well for immediate absorption. Fast-acting means fast-depleting; for sustained but moderate activity, the capsule is best. Echinacea, for example, may be ingested in powdered, encapsulated form for daily maintenance of balance, but can be consumed in liquid extract or tincture form in case of a sore throat or sudden cold, for fast penetration of the tissues in the mouth and throat.

Almost all tonic herbs can be purchased in health food stores, but some brands will have a more extensive list of products than others. Guaranteed potency herbs are the hardest to find, but fortunately, there are a few companies in the United States that are importing these and include them in their product lines.

Teas of yerba maté, licorice root, red raspberry leaves and several other tonics are excellent, pleasant-tasting beverages, and can be utilized in that form to good effect. You may want to experiment a bit to find out which plants are best suited for your own taste buds. Most people avoid teas made from valerian root, gentian root, milk thistle, echinacea and other tonic herbs, though in the 19th century almost all of these plants were gagged down in tea form as medicinal agents. Hence the saying: "If it tastes bad, it must be good for you."

CHAPTER ONE

The Immune System

❧ The term *immune system* is applied to all structures and processes that are involved in defeating the attempts of environmental forces to overrun, destroy or gain control of any part of our body. The environment can be simply defined as everything in the world that is not you. This book, the dirt under your fingernails, the food you eat, the wastes you produce, the air you breathe, a sliver under the skin, the bacteria in your intestines, your dental fillings, the soap you wash with, are all "not-you." Most of the environment that touches you, even when it lives on or in you, is tolerated by your body indefinitely, and some of that environment, such as the bacteria in your intestines that help process food, may actually be beneficial. But things go wrong, "not-you" stuff invades blood and other cells, "friendly" bacteria suddenly turn against you. When that happens, the body automatically initiates a series of reactions to neutralize and eliminate the threat. An immune response is initiated.

Errors may occur and limitations may be seen in the operation of the immune system. It may not react fast enough or strongly enough, and you get a cold or flu. It may not react at all, as in the case of AIDS. It may react too strongly. And it may turn against you, destroying "you" tissues as if they were being processed as "not-you." It may be "faked out" by clever viruses and bacteria such as in malaria.

Herbal medicine includes hundreds of plant materials that can be used to regulate or modulate the functions of the immune system. This chapter will be limited to the immunotonics. These are herbs that restore balance to the immune system, whether it is depleted or overactive. The tonic herbs are well tolerated by the body and can be used on a daily basis, especially during the flu and cold seasons. Immunotonics increase the vigor of the immune response, prolong its action, and help shut it down when it gets out of control.

Herbal medicine has always recognized that the blood could be contaminated with toxins and wastes, and therefore be need of "purification." Modern concepts of the immune system are based on the fact that all "not-you" materials in the blood and other tissues in the body bear structures that do not occur in the body's own cells, structures that can be distinguished by elements of the immune system. These elements include an intricate network of blood, enzymes, cells and hormones, more complex than anything dreamt up by pre-20th century man.

IN THE BEGINNING: ROLE OF THE BONE MARROW

The immune system originates primarily in the bone marrow where white blood cells, or leukocytes, are produced. The bone marrow also produces two other major components of the blood, red blood cells and platelets. The white blood cells are the backbone of the immune system. They circulate in the bloodstream and in the lymphatic system. The lymphatic system has been traditionally ignored by medicine, yet it is involved in an extraordinary number of vital bodily processes, and will be discussed later. There are more than a billion leukocytes in the human body.

Some leukocytes mature in the bone marrow, and some are sent on their way to the thymus gland and mature there. There are two major divisions of leukocytes: phagocytes, or feeding cells, and lymphocytes. In addition there is another key element to the immune system, called the complement system. We will discuss each of these divisions in turn.

PHAGOCYTES, OR FEEDING CELLS

White blood cells called phagocytes are responsible for the nonspecific or general defense of the body. "Nonspecific" means that they attack anything that is not-you. Phagocytes are so named because they generally work by eating their targets, a process called phagocytosis, described later in this section. Phagocytes may attack living organisms such as bacteria, or they may attack a variety of nonliving matter, such as pollen or wastes. They are responsible for keeping the blood and tissues clean. Phagocytes are generally divided into two groups, macrophages and microphages.

Macrophages, or monocytes

These are large cells that feed on everything in their way. They can be considered as the armored units or tanks of the immune system. Even indigestible material can come to an end inside macrophages. It has been observed that some macrophages will tend to preserve some material indefinitely. A swallowed particle finds itself inside what is called a phagosome, a kind of stomach in the cell. Here powerful enzymes (lysosomes) are secreted that devour the material.

Macrophages begin life as monocytes, smaller cells that are like recruits; they become macrophages as the body signals that it needs them. Macrophages can reproduce fairly rapidly, but in pitched battle there are rarely enough of these powerful white blood cells to compensate for the rapidity of a bacterial invasion.

Macrogphages are found in the linings of the lungs and intestines and in almost all mucous membranes of the body. During an infection, macrophages produce substances that prompt bone marrow to produce more monocytes and other white blood cells.

Microphages, or granulocytes

Microphages, as the name implies, are much smaller than macrophages. They are called granulocytes because they contain tiny granules, or sacks in the cell fluid that are filled with potent chemicals and active protein enzymes used to digest and destroy foreign materials. Granulocytes are usually divided into three categories, neutrophils, basophils, and eosinophils.

Neutrophils These are small, nimble phagocytes that are very numerous. These are the "grunts," the foot soldiers of the immune system. They mature fully in the bone marrow, which stores billions of them in tiny sinuses in the marrow. Neutrophils swarm into newly infected or injured areas and hold the lines of defense until the macrophages arrive.

Basophils Because they are relatively immobile, waiting for invaders to brush against them before they are activated, basophils have been likened to mines; in the presence of aliens, they erupt and spew out chemicals that trigger inflammation: vessels swell, other proteins seal off the area, trapping the enemy, and walls of vessels grow sticky.

A basophil resembles a stationary regular tissue cell called the mast cell which mediates the inflammatory response. Mast cells are distributed throughout body tissues. When allergens contact mast cells, the mast cells burst like basophils and dump into the bloodstream chemicals which cause blood vessels to expand and their walls to become leaky, allowing blood to pour out into the tissues, resulting in inflammation; they can also cause asthma attacks. The surface of the mast cell has receptors which attract antibodies. When, in a hypersensitive person, allergens become attached to the antibodies, the mast cell receives a signal to burst.

Eosinophils These white blood cells specialize in devouring complexes of allergens and their reactive molecules (antibodies) in the immune system. They are small and fast-moving, performing blitzkrieg operations. Eosinophils and their targets are what form most of the pus we see in a wound. They are important for initial containment of invading pathogens, and they leave a chemical "scent," a trail that reinforcing immune system components can follow to the battle site.

LYMPHOCYTES

These leukocytes are responsible for the *specific* resistance of the body to disease. Through extremely complex processes, the body learns, even before birth, to recognize families of pathogens and to deal with them effectively. Lymphocytes, so named because of their close relationship to the lymphatic system, are necessary because feeding cells are limited in what they can do. Being nonspecific in nature, feeding cells can be easily deceived by certain kinds of microorganisms. For example, certain bacteria and all viruses are impervious to feeding cells. Pneumococci use cell walls to defend themselves against phagocytes; they cannot be ingested without the aid of antibodies. Some bacteria and all viruses hide inside the body's own cells, enemy troops disguised in friendly uniforms. Situations such as these demand the services of the Green Berets, the special commandos—the lymphocytes. Other terms come to mind: assassins with magic bullets, Tomahawk guided missiles. Lymphocytes have the ability to react specifically against substances foreign to the body.

T Lymphocytes Early in life the thymus is unquestionably the most important organ of the immune system. It is here that about half of the lymphocytes, the T lymphocytes, or T cells, mature and receive valuable training about possible kinds of environmental agents, or antigens, that you will encounter during your life. Several types of T-cells have been discovered, each with its own special action.

Killer cells T cells called killer cells are like a personalized poison gas to invading troops, so to speak. Each killer cell is programmed to poison just one specific antigen, to kill the body's own cells that contain foreign antigens, and to kill tumor cells. Killer cells can be viewed as special combat units in the war against cancer. They hunt through tissues like bloodhounds in search of cells that have separated from an original cancer and are spreading throughout the body. They also have the job of finding cells in which viruses, parasites or bacteria may be hiding.

Helper cells Helper T cells comprise the defense staff unit of the body's immune army. They are the command and control center, directing troop operations, communicating with feeding cells via hormonelike chemical signals transmitted throughout the body, rousing the defenses. Helper cells also help regulate the activities of other T cells.

Suppressor cells Suppressor cells are one of the body's built-in feedback regulating mechanisms for preventing the immune system from overactivity. As the enemy forces diminish, the suppressor cells begin commanding the immune troops to cease fire.

Memory cells Every encounter with an antigen produces T cells whose purpose is to remember for decades to come the disease-producing substance which invaded the body. This information is stored in the vast databases deep within the immune system. When a substance with a mug shot and description stored in the database shows up again, the memory cells guarantee a rapid antibody response to combat it. When this happens, we are immune. Memory cells are the key to vaccination.

B-Lymphocytes

The second important class of lymphocyte, the B cell, matures and is "trained" for battle in lymphoid tissue mainly in adult bone marrow and around the intestines and in fetal liver.

B cells are precursors of plasma cells that eventually produce antibodies. Following training, B cells are dispersed throughout the body. They may circulate in the blood or reside in lymph nodes for years waiting for enemy antigens to come along.

B cells are often activated by macrophages, and under the regulating eye of helper T cells, stimulated to produce millions of antibodies in a very brief time.

Plasma cells　Plasma cells are what B cells turn into in the presence of stimulation from antigens. The function of plasma cells is simple: produce antibodies as fast as possible.

Antibodies or Immunoglobulin　Produced by plasma cells, antibodies are the guided missiles of the immune system. Technically, antibodies are proteins, not cells. They are sometimes called gamma globulins. There are nine different varieties: Immunoglobulin M, IgG1, IgG2, IgG3, IgG4, IgA1, IgA2, IgD, IgE.

Antibodies sabotage viruses' weapons, neutralizing the parts of the virus surface that enable the virus to hook onto and enter a host cell; with attachment sites blocked, the virus is no longer able to invade and take over the host cell.

Antibodies not only neutralize a virus's ability to attach itself to a cell, but also contribute to making the invader more susceptible to the scavenger white cells.

Lymphokines

Lymphocytes and phagocytes release potent humoral substances called lymphokines and monokines respectively, which increase the fury of microscopic combat. They produce interferon, attract all kinds of white cells to the site of an infection or injury, stimulate and activate macrophages, activate additional T cells that are keyed to the invading organism, signal white blood cells to remain at the site of the battle, increase the permeability of capillary walls, help to transform T cell response into a widespread reaction throughout the body, and so forth. Lymphokine activity can be regulated by hormones secreted by the adrenal glands (glucocorticoids), providing a bridge between the immune system and the key central nervous system regulatory mechanisms (e.g., the adrenal-pituitary-hypothalamic axis). Some of the more familiar lymphokines are interleukins, interferons, lymphotoxins, tumor necrosis factor, B cell growth and differentiation factor, colony stimulating factors, and antigen-specific factors.

COMPLEMENT SYSTEM

The complement system is a series of proteins that circulate in the blood waiting for a signal to go into action. They are the minutemen, and they are a deadly lot, skilled in the art of cellular sabotage. The mission of the complement system is to increase the efficiency of antibodies and feeding cells. They also have their own capacity to destroy bacteria by blowing fatal holes in them. The complement system is activated when an antibody finds a bacterium and becomes bound to its antigens. One after another the complement proteins flock to the bacterium and assemble one on top of the other, like the pieces of a puzzle that when completed turns into a powerful drill. The drill bores holes in the cell membrane, resulting in pressurized influx of fluid that causes the cell to swell until it bursts and dies.

Complement proteins also adhere to bacteria already labeled with antibody, marking them and increasing their appeal to any phagocytes in the neighborhood.

ANTIGENS AND ANTIBODIES

An antigen is any substance that elicits a response from a B or T cell: substances on the surface of bacteria, viruses, parasites, yeasts, toxins, living and dead tissue, organic and inorganic debris, and innumerable other substances. Antigens provide the initial signals for all immune reactions, which cease once the antigen has been neutralized, such as when an infection has been resolved. The action of the immune system as a whole can thus be viewed as being directed toward eliminating antigens and producing feedback regulation of continued immune response.

Mature B cells have receptors that can bind to irritants or antigens on the surface of microorganisms and other invaders. Every lymphocyte can bind to only one antigen; this is its specific property. There are around a billion lymphocytes, which among them are specific for about a million different antigens. These can easily take care of all foreign substances we meet in the course of our lives. A healthy immune system knows at the moment of birth how to discover and neutralize foreign substances.

When an antigen encounters a B cell specific for it, the two are bound together and, at that moment, a signal is sent to the nucleus of the lymphocyte: "Produce antibodies against this antigen!" In response, the B cell divides and divides again and again, producing a multitude of clones. The clones are transformed into plasma cells that begin to manufacture antibodies, a couple of thousand per minute, 120,000 per hour. The combined output of all the clones can number in the billions before long. The antibodies neutralize the microorganism and prevent it from entering cells. The process continues until no more antigens can be found.

PHAGOCYTOSIS

When a phagocytic cell encounters an antigen bound to something like a bacterium, it envelops the entire complex, isolates it in a cytoplasmic cavity called a phagosome, and empties enzymes and corrosive hydrogen peroxide into the "stomach" that break down the antigen/bacterium into its constituent parts.

Phagocytes obey three basic signals that keep them from eating everything, including you. The first signal is roughness— only particles with rough texture will automatically be engulfed.

Almost all antigens have rough edges, while your body's own cells are normally smooth. The second signal is ionic charge—only positively charged particles will be engulfed. Most of the body's own substances have a negative charge; this electrical attraction is almost instantaneous. The third signal is chemical—due to the presence of antibodies that mark the invader as a victim.

THE LYMPHATIC SYSTEM

The lymphatic system is a kind of secondary circulatory system, complementing the blood stream. White blood cells, food, fluid and oxygen flow through the bloodstream on their way to the body's tissues. But to reach individual cells, substances in the blood must leave the capillaries and enter the interstitial fluid—the clear, colorless liquid that surrounds and bathes all body cells. The lymph system is composed of millions of tiny ducts or channels in all parts of the body. The fluid flows toward the chest, from which it will eventually flow back into the blood and be transported to the liver and kidneys. Unlike the blood, there is no pump provided to insure lymph flow. Flow depends upon the normal contraction of large muscles and of smooth muscle in the walls of the lymphatic vessels. One-way valves allow lymph to be pumped through the system in only one direction. The rate of flow can be modulated by a variety of nervous, hormonal and physical influences. In the chest, large lymphatic ducts empty into veins near the heart. Fluid, proteins, and lymphocytes pour into the bloodstream, completing a long circuit from the blood, through the tissues, along the lymphatic pathway, and back to the blood.

Immune responses are usually initiated in specific lymphatic organs. Antigens entering any particular part of the body will be transported via macrophages to the appropriate local lymphatic organ where the immune response is initiated. Most lymphocytes constantly recirculate from the blood through secondary lymphoid organs (spleen, lymph nodes, mucosal lymphatic tissues) and back into the bloodstream.

DISORDERS OF THE IMMUNE SYSTEM

Inflammation

Inflammation is a common experience for most of us. It is the body's natural way of responding to a localized invasion of microorganisms or some other form of injury to tissues. Most authorities divide the inflammatory response into four stages: heat, swelling, reddening and pain.

The immune system has several lines of defense. The first is composed of the skin, the mucous membranes and the stomach. The skin and mucous membranes also offer good mechanical protection against most organisms in the respiratory tract. The first line of defense also includes chemical weapons such as sweat and sebum that contain bacterial inhibitors. In addition, the respiratory organs, the intestines and sexual organs are covered with secretions containing lysozyme, an enzyme that can dissolve and break down bacterial protein coverings, thereby denuding the bacteria and robbing them of life. Another form of chemical warfare occurs against bacteria on food entering the stomach, which are annihilated by acid gastric juice.

This first line of defense maintains an uneasy equilibrium with the outside world which can be upset in a number of ways. We can be simultaneously attacked by large quantities of vigorous—or virulent—germs, or we may experience weakened resistance when our defenses have been denied adequate nutrition, or subjected to illness, mental disturbance, stress or advanced age. Breakdowns also occur when the skin is scratched, bruised or punctured. When the first line of defense fails, microorganisms starving on the surface are suddenly exposed to a cornucopia of goodies. Then we have to call upon the second line of defense, a more complicated mechanism and one that carries with it some unpleasant but necessary symptoms.

This second line of defense can be viewed as a series of events that closely resemble a military operation. The enemy attacks, the alarm sounds, the defense forces strike back, the infected or injured area is barricaded, reinforcements are summoned, the enemy is wiped out (hopefully), and order is reestablished.

Injured tissues release substances that sound the alarm to the immune system and pave the way for a counterassault by divisions of white blood cells. The circulation increases and the body broadens the immune system's access routes. The affected area reddens and becomes immersed in blood containing millions of immunological agents, including phagocytes and lymphocytes. As more blood arrives from the interior of the body, where the temperature is 37° centigrade or 98.6° Fahrenheit, to the skin which is 5 to 10° C. cooler, it raises the temperature of the wound area—produces fever. This increases enzymatic activity. Fever may also be a result of rapidly increased production of vast quantities of white blood cells in the bone marrow. Aching bones and sore throat (from lymph node swelling) are signs that the body is busy fighting back. Another heat/fever process is also taking place. During the first phases of an immune response, the body's metabolism generally accelerates, the blood vessels near the surface of the skin constrict, decreasing circulation and heat loss there and driving more of the heated blood to the internal parts of the body. "Chill" is a rough measure of the differential between the higher setting in the brain and the body's lower temperature. Shivering is a rhythmic, involuntary muscle contraction that is the body's attempt to generate heat through motion in order to counteract chills. Chills are generally followed by a changeover to hot skin and a new series of discomforts: dry throat, intense thirst, etc.

Until the end of the 19th century, physicians considered moderate fever beneficial, a natural response to infection that counteracted the disease. Then opinion suddenly reversed, a change that coincided with the discovery of drugs capable of reducing fever. Now the pendulum of medical opinion seems to be swinging back in favor of letting a moderate fever run its course. Medical intervention is reserved for dangerous, life-threatening fevers. The usual herbal approach is to speed up the fever-producing mechanisms while attempting to reduce unpleasant symptoms.

The swelling part of the inflammatory response is due to the accumulation of white blood cells, blood plasma, wastes, and clotting material in the tissues. Pain is the result of nerve endings responding to growing pressure caused by the swelling.

In due course reinforcements arrive at the site of inflammation—large feeding cells, macrophages. As the macrophages begin carrying off antigens and debris of the battle to lymph nodes, we enter the third stage of the war. Lymph nodes are the fortresses of the immune system. During an infection they are a hive of activity. At this point almost all defense forces of the body have been mobilized. Antibodies and killer cells throng the blood and deliver the *coup de grace* to all microorganisms they find.

A postmilitary phase occurs during the healing of the wound. This is an automatic process in which there are thirteen coagulation factors involved. Under the scab, macrophages complete the cleaning up and new skin grows.

Bacterial infection

Occasionally we are assailed by harmful and dangerous bacteria present in the air, in food and in skin wounds. Some of these bacteria are extremely pathogenic. One thousand grams of the toxin produced by the botulin bacterium could, in theory, destroy the entire human race.

The concept of lines of defense is helpful in understanding our natural resistance to bacteria. The first line of defense is mechanical and chemical. Localized defense, the second line, involves the action of phagocytosis and the complement factors.

Some bacteria have adapted themselves to us. They may have a cell surface on which it is difficult for the feeding cell to get a grip; they simply slide out of the way. Others may have a cell surface that is resistant to the shower of enzymes in the phagosome; they hibernate, emerging later to cause infection.

Viral infection

Viruses are truly unique chemical entities. They are the simplest of all existing life forms—a cluster of genes (DNA and RNA) in a protein sheath, composed partly of nonliving and partly of living matter. They are found in water, air, soil, dust, foods; we can inhale them, ingest them or absorb them through our skin. A virus is so simple a structure as to make even its classification as a living body debatable. It has no mechanism for movement, no internal method of reproduction, no equipment for ingesting or digesting food. It cannot even qualify as a cell. It needs a host, yet is even fussy about the host—each kind of virus will accept only one general kind of cell. Viral genes destroy the genes of the host cell and take over control; eventually, the whole apparatus of the cell is working to support the virus. In 12 hours a single virus can produce progeny of astronomical proportions: 10 to the 73rd power, or 10 followed by 73 zeroes. In 12 hours an unprepared immune system cannot possibly mobilize sufficient defensive weaponry: we get sick. To ward off viruses the body needs all the help it can get.

The body's only general defense against viruses is interferon (specific defense can arise from immunity due to a previous infection). Interferon prevents the virus from reproducing and the cell from dividing.

Virtually everyone is infected with *Herpes simplex* virus early in childhood and carries it in a dormant form throughout life; at times of illness, stress and other strains—even too much sun in the spring—the powers of the immune system are reduced and the herpes virus has its chance. Watery blisters or sores around the mouth and nose form.

Acquired immunodeficiency syndrome

Perhaps the most critical epidemic currently facing the world, AIDS is thought to be caused by a virus, or a family of viruses, that dramatically lowers the ability of the body to respond to infection from all other sources. A simple fungal growth in the mouth may end in death. The body seems totally unable to deal effectively with the worsening course of events.

AIDS is associated with the presence of a virus called HIV, or human immunodeficiency virus, but the presence of HIV does not by itself guarantee that full-blown AIDS will soon develop;

it might lie dormant for years and then suddenly erupt into activity. What other factors are involved in AIDS are currently unknown. But certain lifestyle traits have clearly been shown to bear a close association with the acquisition of AIDS: male homosexuality and bisexuality, promiscuity, use of IV drugs, and sexual contact with persons with AIDS or at risk for AIDS. Hemophiliacs and recipients of blood transfusions before transfused blood was screened for AIDS are also at risk. It seems that every year we are discovering additional ways the AIDS virus is being transmitted. It is suspected that there may even be an airborne variety.

Infections that occur as the result of the presence of AIDS are called secondary infections. Among the most prevalent of these are parasitic pneumonia and Kaposi's sarcoma, a cancer of the connective tissues. Other common infectious agents include Epstein-Barr virus, *Herpes simplex* viruses, *Herpes zoster, Papovavirus, Mycobacterium tuberculosis, Salmonella, Candida albicans* and *Toxoplasma gondii.*

The HIV is particularly insidious because it attacks the cells of the immune system itself. It enters the T cell and is able to escape detection by the macrophages at least long enough to replicate a few billion times before bursting the cell and swarming out to find new T cells in which to continue the process. Eventually the population of effective T cells is reduced to a level at which it can no longer respond to pathogenic invasions.

Parasitic infections

Conditions resulting from parasitic infection, such as malaria, trypanosomiasis (sleeping sickness), and schistosomiasis (bilharzia), affect hundreds of millions of people in the Third World. Other examples of common parasites include many kinds of intestinal worms, blood-sucking insects, and insect-borne microorganisms. The relationships between host and parasitic organisms are often extremely complex, as the following examples testify.

Malaria is caused by a microscopic protozoan called a plasmodium. Plasmodia depend on two hosts: the Anopheles mosquito and man. They infest a mosquito's salivary glands and are transferred to man when the mosquito bites. Then parasites penetrate the man's red blood cells, which burst when the plasmodia divide and the result is an attack of fever.

African sleeping sickness is caused by protozoa called trypanosomes, which are transmitted to man by the tsetse fly. Some parasites are adapted to coexisting with human immune defenses, and plasmodia have a suppressive effect on the immune system. Some protozoa can change their coats, as it were—altering their surface antigens—and even doing so several times, playing hide and seek with the immune system. When a host has developed antibodies against the first antigen layer, it is replaced by a new one, with new irritant properties, and so on. Schistosomes can "kidnap" protective antigens from the host organism's cells, thus evading the immune system's attacks. Many protozoa also allow the macrophages to swallow them, continuing their reproduction undisturbed inside their captors. Parasites are masters at deceiving the immune system.

Cancer

Occasionally a cell eludes normal control factors and begins a course of uncontrolled division, the products of which become a lump, and begin to spread through the blood and lymph into other parts of the body. The frequency of cancer would be considerably higher if the body did not possess methods of suppressing unruly cells. The immune system can employ interferon, antibodies, complement, and above all killer cells, in the fight. T cells are the body's principal weapon of defense against tumors.

One of the mysteries of the immune system is its failure to attack all tumor cells. Some deviants seem to be totally ignored by immunoregulators. When that happens, cancer continues, either because these tumor cells lack the antigen properties that normally provoke immune response or because suppressor cells curb the activity of killer cells before they have done their job.

It is becoming increasingly obvious that the role of the immune system in cancer prevention includes the ability to neutralize the activity of free radicals generated during normal metabolism and absorbed from the environment. Free radicals are highly reactive molecules or fragments of molecules that contain one or more unpaired electrons. They roam freely through the body, seeking out tissues to combine with and render morbid. As well as destroying tissues outright, they increase the probability that affected cells will become susceptible to a wide range of infections and diseases such as cancer. The body's main line of defense against free radicals is its supply of free radical scavengers, collectively known as antioxidants, since most free radicals are oxygen radicals. Unfortunately, in the modern world, sources of free radicals from polluted air, food and water have put a great strain on the body's natural antioxidative mechanisms. When our capacity to resist has been exceeded, cell membranes are exposed to the onslaught of free radicals, which combine with lipid portions of the membranes and greatly lower their resistance to nearby carcinogenic pathogens.

Disorders of the respiratory tract

Some of the most potent germs enter the body via the respiratory tract. The proper functioning of the immune system in this part of the body is therefore of great importance. Protection of the body in the respiratory tract is afforded by first-line-of-defense mechanical and chemical devices as well as second- and third-level immune devices.

In the upper airway, the nose is extremely important. Short thick hairs inside the nostril filter out large airborne particles, while smaller particles are trapped by the mucous membranes in the nasal cavity and most of the airway down into the lungs.

There are accessories to the nasal machine:

1) *Sinuses*—cavities in the skull that protect the brain from blows to the front of the head. The sinuses are lined with mucous membranes which serve as a supplemental source of mucus that

drains into the nasal cavity through narrow canals. Colds or allergic reactions can make the membranes swell and block the canals, building up pressure and causing severe headaches.

2) The *pharynx*, which is lined with an abundance of mucous membranes that warm, moisturize and cleanse the air. Myriads of white blood cells are to be found in these tissues. Most airborne antigens come to rest in these tissues and are neutralized by the immune system.

3) The *tonsils* and 4) the *adenoids*, some of the body's largest lymph nodes, located in the pharynx, which can be infected by viruses and bacteria.

5) The *eustachian tubes*, designed to equalize pressure, but during colds, infection can spread up into the tubes and cause earaches.

6) The *larynx* or voice box, that can become inflamed, leading to hoarseness or loss of voice.

The respiratory tract has two more mechanical protective devices, coughing and sneezing.

Certain illnesses assail the defense system of the respiratory tract; chronic inflammations of the respiratory tract—bronchitis and sinusitis—are the result, often with further complications.

A more common consequence is hypersensitivity, or allergies. Allergies are caused by airborne particles that set off a kind of false alarm, causing the immune system to react against itself. These particles are known as allergens; they include pollen, dander, foodstuffs, exhaust fumes and cigarette smoke.

The most common allergy is hay fever, characterized by itching nose and swollen, watering eyes. Asthma is the most troublesome of all allergic ailments; narrow air passages swell, making it difficult to breathe.

The common cold

Remember that all viruses are keyed to one specific kind of tissue. Cold viruses are keyed to attach themselves to the cells of the mucous membranes of the respiratory tract. They destroy these cells one by one, but because the cells are located in tissue that is itself relatively superficial, the loss of these cells brings discomfort but seldom anything worse. There are over 200 different cold viruses known.

The first troubleshooter to arrive at the scene of a viral bridgehead is the nonspecific substance interferon. After several days of holding the line in a lonely battle, the cells and interferon begin to get some help from another nonspecific defense, inflammation, often accompanied by mildly sore throat. These discomforts are usually the first sign that one has a cold, but in fact by this time the cold is already there. The cold sufferer feels just fine while under vicious infectious attack, becomes aware of the cold first when the body is already in the process of curing it, and feels the most miserable during the period his immune system is making him well.

Like the common cold, influenza is strictly a respiratory infection, affecting nose, throat and chest. The terms "stomach flu" and "intestinal flu" are misnomers. These ailments are caused by intestinal viruses or bacteria and are unrelated to true influenza and rarely accompany it in adults; but children often have gastrointestinal upset as a side effect of flu.

While colds are confined to the upper respiratory tract structures such as the nose and throat, classic flu infects the lower respiratory tract also, as well as affecting the entire body and prostrating its victims for days with fever and widespread muscle aches. An influenza virus behaves much like other respiratory viruses. The extent of infection depends primarily on the victim's own supply of antibodies, but is also a function of one's general state of health.

The overactive immune system

In spite of all the inherent checks and balances, the immune process sometimes errs and turns on the body's own cells. Allergies such as eczema, hay fever and asthma are one result. Autoimmune disease is another, more serious outcome.

Autoimmune disease may affect whole organs, or parts of them. Chronic inflammation of the thyroid (Hashimoto's syndrome) is an example of how antibodies attack a vital organ. In insulin-dependent juvenile diabetes, antibodies attack the insulin-producing cell islands of the pancreas. We do not fully understand how such civil wars start. There is good evidence that they may sometimes be initiated by a virus infection.

Systemic lupus erythematosus, multiple sclerosis, myasthenia gravis (weakness of the muscles) and rheumatoid arthritis may also have autoimmune components.

The causal chain of events is probably highly complex. But the end result is sobering: the immune system itself creates disease instead of protecting the body against it.

THE RESPIRATORY SYSTEM

This book lacks a chapter devoted to the respiratory system. This is not an oversight, but an acknowledgement of the difficulties encountered in defining what a respiratory tonic should do, and then finding herbs that meet the criteria decided upon. The reader will have noticed that the respiratory system was mentioned several times in this chapter. That is because it is directly affected by many of the normal immune processes. Much of the "tonifying" of the respiratory system comes, therefore, as a result of a healthy immune system.

Nevertheless, there should be herbs whose application, in small amounts, on a daily basis, would act as tonics directly on the organs of respiration. Such herbs would tend to keep the lungs open and healthy, so that breathing capacity is maximized. But is there such a thing as chronic overbreathing? Tonic respiratory herbs should keep the mucous membranes healthy and able to secrete optimum amounts of mucus to protect the epithelial cells of the organs of respiration. But again, is there such a thing as too much mucus? And if there is, isn't it a sign of healthy processes, either as the result of fighting infection, or soothing inflammation? What would a tonic action be in relation to mucous membranes? These questions and others have yet to be worked out. Until they are, it is difficult, if not impossible to compile a list of respiratory tonic herbs.

In fact, the most benefical of herbs for the respiratory system are ma huang (*Ephedra sinica*) and lobelia (*Lobelia inflata*), both of which are definitely not tonics. Beyond these two respiratory stimulants, there are various other herbs that can affect the quality of respiration, including **mucilaginous** plants such as marshmallow (*Althea officinalis*), coltsfoot (*Tussilago farfara*), mullein (*Verbascum sp.*), and plantain (*Plantago lanceolata*); **expectorant** plants such as ipecacuanha (*Cephaelis ipecacuanha*), primula (*Primula sp.*), elecampane (*Inula helenium*), and hyssop (*Hyssopus officinalis*); **antibiotic** plants such as thyme (*Thymus vulgaris*), and butterbur (*Petasites sp.*); and **cough remedies** such as poppy (*Papaver somniferum*) derivatives and celandine (*Chelidonium majus*).

In addition to the above, there is one other herb that deserves special recognition in regards to its effects on the respiratory system: **Khella (*Ammi visnaga*).** The use of khella in the Middle East dates back centuries, but its use in modern times began in the early 1930s, when it was observed in controlled settings to relax the spasm in muscle fibers induced by kidney stones and thereby reduce the pain. Subsequently, it was found to dilate coronary arteries and thereby reduce the pain of angina pectoris.

The vasodilatory action of khella was eventually investigated by a team of researchers from England who were looking for a good drug for angina. Since khella, in doses strong enough to affect angina, had unpleasant though not dangerous side effects such as nausea and vomiting, these investigators were looking for ways to detoxify the plant. Quite accidentally they discovered that a certain constituent of the plant, khellin, had antiasthma actions. More specifically, it seemed to *prevent* asthma attacks. Further research revealed that the best preparation was simply two chromone molecules hooked together across an oxygen bridge. The chromone molecule was nothing more than the basic molecule of khellin itself. The new substance was called cromolyn sodium.

These findings have spawned a whole era of research on khella, which has culminated in the production of numerous drugs containing cromolyn sodium which have been found to be very effective in preventing asthma attacks, especially in childhood asthma. They are also effective in preventing allergic reactions, hay fever, and related conditions. The operative word is "preventing," since the substance has little effect on an asthma or allergic attack already under way.

The interest in cromolyn has had a good effect on research and development of khella itself. In recent years several European and some American manufacturers have begun producing khella extracts and homeopathic products which purport to be able to prevent asthma and hay fever without the typical side effects of whole plant material.

Khella is not a tonic substance, but its importance in respiratory ailments is strong enough to merit consideration in this chapter. Ma huang and lobelia are very good respiratory stimulants and bronchodilators, and have found widespread application in the treatment of respiratory ailments, especially coughs (lobelia) and asthma (ma huang). But they are also not tonics. Perhaps in some future edition of this book, we will be in a better position to evaluate tonic respiratory herbs.

HERBAL TONICS FOR THE IMMUNE SYSTEM

There is perhaps no other system of the body except the sympathetic nervous system for which tonic herbs are better suited. Because the immune system has to be maintained in a state of readiness, we have to pay some attention to strengthening it. We have to be careful not to overstimulate it, because too many white blood cells can be just as damaging as too few under the proper circumstances. Herbal tonics normalize and balance practically every aspect of immune system function. Plus they can be applied in the case of infection or dysfunction to help speed up and intensify the immune response. Alternatively, they can be applied in case of an overactive immune system to shut down an allergic response. As our understanding of the immune system increases we will probably begin to discover many new and exciting ways that immunotonics increase the health and vitality of human beings.

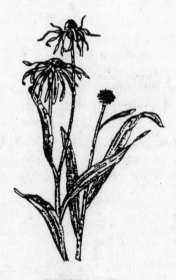

ECHINACEA

ECHINACEA
(Echinacea purpurea, E. angustifolia)

Echinacea is probably the most famous of all immunotonics. During the last 30 years, this herb has been subjected to an incredible amount of research.

The American Indians introduced echinacea to the settlers

during the formative years of modern America. Physicians quickly adopted the herb and during the years of widespread infectious epidemics became quite skilled in its application. By the first decade of the 20th century echinacea had become one of the mainstays of American medicine. Remember that the notion of an immune system was only tenuous at that time. Nevertheless, early researchers accomplished much painstaking work with the use of the microscope, the most advanced medical tool of the time. They were able to determine that echinacea had a profound effect on the number and kind of blood cells in the bloodstream. They found, for example, that the herb tended to keep the ratio of red to white blood cells within acceptable limits, that it promoted the production of white blood cells when the percentage was too low, and that it suppressed the production of white blood cells when there were more of these than was healthy. In this manner, echinacea behaved like a tonic. Not only that, but they determined, without knowing much about the individual leukocytes involved, that echinacea seemed to increase the rate of phagocytosis; what they observed was improved waste elimination and increased destruction of foreign substances in the blood.

Eclectic physicians during this era used echinacea to treat typhoid, meningitis, malaria, diphtheria, severe boils, carbuncles, abscesses of all kinds, reptile and insect bites, cholera, cancer, syphilis, tetanus, impetigo and even rabies. We don't worry much about most of those in our modern society. We can use echinacea to treat much milder kinds of things. It is amazing that early physicians had any luck at all treating such severe conditions, yet old medical journals contain enough positive case histories to convince even the most jaded observer that some degree of protection and curative power was imparted by the herb. Reports resound with enthusiasm and excitement because here was something that really worked.

Interest in echinacea waned in this country with the advent of antibiotics and the ascendancy of the American Medical Association, which successfully routed its traditionally-oriented competitors. We are now witnessing renewed interest in echinacea and herbal medicine in general because we appear to have reached a plateau in orthodox medicine. Immune deficiency and autoimmune disorders, including cancer, AIDS, arthritis, Epstein-Barr virus and others have a lot of people worried. Since plants have historically been the starting place for all new classes of orthodox drugs, it is not surprising that herbal immunomodulators currently hold the most promise for effective therapy.

The frequent administration of small amounts of echinacea seems to impart a degree of immunity against common infectious and allergic ailments. Large daily doses are used to treat an acute infection. The herb increases the body's natural nonspecific resistance to disease, affects the function of phagocytosis, the specific portion of the immune system, and has an immunosuppressive action in some cases.

In the case of nonspecific resistance, echinacea has been shown to improve the first lines of defense, the mechanical resistance, by inhibiting an enzyme called hyaluronidase that can be stimulated by pathogens to break apart the connective tissue surrounding body cells (known as the reticuloendothelial system, or RES). Once the integrity of the RES connective tissues has been compromised, germs can easily latch onto body cells and begin the progressive destruction of cells known as infection. Substances in echinacea combine with receptors on hyaluronidase and neutralize it. The result is a temporary improvement in the skin's and other tissues' ability to keep an army of germs at bay.[1,2]

Interestingly, a mechanism very similar to the action of hyaluronidase on the RES has been proposed as a possible cause of rheumatism and tumor formation.[3]

Echinacea constituents also appear to be involved in the regrowth of connective tissue that has been destroyed during infection. The stimulation of the healing process drastically reduces the degree to which sensitive and vulnerable body cells are exposed to an environment laden with dangerous microorganisms.[4]

During the period of infection, when the body is running low on its resources, echinacea has been found to have a strong and direct activating force on the body's ability to produce macrophages and speed them to the area of infection. Echinacea also stimulates the production of the lymphokines.[5-9]

Another way that echinacea augments immune system function is its ability to exhibit a significant lethal effect on certain forms of cancerous tissue. USDA researchers have isolated a tumor-inhibiting principle in the essential oil of echinacea. The herb may do this by stimulating the production of key lymphocytes which in turn trigger the activation of cells such as the natural killer cells that destroy the cancer.[10]

Factors have been identified in echinacea that both encourage the inflammatory process and inhibit it. Since raising body temperature is a critical part of the body's efforts to mobilize its immune system shock troops, and since an inappropriate release of too much histamine and related inflammatory substances can be counterproductive, perhaps this research has stumbled upon another tonic action of echinacea. The results should also be a warning for all scientists studying this herb to use caution when extrapolating the action of any given set of constituents to the action of the whole plant.[11]

The complement system is also affected by echinacea. Echinacea at first depresses the level of certain complement factors, and then greatly increases the level of those materials. This action would greatly increase the body's specific and non-specific resistance to disease.[12,13]

In 1978, in Germany, another startling aspect of echinacea biochemistry was discovered. Researchers discovered that echinacea behaves in a manner similar to interferon, either by stimulating the production of interferon or by acquiring some of its characteristics. No one knows for sure how it works, but the findings are consistent: in the presence of echinacea, viruses (and bacteria for that matter) had a greatly diminished capacity for causing infections. That means the herb either prevents the virus from reproducing or actively competes with the virus for the receptor sites on the body cells to which the virus is naturally attracted, thereby preventing viruses from gaining entrance to the cell in the first place. Either way, the results are the same—reduced infection![14]

Finally, we must mention that echinacea possesses a mild

but direct antibiotic property of its own against certain kinds of microorganisms, including the notorious *strep* and *staph* germs that plague modern man.[15, 16]

SAFETY DATA

One of the advantages of using echinacea to enhance these aspects of the immune response is that, unlike most drugs used for that purpose, echinacea is completely nontoxic; it is perfectly safe to use every day. Yet a lot of rhetoric is directed at the question of how much and how often and there are as many answers as there are experts. Some people maintain that it should be used in small doses, intermittently. Other experts believe it can be used daily. Everyone agrees that in the case of an ongoing infection large amounts of both powdered encapsulated herb as well as liquid extract should be administered. The best rule of thumb would be to use small daily or semi-daily amounts for immune system enhancement, and larger acute doses during the course of an ongoing infection, cold, flu or fever.

REFERENCES

1. Bonadeo, I., Bottazi, G., and Lavazza, M. "Echinacin B: polisaccaride attivo dell' echiniacea." *Riv. Ital. Essenze Profumi*, 53, 281, 1971.
2. Buesing, K.H. "Inhibition by hyaluronidase by echinacin." *Arzneimittel-Forschung*, 2, 467–469, 1952.
3. Buesing, K.H. "Hyaluronidasehemmung als wirkungsmechanismus einiger therapeutish nuzbarer naturstoffe." *Arzneimittel-Forschung*, 5(6), 320–322, 1955.
4. Tuennerhoff, F.K. and Schwabe, H.K. "Untersuchungen am menschen und am tier ueber den einfluss von echinacea-konzentraten auf de kuesnstliche bindergewebsbildung nach fi-

brin-implantationen." *Arzneimittel-Forschung,* 6(6), 330–334, 1956.

5. Kuhn, O. "Euchinacea and phagocytosis." *Arzneimittel-Forschung,* 3, 194–200, 1953.

6. Stimpel, M., Proksch, A. et al. "Macrophage activation and induction of macrophage cytotoxicity by purified polysaccharide fractions from the plant echinace purpurea." *Infection and Immunity,* 46(3), 845–849, 1984.

7. Wagner, H. et al. "Immunstimulierend wirkende polysaccaride (heteroglykane) aus hoeheren pflanzen." *Arzneimittel-Forschung,* 34, 659–661, 1984.

8. Wagner, H. and Proksch, A. "Isolation of polysaccharide with immunostimulating activity from echinacea purpurea." *Inter. Conf. Chemm. Biotechn. Biol. Act. Nat. Prod. (Proceedings),* Antanasova, B., ed., 3(1), 200–202, 1981.

9. Wagner, H. and Proksch, A. "An immunostimulating active principle from echinacea purpurea." *Zeitschrift fuer Angewandte Phytotherapie,* 2(5), 166–168, 171, 1981.

10. Voaden, D.J. and Jacobson, M. "Tumor-inhibitors III. Identification and synthesis of an oncolytic hydrocarbon from American coneflower roots." *Jour. Med. Chem.,* 15(6), 619–623, 1972.

11. Tragini, E. et al. "Evidence from two classic irritation tests for an anti-inflammatory action of a natural extract, echinacin B." *Food and Chemical Tox.,* 23(2), 317–319, 1985

12. Buesing, H.K. "Die beeinflussung des properdin-spiegels durch extrakte aus echinacea purpurea bei kaninchen." *Zhurnal der Immunitaetsforschung,* 115, 169–176, 1958.

13. Buesing, K.H. "The effect of extracts of echinacea purpurea on the properdin levels in rabbits." *Zhurnal der Immunitaetsforschung,* 115, 169–176, 1958.

14. Wacker, A. and Hilbig, A. "Virus inhibition by echinacea purpurea." *Planta Medica,* 33, 89–102, 1978.

15. Becker, V.H. "Against snakebites and influenza; use and components of echinacea angustifolia and e. purpurea." *Deutsche Apotheker Zeitung,* 122(45), 2020–2023, 1982.

16. Stoll, A. et al. "Antibacterial substances II. Isolation and constitution of echinocoside, a glycoside from the roots of echina-

cea angustifolia." *Helvetic Chimica Acta*, 33, 1877–1893, 1950.

17. Sicha, J., Hubik, J., Dusek, J. "Substances in the echinaceae family which are potential antiviral agents and immunostimulants." *Cesk. Farm.*, 38(9), 424–428, 1989.

GINSENG: CHINESE, AMERICAN, SIBERIAN
(Panax ginseng, P. quinquifolium, Eleutherococcus senticosis)

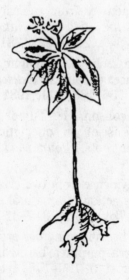

GINSENG

All the major species of plants that go by the name of ginseng have similar effects on the immune system. What goes for one pretty much goes for all. However, the present discussion will be limited to the Chinese ginseng (Panax ginseng); a full discussion of Siberian ginseng (Eleutherococcus senticosis) will be found in the section on the nervous system.

When it comes to the effects of ginseng on the immune system, it has become customary to write and talk in terms of the Russian-born adaptogen hypothesis which was developed to describe the properties of Siberian ginseng. Though basically a circular concept, it does serve the purpose of organizing many apparently contradictory findings on all species of ginseng. For instance, panax ginseng exerts both hypotensive and hypertensive actions. Similar effects are seen with blood sugar. Other characteristics of ginseng are exhibited in unhealthy organisms but are absent in normal healthy organisms.

These findings are not really contradictory, but rather suggest that the guiding principle behind the action of ginseng is to act as a tonic, to "restore" normality and increase the nonspecific resistance of organisms to disease or any other 'change' away from "normal" health. Thereby ginseng increases a person's ability to 'adapt' to changes in the environment. Although the Russians coined the term "adaptogen" to create a market specifically for Siberian ginseng, the term has come to refer to any herb or other agent that increases the ability to adapt. The term is now used to refer to dozens of plants, many of which act in a manner that only vaguely resembles ginseng.

In the chapter on the nervous system I suggest that Hans Selye's model of stress adaptation may be more generally acceptable. Briefly, his model of adaptation, which predates the adaptogenic hypothesis by many years, describes the entire relationship between the nervous system and glands of the body, and the way these interact with environmental, nutritional and physiological stressors ultimately to reduce the impact of stresses on the body. Any substance, including ginseng, that affects those interrelationships will ultimately affect the immune system or the body's ability to deal with stress.

Ginseng affects the body in a very positive manner. It appears to affect the immune control centers of the central nervous system, directly and indirectly through adrenocortical hormones, toning, increasing output, or simply restoring equilibrium. Blood parameters, including pressure, glucose levels, insulin levels and white blood cell count, are stabilized, i.e., reduced or raised as needed in order to restore homeostasis. Analgesic, antipyretic and anti-inflammatory action will occur when needed. Ginseng either thins the blood or increases its clotting ability depending on circumstances. DNA, protein and lipid synthesis are all stimulated when cellular feedback mechanisms signal a state of deficiency. Studies from around the world show that ginseng strengthens the heart, stimulates recovery from surgery and debilitating infectious disease, and otherwise helps people to overcome the effects of physiological stress.

Currently, most plant scientists agree that the immune-stimulating effects of ginseng are the result of a composite of plant chemical groups. We know that the Rb1 and Rg1 ginseno-side fractions carry a good deal of activity, and we know also that these fractions must be present in a certain ratio (Rg1/Rb1 must be no less than 0.5). What we don't know is how important other fractions are, what synergy exists among constituents, what long-term effects are the result of whole root, and what difference all these things make if important stuff is left behind when certain fractions of the plant are extracted.

Space will not permit a comprehensive discussion of the properties of ginseng. The following list summarizes the kind of results appearing in medical journals around the world. But you should use some degree of caution in accepting any of these effects at face value. Much ginseng research is flawed and contradictory. It will take several more years for a clear, valid and reliable picture of ginseng action to emerge. Meanwhile, use the herb as desired, and find out for yourself what it will do.

Properties of Panax Ginseng

1. Stimulation of RNA, DNA and protein synthesis in the liver.[14]
2. Ability to prevent alcohol intoxication.[15]
3. Anticancer properties as shown in studies on animals, humans, and cell cultures.[5, 9]
4. Ability to strengthen the heart muscle and protect it against myocardial ischemia and infarction.[29-31]
5. Ability to reverse essential hypertension.[23, 27]
6. Ability to influence almost all liver functions.[3, 4, 11]
7. Immune-enhancing action, including the stimulation of phagocytosis, modification of interleukin responses, strengthening of the reticuloendothelial system.[9, 18-20, 22, 23]

8. Ability to neutralize free radicals through antioxidative action.[27]

9. Normalizing action on blood sugar levels depending on need.[11]

10. Ulcer-protective properties.[11]

11. Central nervous system depressant or stimulant, anticonvulsant, analgesic, tranquilizing.[15]

12. Antifatigue action in animals and humans.[8, 16, 18, 19]

13. Antipyretic or fever-reducing action.[3, 5, 15]

14. Increases synthesis of cholesterol in liver; enhances cholesterol breakdown into other steroids.[12, 13]

15. Enhances mental acuity and intellectual performance.[1, 2, 7]

16. Stimulates adrenal glands and the entire adreno-hypothalamic-pituitary axis.[16, 20, 21, 24–27]

17. Ability to lower or raise red blood cell count depending on need.[28]

18. Ability to lower or raise white blood cell count depending on need.[15]

19. Healing action on corneal deformities.[15]

20. Has distinct antitoxic action against a wide range of toxins, including radiation, heavy metals and airborne pollutants.[3–5, 15]

21. Has some positive effect on male sterility.[3, 4, 6, 15]

22. Has some female estrogenic hormonal activity.[3, 4, 6, 15]

23. Exerts antipsychotic effects.[6, 7, 15]

SAFETY DATA

Ginseng has a very low toxicity. Some reports appearing in medical journals would have you believe otherwise; but those reports are, unfortunately, in the worst tradition of medical research, not the best. The so-called "ginseng abuse syndrome" hypothesis is based on poorly conducted observations in a highly skewed population whose members bear no similarity to the millions of regular ginseng users throughout the rest of the country and world. Nevertheless, all authorities on ginseng recommend, usually more for philosophical than biological reasons, that the herb be used in moderation. Also, the use of standardized ginseng extracts has the potential of creating imbalances in hypertensive and stressed-out individuals. Whole root should actually be good for these people.[10, 32]

REFERENCES

1. Saito, H., Tsuchiya, M., Naka, S. and Takagi, K. "Effects of panax ginseng root on conditioned avoidance in rats." *Japanese Journal of Pharmacology, 27, 509–516, 1977.*

2. Saito, H., Tsuchiya, M., Naka, S. and Takagi, K. "Effects of panax ginseng root on acquisition of sound discrimination behaviour in rats." *Japanese Journal of Pharmacology*, 29, 319–324, 1979.

3. Takagi, K., "Pharmacological studies of some oriental medicinals." *Yakhak Hoeji*, 17(1), 1–8, 1973.

4. Takagi, K., Saito, H. and Nabatoa, H. "Pharmacological studies of panax ginseng root." *Japanese Journal of Pharmacology*, 22, 245–259, 1972.

5. Petkov, V.W. "Ueber den wirkungsmechanismus des panax ginseng C.A. Meyer." *Arzneimittel-Forschung*, 11, 288–295, 1961.

6. Brekhman, I.I. and Dardymov, I.V. "Pharmacological study of ginseng and related plants." *Proc. Pacific Sci. Cong.*, 11th, 8, 11, 1966.

7. Kim, E.C., Cho, H.Y. and Kim, J.M. "Effect of panax ginseng on the central nervous system." *Korean J. Pharmacol.*, 2, 23–28, 1971.

8. Saito, H., Yoshida, Y. and Takagi, K. "Effects of panax ginseng root on exhaustive exercise in mice." *Japanese Journal of Pharmacology*, 24, 119–127, 1974.

9. Brekhman, I.I. and Dardymov, I.V. "New substances of plant origin which increase non specific resistance." *Annual Review of Pharmacology*, 9, 419–430, 1969.

10. Lewis, W.H., Zenger, V.E. and Lynch, R.G. "No adaptogen response of mice to ginseng and eleutherococcus infusions." *Journal of Ethnopharmacology*, 8(2), 209–214, 1983.

11. Yokozawa, T., Seno, H. and Oura, H. "Effect of ginseng extract on lipid and sugar metabolism. I. Metabolic correlation between liver and adipose tissue." *Chem. Pharm. Bull.* (Tokyo), 23, 3095–3400, 1975.

12. Yamamoto, M., Uemura, T, Nakama, S., Uemiya, M. and Kumagi, A. "Serum HDL-cholesterol-increasing and fatty liver-improving actions of panax ginseng in high cholesterol diet-fed rats with clinical effect on hyperlipidemia in man." *American Journal of Chinese Medicine*, 11(1–4), 96–101, 1983.

13. Qureshi, A.A., Abuirmeileh, N., Din, Z.Z., Ahmad, Y. and Burger, W.C. "Suppression of cholesterogenesis and reduction of LDL cholesterol by dietary ginseng and its fractions in chicken liver." *Atherosclerosis*, 48(1), 81–94, 1983.

14. Iijima, M. and Higashi, T. "Effect of ginseng saponins on nuclear ribonucleic acid (RNA) metabolism. II. RNA polymerase activities in rats treated with ginsenoside." *Chem. Pharm. Bull.*, 27(9), 2130–2136, 1979.

15. Brekhman, I.I. "Pharmacological investigations of glycosides from ginseng and eleutherococcus." *Lloydia.* 32 (March), 46–51, 1969.

16. Petkov, V. and Staneva–Stoicheva, D. "The effect of an extract of ginseng (panax ginseng) on the function of the adrenal cortex." In: Chen and Mukerji, Eds., *Pharmacology of Oriental Plants*, Oxford, Pergamon Press, 1965, pp. 39–50, B 22.

17. Kim, J.Y. "Influence of panax ginseng on the body weights of rats." *Korean Journal of Physiology*, 4, 1–4, 1970.

18. Banerjee, U. and Izquierdo, J.A. "Antistress and antifatigue properties of panax ginseng: comparison with piracetam." *Acta Physiol. Lat. Am.*, 32(4), 277–285, 1982.

19. Wang, B.X., Cui, J.C., Liu, A.J. and Wu, S.K. "Studies on the anti-fatigue effect of the saponins of stems and leaves of panax ginseng." *Journal of Traditional Chinese Medicines*, 3(2), 89–94, 1983.

20. Hiai, S., Yokoyama, H., Oura, H. and Yano, S. "Stimulation of pituitary-adrenocortical system of ginseng saponin." *Endocrinol. Japon.*, 26(6), 661–665, 1979.

21. Hiai, S., Sasaki, S. and Oura, H. "Effect of ginseng saponin on rat adrenal cyclic AMP." *Planta Medica*, 37, 15–19, 1979.

22. Kim, C., Kim, C.C., Kim, M.S., et al. "Influence of ginseng on the stress mechanism." *Lloydia*, 33, 43–48, 1970.

23. Zhang, S.C. and Jiang, X.L. "The anti-stress effect of saponins extracted from panax ginseng fruit and the hypophyseal-adrenal system." *Yao Hsueh Hsueh Pao*, 16(11), 860–863, 1981.

24. Tanizawa, H., Numano, H., Odani, T., Yakino, Y., Hayashi, T. and Arichi, S. "Study of the saponin of panax ginseng C.A. Meyer. I. Inhibitory effect on adrenal atrophy, thymus atrophy and the decrease of serum K+ concentration induced by cortisone in unilateral adrenalectomized rats." *Yakugaku Zasshi*, 101(2), 169–173, 1981.

25. Petkov, V. and Staneva, D. "The effect of an extract of ginseng on the adrenal cortex." *Proceedings of the 2nd International Pharm. Meeting in Prague, 1963*, Pergamon Press, Czech Med. Press. Vol 7: 39–45.

26. Petkov, V. and Staneva, D. "Der einfluss eines ginseng-extraktes auf die funktionen der nebennierenrinde." *Arzneimittel-Forschung*, 13, 1078, 1963.

27. Fulder, S.J. "Ginseng and the hypothalamic-pituitary control of stress." *American Journal of Chinese Medicine.* 9(2), 112–118, 1981.

28. Namba, T., et al. "Hemolytic and protective activity of ginseng saponins." *Chem. Pharm. Bull.*, 21, 459–461, 1973.

29. Zhang, R.B., Li, Z.Y. and Shi, H.T. "Cardiac arrhythmia induced by hypothalamic stimulation in cardiac ischemic rabbits and the antiarrhythmic action of panax ginseng." *Chung Kuo Yao Li Hsueh Pao*, 3(4), 226–230, 1982.

30. Chen, X. "Experimental study on the cardiovascular effects of ginsenosides." *Chung Hua Hsin Hsueh Kuan Ping Tsa Chih*, 10(2), 147–150, 1982.

31. Lee, D.C., Lee. M.O., Kim, C.Y. and Clifford, D.H. "Effect of ether, ethanol and aqueous extracts of ginseng on cardiovascular function in dogs." *Canadian Journal of Comprehensive Medicine*, 45(2), 182–187, 1981.

32. Palmer, B.V., Montgomery, A.C.V. and Monteiro, J.C.M.P. "Ginseng and mastalgia." *British Medical Journal*, 13 May 1978, p. 1284.

GOTU KOLA or CENTELLA
(Hydrocotyle asiatica, Centella asiatica)

Gotu kola, a potent variety of which is known as centella, is a traditional blood purifier, tonic and diuretic hailing from Pakistan, Malaysia, India and parts of Eastern Europe. It is commonly used to help protect and repair or heal the skin, blood and nervous system in the presence of infectious disease. It contains asiaticoside, which has been used for decades in the Far East and for several years in Europe to cure leprosy and tuberculosis. Gotu kola is considered a good herbal tonic because it appears to improve the body's nonspecific resistance to disease. For this reason it is often found in herbal combinations along with ginseng and other adaptogens.

Gotu kola helps purify the blood

The alterative, or blood-purifying, properties of this herb are depended upon very heavily in the practice of herbal medicine, where it is used to treat leprosy, syphilis, psoriasis, cervicitis, vaginitis, blisters, and many other infectious disorders.

Gotu kola enhances mental and behavioral function.

Gotu kola has been cited in Indian sources for its ability to enhance intelligence and improve memory.[1, 2] The herb has been observed in clinical trials to increase the I.Q. and general mental ability and behavioral habits of mentally retarded children in India.[3, 4] In this country it was studied in conjunction with capsicum and ginseng on various indices of activity and fatigue. It was found to contribute to enhanced activity levels and to increase the ability to overcome fatigue. Although the effects of capsicum were separated from those of the other two herbs, the experimental design did not allow for quantifying ginseng's or gotu kola's individual contribution.[5, 6]

Recently an attempt was made to correlate the behavioral effects of consumption of a simple aqueous extract of centella with certain changes in brain chemistry. In animals, trained in a simple behavioral task, centella improved learning and retention. This improvement was correlated with decreased levels of brain neurotransmitters norepinephrine, serotonin and dopamine and their metabolities. Apparently, centella causes an overall decrease in the turnover of central transmitter substances which facilitates learning.[7]

SAFETY DATA

Gotu kola has no known toxicity. Gotu kola is not to be confused with cola acuminata, which contains considerable amounts of caffeine. *The Journal of the American Medical Association*, a few years back, published an article which, among other inexcusable blunders, failed to distinguish adequately between these two species. The resulting confusion is still with us.

REFERENCES

1. *Charaka Smhita Chikitsa Sthana*, 1st Chapter, 3rd Pada, 30th Stanza. (Cited in Naeini, K., et al., *Fitoterapia*, 63(3), 232–237, 1992.)

2. Mukerji, B. *Indian Pharmaceutical Codex*, New Delhi, India, 1953, p. 60.

3. Appa Rao, M.V.R., Srinivasan, K., Koteswara Rao, R., *J. Res. Ind. Med.*, 8, 9, 1973.

4. Swamy, V.N., Gaitonde, M. *Arogya-J. Health Sci.*, XIV, 123, 1988.

5. Mowrey, D.B. "Capsicum, ginseng and gotu kola in combination." *The Herbalist*, Premier issue; 22–28, 1975.

6. Mowrey, D.B. "The effects of capsicum, gotu kola and ginseng on activity: further evidence." *The Herbalist*, 1(1), 51–54, 1976.

7. Nalini, K., Aroor, A.R., Karanth, K.S., and Rao, A. "Effect of centella asiatica fresh leaf aqueous extract on learning and memory and biogenic amine turnover in albino rats." *Fitoterapia*, LXIII(3), 232–237, 1992.

ASTRAGALUS
(Astragalus membranaceous)

Astragalus is a classic Chinese herb, used in several herbal formulas that impact on some of the body's most important systems. Astragalus is most often combined with ginseng, the latter being a *yang* (positive, masculine) substance said to promote the body's aggressive energy, while the former is used to strengthen the defensive energy of the body. In Chinese medicine astragalus is also often combined with Chinese red sage, licorice, codonopsis, schizandra and atractylodes. In Western systems, it occurs with echinacea, ginseng, licorice, schizandra, atractylodes, boneset and garlic.

Strengthening the natural defenses of the body can involve the immune system, the cardiovascular system, and glands from all of the other systems. Astragalus is recommended both to prevent and treat virtually any disease that involves one of those systems or any of those glands; for all immune system breakdowns, including colds, fevers, infections, AIDs, etc; all cardiovascular problems, including heart disease, vascular degeneration and congestion; and all glandular problems, including liver, kidney, spleen and adrenal gland problems.

Considerable research reported in Chinese journals demonstrates that astragalus-containing formulas have effectively inhibited chronic active hepatitis, diabetes, myasthenia gravis, insomnia, hyperthyroidism, and other conditions. Some of these formulas contain more than a dozen different herbs. The therapeutic effect may be the result of the action of one, two, three or more, it may involve interactions, synergisms, meliorating effects, and so forth. At this point in time, it is impossible to know for sure. The patient probably doesn't care.[5-11]

Astragalus has a distinct hypotensive action that is probably due to constituents in its roots which are also probably responsible for vasodilating, antiadrenergic, diuretic and somnolescent effects of the herb. Research has also discovered an anti-inflammatory principle in astragalus. It effectively countered the effects of mast cell substances, thereby providing some support for supposed immunomodulating action of the plant, but it is not certain the plant inhibits the release of substances from the mast cell, or whether it inhibits the interaction between allergen and mast cell. In a routine pharmacological screening trial, astragalus saponins, given intravenously, inhibited the increase in vascular permeability caused by mast cell constituents, thus suggesting another possible mode of action. Administered orally, astragalus saponins exhibited an anti-inflammatory action by reducing experimentally-induced inflammation in rats. And in a recent study, astragalus was found to inhibit the formation of myocarditis (which produces severe lesions of the linings of the heart) caused by Coxsackie B-3 virus.[1, 2, 4, 12]

In one study astragalus saponin induced rapid accumulation of cyclic AMP in rabbit plasma when injected i.p., and enhanced DNA synthesis in the liver. These findings indicate that astragalus probably has an anabolic effect on metabolism; that is, it contributes to the building-up of cell structures and strengthens cell processes.[3]

Astragalus extracts are being used in China to fight several kinds of cancer. Experimentally, the herb has been shown to potentiate killer cell effectiveness. In one model, a lymphokine is used to generate lymphokine-activated killer cells. This process is normally associated with excessive toxicity. Addition of astragalus to the lymphokine significantly decreased the amount needed to activate the killer cells, and hence also reduced toxic side effects to a minimum. Astragalus also significantly boosts the production of macrophages through an action on one of the main components of the complement system.[13, 14]

Astragalus finds application in the treatment and prevention of virally contracted colds and influenza. Studies show that it induces interferon production, which has the end result of preventing viruses from gaining a foothold in the respiratory tract.

One study demonstrated that chronic bronchitis patients experience significant reduction in symptoms when using astragalus. Among 1,137 volunteers, combined astragalus-interferon treatment was significantly more effective in preventing the common cold than interferon alone.[17]

One of the problems of chemotherapy and radiotherapy in cancer patients is a pronounced lowering of the body's already low immune response ability. Some research is being done that strongly indicates a positive role of astragalus administration in these patients. The product enhances natural defense function by stimulating the responsiveness of T cells. In studies recently completed at the University of Texas at Houston, scientists have found that T cells taken from cancer patients with feeble T cell activity became even more aggressive than healthy controls when incubated with astragalus.[15]

SAFETY DATA

Astragalus is a very safe herb. Even very large doses have not produced toxicity in animals and humans.

REFERENCES

1. Hikino, H., Funayama, S.H. and Endo, K. "Hypotensive principle of astragalus and hedysarum roots." *Planta Medica*, 30(4), 297–302, 1976.

2. Zhang, Y., Wang, Y., Shen, J. and Li, D. *Yaoxue Xuebo*, 19, 333, 1984.

3. Zhang, N.D., Wong, Y.L. et al. "Effects of astragalus saponin 1 on cAMP and cGMP level in plasma and DNA synthesis in regenerating rat liver." *Acta Pharmaceutica Sinica*, 19(8), 619–621, 1984.

4. Zhang, N.D., Wong, Y.L. et al. "Effects on blood pressure and inflammation of astragalus saponin 1, a principle isolated from

astragalus membranaceus Bge." *Acta Pharmaceutica Sinica,* 19(5), 333–337, 1984.

5. Yang, G. and Geng, P. "Effects of yang-promoting drugs on immunological functions of yang-deficient animal model induced by prednisolone." *Journal of Traditional Chinese Medicine,* 4(2), 153–156, 1984.

6. Li, G. "Discussions about myasthenia gravis and spleen-kidney theory." *Journal of Traditional Chinese Medicine,* 8(1), 48–51, 1986.

7. Xiao, S. et al. "Hyperthyroidism treated with yiqiyangyin decoction." *Journal of Traditional Chinese Medicine,* 6(2), 79–82, 1986.

8. Xie, Y. et al. "240 cases of insomnia treated by activating circulation and eliminating blood stasis." *Bulletin of Chinese Materia Medica,* 11(5), 58–60, 1986.

9. Zhang, H, et al. "Treatment of adult diabetes with jiangtangjia tablets." *Journal of Traditional Chinese Medicine,* 7(4), 37–39, 1986.

10. Liang, R. and Lui, W. "Clinical study on braincalmin tablets in treating 450 cases of atherosclerosis." *Journal of North Chinese Medicine,* 1, 1985.

11. Zhou, M.X. et al. "Therapeutic effect of astragalus in treating chronic active hepatitis and the changes in immune function." *Journal of Chinese People's Liberation Army,* 7(4), 242–244, 1982.

12. Yang, Y.A., et al. "Treatment of experimental Coxsackie B-3 myocarditis with astragalus membranaceus in mice." *Chin. Med. J.* 103(1), 14–18, 1990.

13. Chu, D., et al. "F3, a fractionated extract of astragalus membranaceous, potentiates lymphokine-activated killer cell cytotoxicity generated by low-dose recombinant interleukin-2" *Chung Hsi I Chieh Ho Tsa Chih,* 10(1), 34–36, 1990.

14. Wang, J., Ito, H. and Shimura, K. "Enhancing effect of antitumor polysaccharide from astragalus or radix hedysarum on C3 cleavage production of macrophages in mice." *Jap. J. Pharmacol.,* 51(3), 432–434, 1989.

15. Wang, D.C. "Influence of astragalus membranaceous (AM) polysaccharide FB on immunologic function of human periphery

blood lymphocyte." *Chung Hua Chung Liu Tsa Chih*, 11(3), 180–183, 1989.

16. Hsu, H.Y. "Application of Chinese herbal formulas and scientific research. (I)." *Oriental Healing Arts International Bulletin*, 11(2), 87–96, 1986.

17. Hou, Y., et al. "Effect of radix astragali seu hedysari on the interferon system." *Chin. Med. J.*, 94(1), 35–40, 1981.

SCHIZANDRA
(Schizandra chinensis)

Schizandra, an Asian herb, is becoming even more popular in the West to which it has been introduced following a centuries-old tradition of use in the East, particularly in China and Japan. The Chinese name for schizandra means five-flavored-fruit (*Wu* = five, *wei* = flavored, tzu = seed, herb or fruit), referring to varying tastes experienced in different parts of the plant. Thus, the skin or peel and pulp are sweet and sour, the kernels are pungent and bitter, and the whole has a salty taste. Since these are the five major tastes in Chinese medicine and philosophy, schizandra is regarded in Chinese medicine as the quintessence of the five elemental energies. The main tastes of schizandra are sour and salty and this herb therefore finds applications as both a *yin* (female, negative) and a *yang* (male, positive) treatment.

The following list of uses and of conditions responsive to this herb show the immense variety of uses to which schizandra is put:

neck and shoulder tension

to beautify skin and protect it from sun and wind

to develop basic life energy

mildly sedative

analgesic

promotes digestion

antitussive

expectorant

promotes circulation of blood

lung diseases

tonic

pectoral

calms anger
astringent
normalizes blood pressure
lung tuberculosis
night sweats
frequent urination from
　deficient kidneys
asthmatic coughs
diarrhea of infants and
　pregnant women and
　dysentery in children
gonorrhea
neurasthenia
neural tonic
stimulating in small
　doses; depressing and
　inhibiting in large
　doses
regulatory to
　cardiovascular system
urticaria

allergic dermatoses
fatigue
mental stimulant
arteriosclerosis
deficient kidney, spleen,
　lungs
nocturnal emission
spermatorrhea
leukorrhea
excessive sweating
deficient yang
　spontaneous sweating
deficient yin night sweats
forgetfulness
insomnia
calming
premenstrual syndrome
stimulates immune
　system
radioprotective

Modern research has provided substantial support for many of the above uses, while others remain to be investigated. Even though we do not yet fully understand the pharmacology of this plant, there are, nevertheless, common threads underlying its mechanism of action, as explored below.

The word is getting out that schizandra probably contains substances that meet the criteria for adaptogens, which means the herb has been found to regulate certain physiological processes or body functions in such a way as to increase the body's natural nonspecific resistance to the effects of stressors. For example, schizandra-fed animals perform significantly better than controls in swimming endurance tests. Schizandra also regulates gastric acidity (both increases and decreases the concentration, depending on the immediate need of the body). In humans, schizandra extract increases muscular endurance. In spite of research along these lines, the ability of schizandra to mediate nonspecific stress appears to be fairly weak when compared to ginseng species. However, according to Chinese medicine, there exists significant synergy between ginseng and schizandra.[1-3]

Many studies have investigated the marked ability of shizandra and its multiple constituents of the lignan class to prevent, treat and cure various kinds of liver disease, and this appears to be the herb's main focus of activity. Whatever effects it may have on the rest of the body, they are all probably mediated by the liver tonic action. In one classic study, 102 patients with hepatitis were successfully treated with schizandra. A full 76 percent of the patients experienced complete recovery within a period of about one month. A cure rate that high suggests strong activity, almost as high as that commonly seen with milk thistle extract.

Significant results have been obtained using a lignan component of schizandra on liver damage induced by several deadly toxins. The schizandra extract not only prevented and inhibited liver damage, but actually cured liver injury caused by the repeated administration of toxins. Among the conditions either prevented or cured were cell death (necrosis), fatty degeneration, inflammatory cell infiltration and hepatitis. Schizandra is a good antioxidant, which means it prevents liver damage through a variety of mechanisms, including the prevention of lesions in liver tissue from the harmful byproducts of free radical damage. Another lignan from schizandra prevents poisoning by facilitating the liver's ability to maintain normal bile production and flow. A diet containing 5 percent schizandra fruit was found to be effective in inhibiting the toxicity of highly carcinogenic and mutagenic substances. Not only does schizandra protect the liver, it also promotes normal liver functioning, including the production of bile, filtration of toxins and the flow of increased quantities of blood. Reported effects of schizandra on digestion may be the direct result of such influences on liver function.[4-16]

The effect of schizandra on the central nervous system is gentle—stimulating but not exciting. It strengthens and quickens reflexes, and increases work efficiency. The stimulating property appears to be adaptogenic: the more you need, the more you get, and when you don't need it, very little is felt. This property may be related to observed tendencies in schizandra to control anger and aggression. An interesting study was carried out on the effects of schizandra extract on neurasthenia. Alcohol extracts were used in 73 cases whose symptoms included headache, insomnia, dizziness and palpitations: 43 were cured, and 13 significantly improved.[17-19]

Schizandra appears to be cholinergic in nature, at least as determined by investigation of its effects in the peripheral nervous system. What remains to be investigated is whether this cholinergic property also applies to the central nervous system. If it does, this would help explain reports of increased cognitive function following schizandra use, including increased memory.[20]

Finally, it should be noted that schizandra has free radical scavenging, antioxidant properties similar to milk thistle; this action alone could account for the herb's incredible effect on liver and immune system.[21]

SAFETY DATA

In the several clinical studies reported to date, no significant side effects were observed. Orally administered, there appears to be no toxicity at normal levels. Severe overdose may produce restlessness, insomnia and dyspnea.

Some persons with peptic ulcers caused by high acidity may experience increased acidity, though the adaptogenic action should prevent this. Epileptics or those with abnormally high intracranial pressure should avoid using schizandra at this time.

REFERENCES

1. Long, Z.Z. and Xie, S.S. "Experimental study on the enhancement of the immunosuppressive effect of cortisone by wurenchum, an extract of schizandra chinensis baill." *Chung Hsi I Chieh Ho Tsa Chih*, 5(6), 361–2, 325, 1985.

2. Salbe, A.D. and Bjeldanes, L.F. "The effects of dietary brussels sprouts and schizandra chinensis on the xenobiotic-metabolizing enzymes of the rat small intestine." *Food Chemistry and Toxicology*, 23(1), 57–65, 1985.

3. Long, Z.Z. "Suppressive effect of wurenchun on the plaque forming cell and specific rosette formation cell of mice." *Chung Hua I Hsueh Tsa Chih*, 64(6), 369–71, 1984.

4. Maeda, S. et al., "Effects of gomisin A on liver functions in hepatotoxic chemical-treated rats." *Japanese Journal of Pharmacology*, 38(4), 347–53, 1985.

5. Liu, G. T. and Wei, H.L. "Induction of hepatic microsomal monoxygenases by schisanhenol in rats." *Chung Kuo Yao Li Hsueh Pao*, 6(1), 41–44, 1985.

6. Takeda, S., et al. "Pharmacological studies on schizandra fruits. III. Effects on wuweizisu c, a lignan component of schizandra fruits, on experimental liver injuries in rats." *Nippon Yakurigaku Zasshi*, 85(3), 193–208, 1985.

7. Xie, J.X., et al. "Studies of antihepatitic drugs. Total synthesis of (+/-) schizandrin C and its analogs." *Sci. Sin. B.*, 26(12), 1291–1303, 1983.

8. Hikino, H., et al. "Antihepatotoxic actions of lignoids from schizandra chinensis fruits.: *Planta Medica*, 30(37), 213–218, 1984.

9. Takeda, S., et al. "Effect of gomisin A (TJN–101), a lignan isolated from schizandra fruits, on liver function in rats." *Nippon Yakurigaku Zasshi*, 91(4), 237–244, 1988.

10. Hernandez, D.E., Hancke, J.S. and Wikman, G. "Evaluation of the anti-ulcer and antisecretory activity of extracts of aralia elata root and schizandra chinensis fruit in the rat." *Journal of Ethnopharmacology*, 23(1), 109–114, 1988.

11. Takeda, S. et al. "Effects of gomisin A, a lignan component of schizandra fruits, on experimental injuries and liver microsomal

drug-metabolizing enzymes." *Nippon Yakurigaku Zasshi*, 87(2), 169–187, 1986.

12. Hendrick, S. and Bjeldanes, L.F. "Effects of dietary schizandra chinensis, brussels sprouts and illicium verum extracts on carcinogen metabolism systems in mouse liver." *Food Chem. Toxicology*, 24(9), 903–912, 1986.

13. Takeda, S. et al. "Effects on TJN-101 on liver regeneration after partial hepatectomy, and on regional hepatic blood flow and fine structure of the liver in normal rats." *Nippon Yakurigaku Zasshi*, 88(4), 321–330, 1986.

14. Takeda, S. et al. "Pharmacological studies on antihepatotoxic action of TJN-101, a lignan component of schizandra fruits. Influence of resolvents on the efficacy of TJN-101 in the experimental acute hepatic injuries." *Yakugaku Zasshi*, 107(7), 514–524, 1987.

15. Takeda, S. et al. "Effects of TJN-101, a lignan compound isolated from schizandra fruits, on liver fibrosis and on liver regeneration after partial hepatectomy in rats with chronic liver injury induced by CC14." *Nippon Yakurigaku Zasshi*, 90(1), 51–65, 1987.

16. Ohkura, Y., et al. "Inhibitory effect of TJN-101 on immunologically induced liver injuries." *Japanese Journal of Pharmacology*, 44(2), 179–185, 1987.

17. Nie, X. Y. Bian, Z. J. and Ren, Z.H. "Metabolic fate of schizandrol A and its distribution in the rat brain determined by thin layer chromatography." *Yao Hsueh Hsueh Pao*, 18(7), 491–495, 1983.

18. Niu, X.Y. et al. "Effects of schizandrol on the central nervous system." *Yao Hsueh Hsueh Pao*, 18(6), 416–421, 1983.

19. Wang, S.H. and Sun, J.T. *Chinese Journal of Dermatology*, 8(1), 14, 1960.

20. Bensky, D. and Gamble, A. *Chinese Herbal Medicine Materia Medica*, Eastland Press, Seattle, 1986, pp. 541–543.

21. Li, X.J. et al. "Scavenging effects on active oxygen radicals by schizandrins with different structures and configurations." *Free Radic. Biol. Med.*, 9(2), 99–104, 1990.

LICORICE ROOT
(Glycyrrhiza glabra)

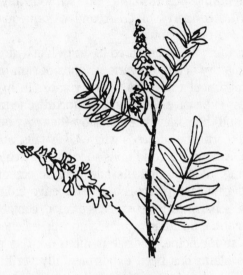

LICORICE

Only the effects of licorice root on the immune system will be reviewed in this chapter. The reader is referred to the chapter on the female reproductive system for a review of the other properties of this plant.

The following discussion of licorice will be short, but should not lead the reader to underestimate the importance of licorice root in immune therapy. To the Chinese, there is no other herb that acts on such a grand scale except, perhaps, ginseng. But the Chinese include licorice root in more combinations than they do ginseng or any other herb. It is considered the key to health. I consider licorice to be one of the two or three most important herbs in the world.

Licorice has anti-inflammatory action

Glycyrrhetinic acid (GLA), an important constituent of licorice root, showed a pronounced anti-inflammatory action by inhibiting the development of histamine-, serotonin-, bradykinin- and formalin-induced edemas, comparing very favorably to orthodox anti-inflammatory drugs such as butadione and hydrocortisone, and resembling prednisolone, but without any side effects. The antiarthritic property of GLA and of aqueous extracts of licorice have also been shown.[1-7]

GLA has often been compared to drugs like hydrocortisone for its anti-inflammatory action on various kinds of skin problems. A 2 percent GLA ointment compares very favorably to hydrocortisone, and is much less expensive. GLA and hydrocortisone may not act in the same way, and there is evidence to show they may be complementary; thus hydrocortisone succeeds where GLA fails, and the reverse is equally true. Among the conditions successfully treated with GLA are the following: atopic, subacute and chronic eczematous conditions; itching dermatoses; pruritus; acute impetigo; infantile eczema; flexural eczema; seborrheic, infective, sensitization, contact, neuro-, and exfoliative dermatitis; pustular psoriasis; impetigo; lichen simplex.[4]

In Chinese medicine, licorice is often used as a remedy for jaundice. This claim has been experimentally verified in studies showing that licorice has a significantly beneficial action on the course of obstructive jaundice. GL and GLA have both been shown to prevent the development of experimental cirrhosis in animals treated with liver toxins such as carbon tetrachloride.

The demulcent and expectorant properties of licorice are well accepted as a matter of course by most medical experts. And the antitussive activity of GLA has been experimentally validated.

There is some evidence that the anti-inflammatory properties of licorice and GLA include some effect on the course of asthma. GLA has also proven a viable treatment for tuberculosis, in which its action was comparable to commonly-employed steroids like deoxycorticosterone.[8, 9]

Immunosuppressive action

GLA stimulates the immunosuppressive property of cortisone, while exhibiting an immunosuppressive action of its own.

Whole licorice root potentiates immune activity when necessary and also suppresses it when needed.[10]

Licorice root has anticancer properties

Several licorice compounds have been tested in rats and mice and various experimental and clinical tumors. Some of these constituents slightly inhibited the growth of tumors even at submaximal doses and after oral administration. In vitro tests with all components were weak. Inhibition of the catabolism of corticosteroids is thought to be the mechanism of action.[11]

Licorice root activates and mimics interferon

Glycyrrhizin (GL), a constituent of licorice, and, to a lesser extent, GLA have been found to induce interferon production in mice. A preparation of GL combined with glycine and cysteine has been widely and successfully used in Japan as an antihepatitis drug. Interferon has also been used to treat hepatitis B patients. It may be that licorice is an effective antihepatitis drug because it induces interferon. Another study, however, found that GL is also effective against alcoholic hepatitis. Therefore, the antihepatitis effect of GL may involve more than just interferon induction.[12, 13]

Glycyrrhizic acid, at concentrations well tolerated by uninfected cells, inhibits both growth and cytopathic effect of vaccinia, herpes simplex, Newcastle disease, and vesicular stomatitis viruses while being ineffective on poliovirus. It is suggested that glycyrrhizic acid interacts with virus structures (conceivably proteins) producing different effects according to the viral stage affected: inactivation of free virus particles, extracellularly; prevention of intracellular uncoating of infecting particles; impairment of the assembling ability of virus structural components.[14]

Ethanol extracts of the powdered roots of commercial licorice showed reproducible antimicrobial activity in vitro against

Staphlyococcus aureus, Mycobacterium smegmatis and *Candida albicans*.[15]

Recent findings show that licorice root has a potentiating effect on the reticuloendothelial system, the first line of defense against micro-organisms.[16]

SAFETY DATA

See the chapter on the female reproductive system for a full discussion of licorice's safety.

REFERENCES

1. Nasyrov, K.M. and Lazareva, D.N. "Study of the anti-inflammatory activity of glycyrrhizin acid derivatives." *Farmak-i Toksikol.*, 43(4), 399–404, 1980.

2. Gujral, M.L. et al. "Antiarthritic activity of glycyrrhizin in adrenalectomized rats." *Ind. J. Med. Sci.*, 15(8), 625–629, 1961.

3. Parmar, S. S. et al. "Biochemical basis for anti-inflammatory effects of glycyrrhetic acid and its derivatives." *Int. Cong. Biochem.*, 6(5), 410, 1964.

4. Sommerville, J. "Glycyrrhetinic acid." *British Med. J.*, Feb. 2, 1957, pp. 282–283.

5. Ichioka, H. "The pharmacological action of glycyrrhizin. I. The effect on the blood bilirubin level in rabbits with ligated common bile duct." *Gifu Daigaku Igakubu Kiyo.* Gifu University School of Medicine. 115(3), 792, 1968.

6. Zhao, M.Q. et al. "The preventive and therapeutic actions of glycyrrhizin, glycyrrhetic acid and crude saikosides on experimental cirrhosis in rats." *Yao Hsueh Hsueh Pao*, 18(5), 325–331, 1983.

7. Anderson, D. M. and Smith, W. G. "The antitussive activity of glycyrrhetic acid and its derivatives." *J. Pharm. Pharmacol.*, 13, 396–404, 1961.

8. Miyoshi, H. "Antidotal value of glycyrrhizin." *Nisshin Igaku,* 39, 358–365, 1952.

9. Chang, L. "Preliminary report on using glycyrrhiza in combination with antituberculosis drugs in pulmonary tuberculosis." *Jen Min Pao Chien,* 3, 235–238, 1959.

10. Takagi, K., Watanabe, K. and Ishi, Y. "Peptic ulcer inhibiting activity of licorice root." *Proc. Int. Pharmacol. Meeting* 7(2), 1–15, 1965.

11. Shvarev, I.F., et al. "Effect of triterpenoid compounds from glycyrrhiza glabra on experimental tumors." *Voprosy Izuch Ispol'z Solodki SSR, Akad. Nauk SSR,* 1966, p., 167–170.

12. Fujisawam, J. et al. "Therapeutic approach to chronic active hepatitis with glycyrrhizin." *Asian Med. J.,* 23. 745–756, 1980.

13. Greenburg, H.B. et al. "Effect of human leukocyte interferon on hepatitis B virus infection in patients with chronic active hepatitis." *New Eng. J. Med.,* 295, 517–522, 1976.

14. Pompei, R. et al. "Antiviral activity of glycyrrhizic acid" *Experientia,* 36, 304, 1980.

15. Mitscher, L.A., et al. "Antimicrobial agents from higher plants. Antimicrobial isoflavonoids and related substances from glycyrrhiza glabra L. var. typica." *J. Natural Products,* 43(2), 259–269, 1980.

16. Tomoda, M. et al. "Characterization of two polysaccharides having activity on the reticuloendothelial system from the root of glycyrrhiza uralensis." *Chem. Pharm. Bull.,* 38(6), 1667–1671, 1990.

LAPACHO
(Tabebuia avellandedae, T. impetiginosa)

Lapacho is found in the rain forests and mountains of Paraguay, Argentina and Brazil. This plant holds great promise for the effective treatment of cancers, such as leukemia, and of *Candida* and other troublesome infections, as well as debilitating diseases (including arthritis), and a host of other complaints.

The medicinal part of the tree is the bark, specifically the inner lining of the bark, called the phloem (pronounced floam). The use of whole bark, containing the dead wood, naturally dilutes the activity of the material. Lapacho is also known by the Portuguese name of Pau d'arco, and by tribal names such as *taheebo* and *ipe roxo*. Some texts distinguish between *lapacho colorado* (red lapacho = ipe roxo) (scarlet flowers) and *lapacho morado* (purple lapacho), which grows in cooler climates such as high in the Andes, and high places in Paraguay. Recent evidence suggests that these two varieties of lapacho possess superior medicinal properties, with a slight bow going to the purple as the best of all.

Most of the chemical analyses of lapacho have been performed on the heartwood of the tree, rather than on the phloem, or inner lining of the bark, which is used medicinally. It is unclear why this has occurred. One reason may be that the heartwood contains enough quantities of a couple of important constituents, mainly lapachol and tabebuin, to satisfy current research interests. It is probably safe to assume that the living bark contains a similar set of active constituents to the heartwood plus some others that make it more effective and would account for the living bark's greater popularity as a folk medicine. Traditionally, as anyone who chooses to examine the herbal literature of the world can verify, it is the living bark of a plant, especially a tree or shrub, that is used medicinally, not the heartwood. The reason is simple: the nutrients and representative families of chemical substances used to sustain the life of the tree are found in greatest concentration in the cambium layer and phloem of the living bark.

The life processes of a mature tree are carried out in the thin corridor lying between the outer bark and the inner heartwood. Pull the bark off of a tree and you will notice moist, very thin layers of tissue that seem to shred when picked at with the hands. This is the cambium layer. Its purpose is to create new tree tissues, such as phloem, through cell division. The newest, youngest phloem cells are just outside the cambium. As new phloem is added, older cells are crushed and pressed into the bark. Younger, newer cells added to the inside of the cambium layer are called xylem. Newer xylem is called sapwood; older xylem is crushed and pressed into the heart of the tree. It is therefore known as heartwood. The actively conducting tissues of a tree are the thin layers of fresh xylem and phloem on each side of the cambium. The outer bark and heartwood are, essentially, inactive materials that only serve to provide strength to the tree. Indiscriminate combining of older, less active layers of bark and tree with the younger, living tissues results in a dramatic dilution of active principle and medicinal value. Yet it is a common practice of commercial lapacho suppliers.

Lapachol is just one of a number of plant substances known as napthaquinones (N-factors) that occur in lapacho. Anthraquinones, or A-factors, comprise another important class of compounds. The N-factors are not common except in herbal tonics. Seldom do both N- and A-factors occur in the same species. Several of the remarkable properties of lapacho may be due to a probable synergy between A- and N-factors.

Quercitin, xloidone and other flavonoids are also present in lapacho; these undoubtedly contribute to the plant's effectiveness in the treatment of tumors and infections.

The native Indians of Brazil, northern Argentina, Paraguay, Bolivia and other South American countries have used lapacho for medicinal purposes for thousands of years; there are indications that its use may actually antedate the Incas. Before the advent of the Spanish, the Guarani and Tupi-Nambo tribes in particular used great quantities of lapacho tea. In the high Andes, the Calawaya, the Quechua, Aymara and other tribes used lapacho (taheebo to them) for many complaints.

Lapacho is applied externally and internally for the treatment of fevers, infections, colds, flu, syphilis, cancer, respiratory problems, skin ulcerations and boils, dysentery, gastrointestinal problems of all kinds, debilitating conditions such as arthritis and prostatitis, and circulation disturbances. Other conditions reportedly cured with lapacho include lupus, diabetes, Hodgkin's disease, osteomyelitis, Parkinson's disease and psoriasis.

Lapacho is used to relieve pain, kill germs, increase the flow of urine, and even as an antidote to poisons. Its use in many ways parallels that of echinacea on this continent and ginseng in Asia, except that its actions appear to exceed them both in terms of its potential as a cancer treatment. The Guarani, Tupi and other tribes called the lapacho tree *tajy*, meaning "to have strength and vigor," or simply "the divine tree." Modern Guarani Indians prefer the purple lapacho, but also use the red lapacho. And they use only the inner linings of the bark.

Research on lapacho has been going on for a long time. E. Paterno isolated the active constituent, lapachol, in 1884. In 1896, S.C. Hooker established the chemical structure of lapachol, and L.F. Fieser synthesized the substance in 1927! So it would be a mistake to call lapacho a modern discovery.[1-3]

As early as 1873, physicians were aware of the healing action of lapacho. Dr. Joaqin Almeida Pinto wrote during that year, "Pau D'Arco: Medicinal Properties: prescribed as a fever-reducer; the bark is used against ulcers; also used for venereal and rheumatic disorders and especially useful for skin disorders, especially eczema, herpes, and the mange."[4] Another physician, Dr. Walter Accorsi, reported that lapacho, "eliminated the pains caused by the disease [cancer] and multiplies the body's production of red corpuscles."

However, the science of lapacho began properly with the work of Theodoro Meyer in Argentina, who tried for decades with little success to convince the medical world of the value of lapacho for infections and cancer. Data from his laboratory are astounding in terms of the success rate observed when applying the herb to dozens of different kinds of cancer. Much of Meyer's work was primitive by modern research standards; most of it lacked adequate controls and statistical evaluation. But the sheer bulk of it is good evidence for the efficacy of lapacho. The Meyer era ended at his death in 1972, with the scientific world left still largely unconvinced of the usefulness of lapacho as a modern medicinal agent. Perhaps the most important thing Meyer accomplished, from a scientific point of view, was to bring lapacho to the attention of the rest of the world, to extract the plant from the jungles of the Amazon, and announce, "Here is a folk remedy with great promise for all mankind."

Independent of Meyer, a physician in Brazil, about 1960, after hearing a tale of its miraculous curative powers, used lapacho to treat his brother who was lying in a Santa Andre, Brazil hospital, dying of cancer. His brother recovered, and the physician, Dr. Orlando dei Santi, began to use the herb to treat other cancer patients at the hospital. Other physicians joined the team, and after a few months, several cures were recorded. In the typical case, pain disappeared rapidly and sometimes complete remission was achieved in as little as four weeks.

Because of the work at the Municipal Hospital of Santo Andre, lapacho has become a standard form of treatment for some kinds of cancer and for all kinds of infections in medical establishments throughout Brazil. It should be noted that after the first reports of "miraculous" herbal cures appeared in Brazil, the national government ordered a blackout of any more public statements by doctors involved in the research. The silence was finally broken by Alec De Montmorency, who in 1981 published a lengthy review of the ongoing clinical work in Brazil. This report succeeded in stimulating worldwide interest in the plant.

In 1968, Dr. Prats Ruiz of Concepcion, Paraguay, successfully treated three cases of leukemia in his private clinic. Some of these results were widely published and also helped to establish the popularity of lapacho among the "civilized" inhabitants of South American countries.

American physicians, of course, tend to look disparagingly upon clinical evidence from backward areas of South America, preferring instead sanitized evidence from their own brightly lit laboratories. The weight of the South American clinical evidence has not been sufficient to cause widespread acceptance of the treatment outside South America, but it has stimulated research interest abroad. Pharmaceutical companies regularly screen lapacho for the presence of substances that could be the basis for new drug applications. As we shall see, however, no isolated component of lapacho comes anywhere close to being equal to the combined activity of all constituents, or, in other words, to the whole herb.

A common thread that runs throughout early and current empirical and clinical reports of lapacho treatment is the consistent observation that the herb eliminates many of the common side effects of the orthodox medications. There is no explanation of this action, but it is so often seen that one cannot easily doubt its validity. Pain, hair loss and immune dysfunction are among the symptoms most commonly eliminated.

While scientific research on lapacho has been going on for decades, most of it is worthless from a medicinal point of view. Some of it, however, is very good, and has resulted in the isolation of several individual medicinally active constituents and in the analysis of their properties. The current interest in AIDS has stimulated renewed interest in lapacho since the herb is such an effective antiviral substance.

EFFECTS OF LAPACHO

The following is a summary of some of the effects of lapacho and/or any of its constituents that have been validated by modern research:

Laxative effect

Regular use of lapacho will maintain regularity of bowel movements. This property is undoubtedly due to the presence of the naphthoquinones and anthraquinones. Users of lapacho universally report a pleasant and moderate loosening of the bowels that leads to greater regularity without any unpleasant side effects such as diarrhea.

Anticancer effect

The greater part of the basic research on lapacho, both in the United States and in other countries, has dealt directly with the cancer question. Obviously, this issue is of great importance. Any tendency of lapacho to ameliorate the course of cancer should be made known to all persons likely to benefit from it. The absence of side effects makes lapacho a treatment of choice, even in conjunction with standard forms of therapy. The user has nothing to lose and much to gain from the judicious use of lapacho.

Naturally, any and all treatment of a cancerous condition should be done under the supervision of a qualified physician.

Some constituents or groups of constituents of lapacho have indeed been found to suppress tumor formation and reduce tumor viability, both in experimental animal trials and in clinical settings involving human patients. In addition, anecdotal data abounds to such an extent that to overlook its importance is to turn one's back on a potentially invaluable source of aid and health. Leukemia has proven particularly susceptible to the application of lapacho and several of its constituents. Some researchers feel that lapacho is one of the most important antitumor agents in the entire world.

Part of the effectiveness of lapacho may stem from its observed ability to stimulate the production of red blood cells in bone marrow. Increased red blood cell production would improve the oxygen-carrying capacity of the blood. This, in turn, could have important implications for the health of tissues throughout the body. Also needed for oxygen transport by red cells is iron. This might explain the augmentation in lapacho's therapeutic properties when it is combined with iron-rich yerba mate, another South American plant; in fact, it is native practice to almost always combine these two plant species.

National Cancer Institute research on the anti-cancer action of lapacho has been disappointing. Unfortunately, the NCI restricted its investigations to lapachol, and once it found that this substance had side effects that offset its potential therapeutic benefits, it abandoned the project. From the perspective of a tonic, one can readily perceive the fallacy of that approach, and would suspect that the problems in the research stemmed directly from employing isolated herbal constituents. As one might also suspect, research that utilized whole lapacho has produced clinical anticancer effects without side effects.[29, 30]

Animal research in the United States made a gigantic stride forward when it was discovered that lapachol inhibited solid tumors (Walker carcinosarcoma 256 and Ehrlich solid carcinoma) and Ehrlich ascites cell tumors.[31] Such research then took a gigantic stride backwards when clinical toxicity of lapachol prematurely ended those investigations.

One interesting line of research has shown that lapachol is more effective when ingested orally than when injected into the gut or into the muscles. These results contradict a substantial amount of research on orthodox drugs that indicates the superiority of injectable routes. What is the meaning of this anomaly? Could it be a sign that natural routes of administration (i.e., oral) are better suited for natural substances? The further removed from the natural state, the more active substances become when injected directly into the blood stream, and the less able the natural processes of the body are in dealing with them.

Using the wood of the plant, several researchers have studied the effects of lapachol, alpha- and beta-lapachone and xyloidone on experimental cancer (Yoshida's sarcoma and Walker 256 carcinosarcoma). As high as 84 percent inhibition was observed on Yoshida's sarcoma, and no toxicity was found.[32]

In one clinical study,[33] South American researchers administered lapachol to patients with various forms of cancer, including adenocarcinoma of the liver, breast and prostate, and squamous-cell carcinoma of the palate and uterine cervix. Taken orally, the substance resulted in temporary reduction of all conditions and in significant reduction in pain. Duration of treatment was anywhere from 30 to 720 days, with an average of about two months. For example, one patient with liver cancer experienced a significant reduction in jaundice accompanied by other signs of improvement after eight days of therapy. These results were in close accord with results obtained by the same researchers in animal studies.[34] One wonders what the administration of whole purple lapacho phloem might have accomplished in this setting; other lines of evidence suggest that even better results might have been obtained.

A note on nausea: In the human study reported above, some patients dropped out of the experiment due to nausea. This is a common observation in some, but certainly not all, people who begin to experience the cleansing action of lapacho (and other healthful herbs). As toxins (and toxic medicines) and wastes are drawn out of the cells, or flushed out, or are physiologically drawn out of the cells, through the action of the herb, they tend at times to accumulate in the blood, lymph, lymph nodes, skin, liver and kidneys awaiting the opportunity to be expelled from the body. Backing up, they can on occasion produce sensations such as nausea; the body may even try to rid itself of some toxic substances by vomiting. Not to worry. These transient signs dissipate once the toxins are moving freely from the body. They are a positive sign that the herb is working. Remember the body only has three basic processes for getting rid of wastes: lower bowel movement, sweating, urinating. The use of lapacho can so overload these processes in the early stages that discomfort may be produced.

Antioxidant effect

In vitro trials show definite inhibition of free radicals and inflammatory leukotrienes by lapacho constituents. This property might underlie the effectiveness of lapacho against skin cancer, and definitely helps to explain observed anti-aging effects. Modern science has recently uncovered the importance of free radicals in the generation of many debilitating diseases, from cancer to arthritis. These molecules are even heavily implicated in the normal aging process. Reversing their action has become big business in world health circles. Antioxidants, or free-radical scavengers, have emerged as premier candidates for the role of healers and disease preventers. Among the anti-oxidants few have greater potency than lapachol.

Analgesic effect

The administration of lapacho is consistently credited in reports issuing from South American clinics as a primary modality for lessening the pain associated with several kinds of cancer, especially cancer of the prostate, liver or breast. Arthritic pain has also been relieved with lapacho ingestion.

Antimicrobial/antiparasitic effects

Includes inhibition and destruction of gram positive and acid-fast bacteria (*B. subtilis, M. pyogenes aureus*, etc.), yeasts, fungi, viruses and several kinds of parasites.[5-8] Two troublesome families of viruses inhibited by lapachol are noteworthy, herpes-viruses and HIV's. Together these viruses account for much of the misery of mankind. The antimalarial activity of lapacho spawned a great deal of research interest in the early decades of this century. A 1948 article reviewed the progress and indicated that the N-factors, especially lapachol, were among the most promising antimalarial substances known at that time. Lapacho's immunostimulating action is due in part to its potent antimicrobial effects.

One of the strongest actions of lapacho is against viruses. The range of viruses inactivated by lapacho extends from those that cause the common cold to those that are responsible for AIDS. It has been shown to actively inhibit, kill or stunt the growth of several dangerous viruses, including herpesvirus hominis types I and II, polio virus, vesicular stomatitis virus, avian myeloblastosis virus, murine leukemia virus, Friend virus, and Rous sarcoma virus.[20-24] Several other viruses are also inhibited by lapacho's N- and A-factors.

One N-factor, beta-lapachone, inhibits enzymes in virus cells that directly affect the synthesis of DNA and RNA. It is also a potent inhibitor of the enzyme reverse transcriptase, involved in RNA/DNA relationships. Once these processes are inhibited, the virus is unable to take over the reproductive processes of the cell and cannot, therefore, replicate itself and infect other cells. Such inhibition is a characteristic of most substances that are being tested for activity against AIDS and Epstein-Barr. The enzyme in question is a key to the action of retroviruses. These viruses, also known as ribodeoxyviruses or oncornaviruses, have been implicated in the development of several kinds of experimental cancers. Beta-lapachone is obtained simply by treating lapachol with sulfuric acid, and tests show that it has a unique method of action vis-a-vis the reverse transcriptase inhibition.[25]

Note: Sulfurous compounds in some plants, especially

yerba maté, when combined with lapacho, might provide a catalytic base for the transformation of lapachol to beta-lapachone, and hence increase the effectiveness of the lapacho. In this light, it is interesting to note that native folklore teaches that yerba mate is a catalyst for lapacho; yerba mate becomes the foundation for lapacho therapy.

Lapacho components have been intensively studied in terms of their action against two rather nasty parasites: *Schistosoma mansoni* and *Trypanosoma cruzi*, both responsible for considerable disease and misery in tropical countries. Lapacho was effective against both.[26–28] Taken by mouth, lapachol is eventually secreted onto the skin via the sebaceous glands where it acts as a topical barrier, inactivating microorganisms soon after they contact the skin. Meanwhile, throughout the GI tract, it is performing the identical function on the mucous membranes, preventing the penetration of parasites. The mechanism of action is not well understood, but is felt to involve the uncoupling of cellular respiration (see the following section on mechanisms of action), the stimulation of lipid peroxidation and superoxide production, and the inhibition of DNA/RNA biosynthesis.

Antifungal effect

Lapacho is often singled out as the premier treatment for Candida or yeast infections. Lapachol, N-factors and xyloidone appear to be the primary active principles.[9–10] By the mid-70s the list of N-factors that inhibited *Candida albicans* and other fungi had grown to several dozen.[11–15]

It would be misleading to categorically state that the N-factors in lapacho have proven antimicrobial and antifungal activity in and of themselves. Studies have shown that the manner in which they occur in the plant must be taken into consideration. We know, for example, that antifungal activity is lost when the N factors are tightly bound to highly water-soluble or highly fat-soluble groups. It has not been clearly determined how the N-factors occur in lapacho.[16]

N-factors, obtainable from various chemical supply companies, have become favorite testing agents in government and university labs due to the rise in yeast infections resulting from increased use of cytotoxic drugs, corticosteroids, antibiotics and immunosuppressants.[17,18]

An interesting application has been reported in which toe and fingernail fungal infections are relieved by soaking these appendages in lapacho tea off and on for a couple of weeks.

Anti-inflammatory

The anti-inflammatory and healing action of lapacho extracts was demonstrated in a study in which purple lapacho extract was administered to patients with cervicitis and cervicovaginitis, conditions resulting variously from infections (*Candida albicans*, *Trichomonas vaginalis*), chemical irritations and mechanical irritation. The lapacho extract was applied intravaginally via gauze tampons soaked in the extract, and renewed every 24 hours. The treatment proved to be highly effective.[19] One wonders what might happen were the tampon method combined with the ingestion of strong teas.

The anti-inflammatory action of lapacho might also account for its observed tendency to reduce the pain, inflammation and other symptoms of arthritis. Anecdotal accounts of complete cures are even available. As yet virtually untested in research settings, the purported ability of this plant to reduce symptoms of joint disease may be ultimately validated and added to the growing list of benefits to be enjoyed by the daily ingestion of lapacho tea.

Other beneficial effects

Routine screenings have revealed several minor properties of lapacho that might occur if needed in certain individuals: diuretic, sedative, decongestant, and hypotensive, to name a few.

Unfortunately, space limitations preclude a lengthy discussion of all the benefits of lapacho, but some of the major actions listed above require further elaboration, which will be given in the next section.

MECHANISMS OF ACTION

Every cell of the body requires oxygen and glucose to obtain energy for life-sustaining functions. The oxygen and glucose are subjected to a fairly complex metabolic process in the tiny energy-producing structures in the cell called mitochondria. This process requires numerous enzymes and coenzymes. The oxygen and glucose are converted to carbon dioxide and water which are then returned to the blood. The CO_2 is exhaled by the lungs (hence this metabolic process is often called respiration); excess water is eventually drawn off through perspiration or through the kidneys. During this conversion, several electrons are freed, which are immediately utilized by another pathway to produce ATP (adenosine triphosphate), the energy currency of the cell. ATP is the molecule every cell is required to utilize, or spend, to obtain energy. The two paths, one for breakdown of glucose, and one for synthesis of ATP, are tightly coupled together. Should they become uncoupled, the cell can no longer obtain energy, and it dies, a process referred to as uncoupling of oxidative phosphorylation.

Many agents have been found that uncouple oxidative phosphorylation; many of them resemble the N-factors in lapacho. In fact, it has been found that lapacho works like other benzoquionones, i.e., it uncouples the mitochondrial oxidative phosphorylation occurring in cancerous cells, but not in healthy ones.[35] This selective killing (cytotoxicity) of tumor cells is what makes lapacho such a potentially valuable agent for the treatment of cancer.

One of the games science plays is attempting to discover at what point cellular respiration is broken up by chemical agents. The components of lapacho seem to interrupt the process at several points, usually by inhibiting an enzyme or coenzyme that is required for the next step in the chain to occur properly.[36–38] For instance, lapacho inhibits the proper functioning of ATPase, the enzyme that catalyzes the final step in the formation of ATP.[39]

Lapachol has also been shown to inhibit the amount of another substance required for cellular reproduction: uridine triphosphate.[40] This molecule is the main source of substances (called pyrimidine nucleotides) that are required by cells in order to build DNA, RNA and most other important proteins of the body. Lapacho may actually block the synthesis of pyrimidines in cancer cells (by inhibiting the enzyme dihydroorotate dehydrogenase).[41] The result would be certain cellular death.

There is also evidence that lapacho interacts directly with the nucleic acids of the DNA helix in cancerous cells.[42] If such interaction, or bonding, takes place, DNA replication would be impossible. The result is also eventual death of the cell.

Finally, the lapacho constituent beta-lapachone has been shown to weaken malignant cells, even to the point of cellular death, by stimulating a process known as lipid peroxidation, which produces toxic molecules.[43]

SAFETY DATA

While there can be no doubt that lapacho is highly toxic to many kinds of cancer cells, viruses, bacteria, fungi, parasites and other kinds of microorganisms, the substance appears to be without any kind of significant toxicity to healthy human cells. The side effects mainly encountered (and usually with isolated lapacho constituents) are limited to nausea and anticoagulant effects in very high doses, a tendency to loosen the bowels, and diarrhea in very high doses. As indicated earlier, some nausea should be expected as a natural consequence of the detoxification process. The FDA gave lapacho a clean bill of health in 1981.

Some trials have indicated that lapachol has antivitamin K action. Other constituents have a provitamin K action; it is likely, therefore, that the two actions cancel each other out (except possibly when one or the other is necessary, as one would expect from an herbal tonic).

Perhaps the most significant study on toxicity was published in 1970 by researchers from Chas Pfizer & Co., Inc. Looking specifically at lapachol, these investigators found that all signs of lapachol toxicity in animals were completely reversible and even self-limiting, i.e., over time the signs of toxicity decreased and even disappeared within the time constraints of the study.

The most severe kinds of self-limiting side-effects they observed were an antivitamin K effect, anemia, and significant rises of metabolic and protein toxins in the bloodstream. The diminuation of these signs indicates that lapacho initiates an immediate alterative or detoxification effect on the body's cells. Once the cells are "cleaned up," the signs of toxicity disappear. This effect is quite common among herbal tonics.

REFERENCES

1. Paterno. E. "Richerche sull'acido lapico." *Gazz. Chim. Ital.* 12, 227–392, 1882.

2. Hooker, S.C. "Constitution of lapachol and its derivatives. The structure of the anylene chain." *J. Chem. Society,* 89, 1356, 1896.

3. Fieser, L.F. "Alkylation of hydroxynaphthoquinone. A synthesis of lapachol." *J. Am. Chem. Soc.*, 49, 857, 1927.

4. Pinto, J. de Al. *Dictionary of Brazilian Botany or Compendium of Brazilian Vegetation. Indigenous and Introduced.* Entry for Lapacho. Rio de Janeiro, 1873.

5. Concalves de Lima, O., D'Albuquerque, I., et al. "Primeiras observacoes sobre a acao antimicrobiana do lapachol." *An. Soc. Biol. PE,* 14(1/2), 129–135, 1956.

6. Concalves de Lima, O., D'Albuquerque, I. et al. "Uma nova substancia antibiotica isolada do 'pau darco', tabebuia sp." *An. Soc. Biol. PE,* 14 (1/2), 136–140, 1956.

7. Concalves de Lima, O., D'Albuquerque, I. et al. "Substancias antimicrogianas de plantas superiores. Comunicacao XX. Atividade antimicrobiana de alguns derivados do lapachol em comparacao com a xiloidona, nova orto-naftoquinona natural

isoladada de extratos do cerne do pau d'arco roxo, tabebuia avellandae Lorl. ex Griseb." *Rev. Inst. Antibiot., Recife,* 4 (1/2), 3–17, 1962.

8. Concalves de Lima, O., D'Albuquerque, I. et al. "Substancias antimicrobianas de plantas superiores. Comunicacao XXV. Obtencao dxiloidona (Desidrolapachona por transformacao de Lapachol em presenca de piridina." *Rev. Inst. Antibiot., Recife,* 6 (1/2), 23–34, 1966.

9. Duke, J. *CRC Handbook of Medicinal Herbs.* CRC Press, Boca Raton, Florida, 1985, p. 470.

10. Kumazawa, Y., Itagaki, A. Fukumoto, M. et al. "Activation of peritoneal macrophages by berberine-type alkaloids in terms of induction of cytostatic activity." *Int. J. Immunopharmac.,* 6, 586–92, 1984.

11. Ambrogi, V., Artini, W. et al. "Studies on the antibacterial and antifungal properties of 1,4-naphthoquinones." *Br. J. Pharmacol.,* 40, 871–880, 1970.

12. Oster, K.A. and Golden, M.J. "Studies on alcohol-soluble fungistatic and fungicidal compounds. III. Evaluation of the antifungal properties of quinones and quinolines." *J. Am Pharm. Assoc.,* 37, 429–434, 1948.

13. Popov. L., Ivanov, Ch. et al. "Synthetic fungicides. I. Antimycotic action of phytohormonal-type substances and of beta-naphthalenic derivatives." *C.R. Acad. Bulg. Sci.,* 6, 37–40, 1953.

14. Vladimirtsev, I.F., Bilich, B.E. et al. "Antimicrobial properties of some naphthoquinones." *Fiziol. Akt. Veshchestva,* 2, 121–124, 1969.

15. Zsolanai, T. "Versuche zur entdeckung neurer fungistatika." *Biochem. Pharmacol.,* 11, 515–534.

16. Gershon, H. and Shanks, L. "Fungitoxicity of 1,4-napthoquinones to candida albicans and Trichophyton mentagrophtes. *Can. J. Microbiol.,* 21, 1317–1321, 1975.

17. Hart, P.D., Russell, E. and Remington, J.S. "The compromised host and infection. II. Deep fungal infection." *J. Infect. Dis.,* 120, 169–191, 1969.

18. Rifkind, D., Marchioro, L., Schneck, A. and Hill, B. "Systemic fungal infections complicating renal transplantation and immunosuppressive therapy." *Am. J. Med.,* 43, 28–38, 1967.

19. Wanick, M.C., Bandeira, J.A. and Fernandes, R.V. "Acao anti-inflamatria e cicatrizante do extracto hidroalcoolico doliber do pau d'arco roxo (tabebuia avellanedae), em pacientes portadoras de cervicites e cervico-vaginites." *Revista do Instituto de Antibioticos*, 10(½), 41–46, 1970.

20. Lagrota, M. et al. "Antiviral activity of lapachol." *Rev. Microbiol.*, 14, 21–26, 1983.

21. Wanick, M.C. et al. "Acao antiinflamátoria e cicatrizante do extrato hidroalcoolico do liber do pau d'arco roxo (tabebuia avellanedae), em pacientes portadoras de cervicites e cervico-vaginites." *Separata da Revista do Insituto de Antibioticos*, 10, 41–46, 1970.

22. Gilber, B., de Souza, J.P., Fascio, M. et al. "Schistosomiasis. Protection against infection by terpenoids." *An. Acad. Brasil Cienc.*, 42(suppl), 397–400, 1970.

23. Lihares, MIS and de Santana, C.F. "Estudo sobre ofefeito de substancias antibioticas obtidas de streptomyces e vegetais superiores sobre of herpesvirus hominis." *Revista Instituto Antibioticos, Recife*, 15, 25–32, 1975.

24. Schaffner–Sabba, K. et al. "B-lapachone: synthesis of derivates and activities in tumour models." *J. Medicinal Chem.*, 27, 990–994, 1984.

25. Schuerch, A.R. and Wehrli, W. "Beta-lapachone, an inhibitor of oncornavirus reverse transcriptase and eukaryotic dna polymerase-alpha." *Eur. J. Biochem.*, 4, 197–205, 1978.

26. Austin, F.G. "Schistosoma mansoni chemoprophylaxis with dietary lapachol." *Am. J. Trop. Med. Hygiene*, 23, 412–419, 1974.

27. Giojman, S.G. and Stoppani, A.O.M. "Oxygen radicals and macromolecule turnover in trypanosoma cruzi." *Life Chem. Rep.*, (suppl 2), 1984, 216–221.

28. Boveris, A., Stoppani, A.O.M., Docampo, R. and Cruz, F.S. "Superoxide anion production and trypanocidal action of naphthoquinones on trypanosoma cruzi." *Comp. Biochem. Phys.*, 327–329, 1978.

29. Linardi, M.C.F., de Oliveira, M.M. and Sampaio, M.R.P. *J. Med. Chem.*, 18, 1159, 1975

30. Hartwell, J.L. and Abbott, B.J. *Adv. Pharmacol. Chemother.*, 7, 170, 1969.

31. de Oliveira, M.M., Linardi, M.C.F. and Sampaio, M.R.P. "Ef-

fects of quinone derivatives on an experimental tumor." *J. Pharm. Sci.* 67, 562–563.

32. de Santana, C.F., de Lima, O. et al. "Observacoes sobre as propriedades antitumorais e toxicologicas do extrato do liber e de alguns componentes do cerne do pau d'arco (tabebuia avellanedae)." *Revista do Instituto de Antibioticos, Recife*, 8(½), 87–94, 1969.

33. de Santana, C.F., Lins, L.J.P. et al. "Primeiras observacoes com emprego do lapachol em pacientes humanos portadores de neoplasias malignas." *Revista do Instituto de Antibioticos, Recife.* 20(½), 61–68, 1980/1.

34. Santana, C.F., Concalves de Lima, O. et al. "Observacoes sobre as propriedades antitumorais e toxicologicas do extrato do liber e de alguns componentes do cerne do pau d'arco (Tabebuia avellanedae)." *Rev. Inst. Antibiot. Recife.* 8(½), 89–94, 1968.

35. Hartwell, J.L. *Plants Used Against Cancer. A survey.* Graterman Publications, Lawrence, Mass. 1982, Citation for Lapachone.

36. Bachur, N.R., Godon, S.L., Gee, M.V. and Kon, H. "NADPH cytochrome p-450 reductase activation of quinone anticancer agents to free radicals." *Proc. Natl. Acad. Sci. USA,* 76, 954–957, 1979.

37. Bachur, N.R., Gordon, S.L. and Gee, M.V. "A general mechanism for microsomal activation of quinone anticancer agents to free radicals." *Cancer Res.,* 38, 1745–1750, 1978.

38. Iwamoto, Y., Hansen, I.L., Porter, T.H. and Folkers, K. "Inhibition of coenzyme Q10-enzymes, succinoxidase and NADH oxidase, by adriamycin and other quinones having antitumor activity." *Biochem. Biophys. Res. Com.,* 58, 633–638, 1974.

39. de Lima, O.G., d'Albuquerque, I.L., et al. "Uma nova substancia antibiotica isolado do pau d'arco tabebuia sp." *Annais da Sociedade de Biologica de Pernambuco.*, XIV, 136–140, 1956.

40. Bennett, L.L., Smithers, D., Rose, L.M. et al. "Inhibition of synthesis of pyrimidine nucleotides by 2-hydroxy-3 (3,3-dichloroallyl)-1, 4-naphthoquinone." *Cancer Res.,* 39, 4868–4874, 1979.

41. Howland. J.L. "Uncoupling and inhibition of oxidative phosphorylation by 2-hydroxy-3-alkl-1, 4-naphthoquinones." *Biochim. Biophys. Acta.* 77, 659–662, 1963.

42. Lee, S.H., Sutherland, T.O., Deves, R. and Brodie, A.F. "Respiration of/active transport of solutes and oxidative phosphorylaton by naphthoquinones in irradiated membrane vesicles from mycobacterium phlei." *Proc. Natl. Acad. Sci. USA,* 77, 102 106, 1980.

43. Docamp, R., Cruz, F.S., Boveris, A. et al. "B-lapachone enhancement of lipid peroxidation and superoxide anion and hydrogen peroxide formation by sarcoma 180 ascites tumor cells." *Biochem. Pharmacol.,* 28, 723–728, 1979.

CHAPTER TWO

The Cardiovascular System

❧ The cardiovascular system consists of blood, the heart and the vessels. The blood is the liquid carrier of all life-giving substances. The vessels are the pipes in which the blood flows and from which it emanates to the body's billions of cells. The heart is the pump that keeps the fluid moving.

Here is a partial list of what the blood does for us:

1. It carries the materials of digestion from the small intestine.
2. It carries oxygen from the lungs.
3. It carries hormones from the endocrine glands.
4. It controls the amount of water and the relative pH inside of body cells; it is a necessary component of the lymph system.

5. It is the home of antibodies, white blood cells and other immune system components, and makes certain they get to the site of an infection.

6. It carries blood clotting agents which assure that vessels get repair quickly when they are damaged.

7. It carries enzymes.

8. It distributes the heat produced during cell metabolism.

9. It carries away waste products of cell matabolism and delivers them to the lungs, kidneys and skin for elimination from the body.

Should any of the above processes become seriously disturbed, death ensues more or less rapidly.

Whole blood contains its own kinds of cells, which are generally divided into three types: red cells, white cells and platelets. Together, these cells account for 45 percent of blood. The remaining 55 percent is a liquid composition called plasma. Plasma is 91 to 92 percent water. About 7 percent is made up of proteins such as albumin, globulin and fibrin. The plasma also contains very small amounts of sugars, salts, and fats.

Red blood cells are also known as red corpuscles or erythrocytes, while white blood cells are sometimes called white corpuscles or leukocytes. The platelets are also called thrombocytes.

Red blood cells are really not cells but corpuscles, because they lack the nuclei that are required for cell division. A red blood corpuscle is about one-third hemoglobin, an iron-rich protein that captures oxygen as the blood flows through the lungs. Red blood cells are produced in the red marrow of the bones, live for about 110 days and are then removed from the blood by the liver and spleen.

White blood cells are larger than red corpuscles. They have distinct nuclei. Red cells outnumber the white by about 600 to one. White cells are the body's main defense system against disease. These are discussed more fully in the chapter on the immune system. Briefly, white cells can move around, attach and detach themselves from vessel walls, surround and attack bacteria, and remove waste from the site of infection.

Platelets are very small granular fragments of cells that float about in the blood waiting for a chance to help in the repair of vessels. Sometimes fragments clump together when they shouldn't, forming dangerous blood clots.

How blood clots

One of the most rapid and amazing processes in physiology is the repair of a broken blood vessel. During bleeding, platelets flow through the cut along with the other components of blood; but as they bump against the jagged edge of the vessel, they rupture, spilling out a substance called thromboplastin. This substance, in the presence of blood-borne calcium, reacts with a blood protein known as prothrombin to form another substance called thrombin. Thrombin then reacts with another protein called fibrinogen to form fibrin. It is fibrin that actually begins to seal off the blood flow by forming long, thin strands of material across the wound like a net. The net traps red blood cells, forming a clot. As the clot dries, it turns into a scab. The clot traps the blood inside the vessels, which then undergo a more systematic repair process of the vessel wall itself.

How blood is made

Blood cells are produced from special stem cells in the marrow of long bones. Stem cells differentiate into either red or white blood cells as required by the body at any given point in time. From the marrow they enter the bloodstream, where they mature. Red cells lose their nuclei and gain the hemoglobin molecule during maturation.

Some of the factors that stimulate the production of red

cells are strenuous exercise, emotional stress, high temperatures, high altitudes and loss of whole blood.

White cells are not only produced in bone marrow, they are also formed in special lymphoid tissues throughout the body. Factors that stimulate the production of white cells are disease and infection. The lifespan of white cells is highly variable, depending upon the type of white cells, from a few days to several months.

Platelets are also produced in the bone marrow, but they do not come directly from stem cells. Instead they are formed from small bits of cytoplasm that break off from stem cells. Platelets only live for about ten days.

THE CIRCULATORY SYSTEM

Blood moves throughout the body as the heart pumps. It is carried in the blood vessels. Blood vessels that carry blood away from the heart are called arteries, while those that carry blood toward the heart are called veins. Vessels that help link arteries with veins are called capillaries.

The largest blood vessel in the body is the aorta. It is an artery. It branches into smaller arteries, and these in turn branch into yet smaller arteries called arterioles. The arterioles branch finally into the smallest arteries of all, the capillaries.

Capillaries are microscopic, invisible to the naked eye. Their walls are only one cell thick and are highly permeable; that is, they have holes in them. This allows oxygen and small bits of nutrients, enzymes, hormones and other substances to pass out easily from the vessel. Every single cell of the body is fed by one or more capillaries. The capillary has to be very close to the cell because the nutrients that flow from the vessels need to be rapidly taken up by the cell.

As the tissue cells breathe and undergo their individual cellular processes, they create wastes in the form of acids, carbon dioxide, and other substances. These pass out through the permeable membrane of the cell and in through the permeable membrane of capillaries on the venous side of the circulatory system.

You can see that arteries do not directly connect to veins. Fluids from arteries pass into the spaces between tissue cells (called interstitial space), are absorbed by cells, flow out from cells and are taken up by veins. All of these actions are controlled by critical differences in pressure that exist in the artery/cell/vein network.

Capillaries on the return side connect with venules, similar in size to arterioles, which run into veins. The veins empty into the venae cavae that return the blood to the heart. The entire cycle of blood from the heart through the body and back to the heart takes about 20 seconds.

STRUCTURE AND FUNCTION OF BLOOD VESSELS

In structure, arteries, veins and capillaries differ from one another in some critical ways. The walls of arteries are made of three layers. The outermost is a tough, fibrous tissue with little elasticity. The middle layer is elastic smooth muscle; this layer expands as blood surges through, but only as much as the outer layer will allow. The inner layer is a thin, smooth sheet of cells called the endothelium.

The walls of veins consist of the same three layers as arteries, but they are much thinner. The outer layer is actually much more developed in veins than in arteries, while the middle layer has much less smooth muscle.

Capillaries, as mentioned above, are made up of a single layer of cells, the endothelium.

Blood flow in the arteries is directed by muscular contractions of the heart; hence it can be under a great deal of pressure. Blood flow in the veins, however, is not affected by heart activity. It is the result of contractions in muscles that surround the veins. Venous flow is assisted by one-way valves in the larger veins that prevent the blood from backing up due to gravity and sluggish muscular effort.

Of major importance to health is the fact that there is not enough blood in the body to fill up all of the body's capillaries at the same time. Which capillaries receive the most blood at any one time is determined by the demands being placed on the body from the person or his environment.

There are actually muscles in the walls of arterioles that open and close the vessel and thereby regulate how much blood will be allowed to flow in the capillaries beyond. As an example of how this affects the quality of life, consider what happens when you exercise after eating a big meal. Muscular work puts large demands on the body's ability to deliver oxygen and nutrients to the muscle cells. Therefore, the muscles in the arterioles open up to allow blood to flow into the capillaries that feed the muscles. Meanwhile, they shut down the flow of blood into the capillaries that feed the digestive system, thereby inhibiting digestion.

What causes blood pressure

Systolic arterial blood pressure results from cardiac contraction of the ventricles of the heart. Diastolic pressure results from the resting stage of the heart's rhythm. Normal systolic/diastolic blood pressure in a healthy adult of average size and weight is about 120/70mm.

THE HEART AND BLOOD FLOW

The heart is composed of cardiac muscle, held together by thick connective tissue called the pericardium. The heart has four chambers, the left and right atria and the left and right ventricles, separated by a thick piece of muscle called the septum. The inside of the heart, like the vessels, is lined by a thin layer of endothelium. The upper chambers of the heart are the atria. They are the receiving chambers for returning blood. They move the blood into the ventricles. The ventricles pump the blood away from the heart to the lungs and body.

Blood flow would be very straightforward were it not for one thing: Blood returning from the extremities of the body has very little oxygen in it, and a lot of carbon dioxide. Before it can be recirculated, it must be returned to the lungs where the necessary gaseous exchange can take place. As the blood empties into the right atrium from the venae cavae, it is pumped into the left ventricle, from which it is pumped directly to the lungs through the pulmonary artery. In the lungs it circulates through a very dense capillary bed lined with microscopic air sacs. Here the red blood cells exchange carbon dioxide for oxygen. The oxygenated blood then returns to heart via the pulmonary vein. The circulation of blood from heart to lungs and back to the heart is called the pulmonary system.

Blood from the pulmonary vein enters the left atrium and is pumped from there into the left ventricle, whence it is pumped into the aorta. The circulation of blood from the left ventricle through the body and back to the heart is called the systemic system.

Blood flow in the heart itself is controlled by valves that allow flow in one direction only, in a coordinated effort that gives rise to the characteristic "lub-dup" sound. During the pause between "lub-dups" the heart is at rest.

DISORDERS OF THE CARDIOVASCULAR SYSTEM

While the heart is an extraordinary pump, capable of years of uninterrupted activity under the most trying of circumstances, it is still subject to a variety of problems. Likewise, the tubes of the circulatory system are also subject to deterioration over time. Some of the problems that can be encountered are listed below.

Stroke

A rupture (hemorrhage) or blockage (thrombosis or embolism) of a blood vessel in the brain; results in loss of oxygen to various parts of the brain. Symptoms include loss of consciousness, paralysis, slurred speech, visual disturbances. Also called cerebral vascular accident or cerebral apoplexy. Tissue death (infarction) is a common result of a stroke.

Thrombosis

A common cause of strokes, thrombosis is the formation of a clot (thrombus) that blocks an artery. These clots build up on artery walls until total blockage occurs. Thrombosis can occur in any blood vessel. It is an abnormality of the normal clotting process. Thrombi in arteries severely affect the health of the organ normally supplied with blood by that artery. Thrombi in veins are not immediately life-threatening, but they can cause pain, tenderness, swelling, and discoloration. The main threat from a thrombus in a vein is that a piece (an embolus) will break off, travel to the heart and from there to the lungs where it will block an artery, resulting in a pulmonary embolism.

Cerebral thrombosis

As the name implies, this ailment is caused by the formation of a thrombus in one of the arteries supplying the brain.

Acute myocardial infarction or heart attack

Results from a thrombus forming in one of the coronary arteries.

Embolism

Common cause of strokes. Blockage by an embolus (usually a piece of a clot that has broken off of a thrombus somewhere in the body) that has found its way into an artery to the brain, where it lodges.

Atherosclerosis

A disease of the arterial wall in which the normally thin inner layer (endothelium) grows thicker due to the buildup of plaque, causing a constriction of the channel and thereby inhibiting the free flow of blood. Plaques (or raised patches) consist of low-density lipoproteins, decaying muscle cells, fibrous tissue, clumped-up platelets, cholesterol and even mineral deposits. Plaque formation increases with age and is a function of diet and other factors; it encourages formation of thrombi and emboli.

Hyperlipidemia

Metabolic disorder involving high levels of lipids in the blood. These lipids include cholesterol, triglycerides and lipoproteins. There are LDLs (low-density lipoproteins), VLDLs (very low-density lipoproteins) and HDLs (high-density lipopropteins). There are several types of hyperlipidemia. The HDLs are not considered a cause of hyperlipidemia. Hyperlipidemia may have genetic origins, or be caused by disease such as lupus, nephrotic syndrome, Cushing's disease, hypothyroidism, diabetes mellitus, obesity, alcoholism, renal failure or estrogen therapy. The condition can lead to atherosclerosis and coronary heart disease.

Angina pectoris

Antherosclerosis in arteries leading to the heart muscle.

Intermittent claudication

Atherosclerosis in vessels leading to the muscles of the legs. Produces pain during walking.

Transient ischemia

Atherosclerosis in vessels leading to the brain. Signs and symptoms resemble those of stroke, plus episodes of dizziness.

Pulmonary embolism

Lodging of an embolism, a fragment of a blood clot, in an artery of the lungs.

Congestive heart failure, congestive cardiomyopathy

The heart's inability to keep up its work load of pumping blood through the body and lungs. Either side of the heart may be affected. Increasing demands on the left side can result from hypertension, anemia, hyperthyroidism, heart valve defects, congenital heart defects, arrhythmias, myocardial infarction and cardiomyopathy. Unusual demands on the right side are caused by pulmonary hypertension, bronchitis, emphysema, valve defects, congenital heart defects and left-sided failure. In all these conditions, the inability of the heart to meet the demands placed on it results in back pressure and congestion of blood in areas such as the lungs (left-sided failure) or the venous system (right-sided failure). Symptoms include difficulty in breathing, distended neck veins, enlarged liver, edema, fatigue, swelling in ankles and legs and indigestion (from congestion in intestines).

Congenital heart disease

Refers to any of a multitude of structural defects that have been present from birth, usually affecting septum and valves.

Rheumatic fever

A disease characterized by inflammation in tissues throughout the body. It attacks the joints but is rarely crippling. Of greater concern is its effect on the heart muscle. Follows strep throat infections, but appears to be some kind of autoimmune disorder, i.e., in its efforts to fight the strep, the immune system begins to turn on the body itself.

Mitral stenosis

A narrowing of the orifice of the mitral valve in the heart, which causes the atrial portion of the left side to work harder in order to move blood through the narrowed opening. Usually due to scarring of valve from an attack of rheumatic fever. Causes shortness of breath that worsens over time, palpitations, atrial fibrillation (rapid, irregular heartbeat), flushed cheeks, chest infections, coughing of blood and fatigue. Treated with digitalis and diuretics.

Mitral valve prolapse

A slight deformity of the mitral valve that can produce leakage of the valve and a characteristic heart murmur. Cause is not known, but it may be inherited or result from rheumatic fever, coronary heart disease or cardiomyopathy. May produce chest pain, arrhythmias, or heart failure.

Endocarditis

Refers to an infection of the heart valves. Usually occurs in people with rheumatic fever, in drug addicts using unsterile needles, or from a viral infection.

Cardiomyopathy

A general term for disease of the heart muscle. Can be inherited, or the result of vitamin deficiency or alcoholism. A viral infection can also produce this condition.

Myocarditis

A general term for inflammation of the heart muscle. Viral infections and toxicity from bacterial infections are the primary causes.

Arrhythmias

Abnormalities in the rhythm or rate of the heartbeat caused by some kind of irregularity in the electrical impulses to the heart or in the transmission of impulses through the heart's electrical conducting pathways. There are two main groups of arrhythmias: tachycardias, in which the heart rate is faster than normal, i.e., faster than 100 beats per minute; and bradycardias, in which the rate is slower than 60 beats per minute. The beat may be normal (as in sinus tachycardia or supraventricular tachycardia) or irregular (as in ventricular tachycardia). Arrhythmias are usually caused by coronary heart disease, with the vessels bringing blood to the heart becoming too narrow, due to atheroma (fatty deposits), to supply the conducting tissue of the heart with enough blood to assure efficient operation. Sinus tachycardia may result after exercise or stress, and sinus bradycardia often appears in athletes. Tachycardias are also caused by caffeine in sensitive persons. Arrhythmias give rise to the common feeling of palpitations, and may cause dizziness or faintness due to a reduction in blood flow to the brain, or breathing difficulty if the blood supply to the lungs is reduced. Arrhythmias also cause bouts of angina pectoris.

Varicose veins

Swelling, distortion and twisting of a vein, usually in the legs. Caused by lack of tone in tissues supporting the vein and subsequent failure of valves further up the leg. Blood pools under the force of gravity in superficial veins, causing them to swell and twist. Obesity, menopause, pregnancy, PMS (premenstrual syndrome) and standing for long periods are aggravating factors.

Phlebitis

Inflammation of a vein, normally associated with a tendency to blood clotting in the affected vein (called thrombophlebitis).

Hemorrhoids

Varicose veins of the anus.

Ischemia and/or vascular insufficiency

Insufficient supply of blood to a specific organ or tissue. Injuries to vessels, constriction to spasm of vessel muscles, sitting too long in one position, atherosclerosis, or cardiac inadequacy are some causative factors. With age comes the gradual deterioration of capillaries throughout the body, especially those feeding the brain, the eyes, the extremities and the ears. The vessel walls become brittle, fragile and hyperpermeable—too leaky—allowing nutrients and toxins to pass through to the wrong places in the wrong amounts. Such damage to the capillaries is not dangerous in itself, but it means that any cells depending on those capillaries for nutrients and oxygen will certainly die.

❧ HERBAL TONICS FOR THE CARDIOVASCULAR SYSTEM

The purpose of consuming herbal cardiotonics is to prevent the premature and unnecessary degradation of the cardiovascular system. The use of these tonics from an early age will help delay the onset of free radical damage, plaque buildup, muscular degeneration and fatigue, capillary rigidity, fragility and hyperpermeability, cholesterol buildup, arthritic lesions, and any of the other numerous defects that lead to cardiovascular problems.

Cardiotonics are widely used in Europe, especially Germany, throughout a person's adult life. A routine checkup in Germany will often produce some sign that cardiovascular disease is a potential problem. Instead of waiting until the condition gets markedly worse, and then administering a powerful, habituating drug such as the digitalis derivatives, German physicians will prescribe a simple herbal tonic, perhaps hawthorn. American physicians, without recourse to mild cardiotonics, can only recommend drugs. The difference between using a cardiotonic and not using one may be counted in the number of decades of good cardiovascular health you have left to enjoy before you succumb to drug therapy or surgery.

HAWTHORN BERRY
(Crataegus oxyacantha)

Hawthorn berry is perhaps the world's best cardiotonic. It dilates peripheral blood vessels, increases metabolism in the heart muscle, dilates coronary vessels and improves the blood supply to the heart. Some research suggests it also helps stabilize cardiac activity by abolishing tachycardia and other arrhythmias. It is hypotensive, and has an anabolic effect on metabolism. Compared to digitalis, it is much safer to use and milder in activity. The use of hawthorn tends to help normalize both high and low blood pressure. Antispasmodic and sedative properties along with stimulant activity, have been observed with hawthorn, though they have not been the subject of much experimental investigation. Mild antiarteriosclerotic principles have also been identified in hawthorn.

Hawthorn functions by peripheral vasodilation, very mild dilation of coronary vessels, increased enzyme metabolism in the heart muscle, and increased oxygen utilization by the heart.

One way of organizing the healing properties of hawthorn has been supplied by a noted European expert in hawthorn research, R. F. Weiss, who maintains that hawthorn products are characterized by three basic healing properties which complement one another:

(1) Improvement of coronary blood supply, which leads to lessening of anginal attacks and general lessening of subjective complaints.

(2) Improvement of the metabolic processes in the myocardium, which results in an improvement of the functional heart activity.

(3) Abolishment of some types of rhythm disturbances.[1]

In patients with perfusion disorders of the coronary arteries that are mainly due to coronary sclerosis, hawthorn significantly decreased oxygen utilization during exercise. In 40 of 52 patients, intravenous administration of hawthorn extract for a mean period of 13.4 days produced a noticeable decrease of the ischemia reaction in the exercise EKG. In patients undergoing standard therapies, an improvement could be seen in only 25 percent of the cases.[2]

In another study on subjects with primary heart disease, intravenous hawthorn extract produced a rapid improvement in almost all cases, as determined by an increase in the mechanical efficiency of the heart muscle. In patients with secondary heart disease, the effect was not as great in terms of the number of cases helped, but significant effects were seen in those cases that were helped. The herb also helped patients whose heart disease was caused by hepatitis or other liver disease. These results taken together suggest a positive inotropic action.[3]

Similar findings have been reported by several other investigators.[4]

Recently, excellent results on a wide variety of coronary problems were obtained utilizing an exacting crossed, double-blind procedure. The substance used was a German drug called

Corguttin, which is composed of hawthorn, *Convallaria majalis*, *Primula officinalis* and *Valeriana officinalis*. This product proved extremely effective in taking care of the routine, daily needs of patients with minor heart problems.[5]

Hawthorn has vasodilatory action

In dogs and guinea pigs, hawthorn had a marked and prolonged ability to dilate blood vessels, and an ability to lower peripheral resistance to blood flow. The extract was injected directly into the coronary artery. It caused no change in the volume of coronary blood flow, but still showed lowering of peripheral resistance. The blood supply of the central nervous system was influenced in the same manner as that of the coronary vessels: the resistance to blood flow was lowered, and the blood volume passing through the carotid artery was also increased.[7,8]

Hawthorn successfully destroys experimentally-induced blockade of anaerobic glycolysis, a condition that typifies some forms of heart disease caused by enzyme insufficiency.[9]

In patients with chronic cardiac insufficiency, hawthorn has produced a quickening of the heartbeat. It increased coronary blood flow by increasing the cardiac output and by direct influence on the smooth muscles of the vessels. Arterial and venous blood pressure were not affected, the EKG was not influenced and no pulmonary damage was observed.[10-12]

Hawthorn is hypotensive

A fraction of the hawthorn extract containing flavone polymers had a low toxicity in the mouse, a pronounced hypotensive activity in the cat, and strong and prolonged cardiotonic action and detoxifying properties in the rabbit.[12] Oligomeric procyanidins isolated from hawthorn extract decreased blood pressure in cats, decreased aggression in mice, decreased body temperature in mice, and prolonged hexobarbital narcosis in mice.[11]

Hawthorn versus digitalis

It used to be assumed that hawthorn and digitalis belonged to the same class of agents, but that hypothesis has been totally refuted by studies showing that, for example, hawthorn may partly antagonize undesirable properties of digitalis. In addition, hawthorn enhances pulse and positively potentiates the force of muscular contractions. It also enhances cardiac output or performance in rats measured by stress swimming trials. On isolated frog heart, it has a tonic and normalizing action. Hawthorn also differs from digitalis in that it lowers the blood pressure through dilation of peripheral vessels, not through a direct action on the heart. Hence it preserves critical reflexive blood pressure regulation.

In man, hawthorn acts even on the healthy heart to increase cardiac activity. Hawthorn appears to have a less immediate effect than digitalis. After longer periods of use, subjective betterment accompanied by objective measurable improvement in tonus and regulation of cardiac activity are observed with hawthorn. Unlike digitalis, hawthorn exhibits an absence of cumulative activity. [10, 13–17]

There exists an apparent synergism between hawthorn and digitalis, as suggested by the fact that heart tissue pretreated with either one of the substances becomes sensitized to the other, so that only about one-half the normal dose of the second is required to obtain normal results. [18]

Hawthorn has an anabolic effect on metabolism

One of the more important effects of hawthorn is on metabolism in the heart muscle itself. In one trial, after 14 hours of abstinence from food, the concentrations of free fatty acids, free glycerol, triglycerides, glucose, lactate and pyruvate were determined in the blood of ten human subjects, whereupon hawthorn extract was injected intravenously. After 30, 60, and 120 minutes, further determinations were made. At the 30 and 60 minute intervals, a significant decrease in free fatty acids and in lactate was observed. Glucose and pyruvate also decreased, whereas the concentration of triglycerides increased. The observed alterations in fat and carbohydrate metabolism suggest that hawthorn has an anabolic (or upbuilding) effect on metabolism, presumably by an influence on the enzymatic system. By this means, a decrease in oxygen and energy consumption would occur. The implication is that under stress (as in exercise or physical labor), the heart would have a greater capacity for work than normal.[9]

Much more research could be reviewed, but the above is sufficient to demonstrate the ability of hawthorn to help maintain a strong and efficient heart and vascular system.

SAFETY DATA

No toxicity has ever been attributed directly to hawthorn. However, since it is an active cardiotonic herb, users should exercise extreme caution when combining this herb with other cardiac drugs. For example, it is known that the action of digitalis is markedly enhanced when combined with hawthorn.

REFERENCES

1. Weiss, R. F. *Lehrbuch Der Phytotherapie*, Stuttgart, Hippokrates Verlag: 1960, p. 408.
2. Kandziora, J. "Crataegutt-wirkung bei koronarendurchblutungsstoerungen." *Muenchener Medizinischer Wochenschrift*, 6, 295–298, 1969.
3. Echte, W. "Die einwirkung von weissdornextrakten auf die dynamik desmenschlichen herzens." *Arztliche Forschung*, 14(11), I/560–566, 1960.
4. Ullsperger, R. "Vorlaufige mitteilung ueber den coronargefaesseerweiternden wirkkoerper aus weissdorn." *Pharmazie*, 6(4), 141–144, 1951.

5. Hanak, T. "Phytotherapie in der kardiologischen alltagspraxis." *Zhurnal der Allgemein Medizin*, 56, 276–283, 1980.

7. Kovach, A.G.B., Foeldi, M. and Fedina, L. "Die wirkung eines extraktes aus crataegus oxyacantha auf die durchstroemung der coronarwirkung von hunden." *Arzneimittel-Forschung*, 9(6), 378–379, 1959.

8. Haireddin, J., Oberdorf, A. and Rummel, W. "Zur frage der coronarwirkung von crataegus extrakten." *Arzneimittel-Forschung*, 6(2), 1956.

9. Koehler, U. "Die hepatogene herzmuskelschwaeche." *Cardiologia*, 31, 512–522, 1957.

10. Hockerts, Th. and Muelke, G. "Beitrag zur frage einer coronarwirkung von wasserigen extrakten aus crataegus droge." *Arzneimittel-Forschung*, 5(12), 755–757, 1955.

11. Rewerksi, W., Tadeusz, P., Rylski, M. and Lewak, S. "Einigepharmakologische eigenschaften der aus weissdorn (crataegus oxyacantha) isolierten oligomeren procyanidine." *Arzneimittel-Forschung*, 21(6), 886–888, 1971.

12. Rewerksi, W. and Lewak, S. "Einige pharmakologische eigenschaften deraus weissdorn (crataegus oxyacantha) isolierten flavanpolymeren." *Arzneimittel-Forschung*, 17(4), 490–491, 1967.

13. Wezler, K. "Zur herzwirkung der crataeguswirkstoffe." *Arzneimittel-Forschung*, 8(4), 175–181, 1958.

14. Boehm, K. "Results of investigation on crataegus. II. Animal experiments with total extracts and isolated active compounds." *Arzneimittel-Forschung*, 6, 35–38, 1956.

15. Muth, H. W. "Studies on the vasoactive effects of cratemon preparations." *Therapie der Gegenwart*, 115(2), 242–255, 1976.

16. Boehm, K. *Arztliche Forschung*, 9, 442–445, 1955.

17. Fiedler, U., Hildebrand, G. and New, R. "Weitere inhaltsstoffe des weissdorns: der nachweis von cholin and acetylcholin." *Arzneimittel-Forschung*, 3(8), 436–439, 1953.

18. Bersin, T., Mueller, A. and Schwarz, H. "Substances contained in crataegus oxyacantha. III. A heptahydroxyflavan glycoside." *Arzneimittel-Forschung*, 5, 490–491, 1955.

19. Hammerl, H., Kranzl, C., Pichler, O. and Studlar, M. "Klinischexperimentelle stoffwechseluntersuchungen mit einem crataegus extract." *Arztliche Forschung*, 21(7), 261–264, 1967.

BUTCHER'S BROOM
(Ruscus aculeatus L.)

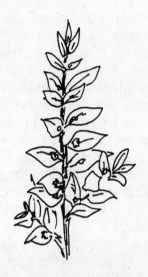

BUTCHER'S BROOM

In recent years, butcher's broom has risen to prominence in European medical care as a primary treatment for vascular disorders of all kinds. Before it was standardized and made into a guaranteed potency form, it was of limited usefulness due to variations in the concentration of active constituents. Now it has been standardized to contain guaranteed levels of the principle components, called ruscogenins. Butcher's broom products that are not carefully manufactured are often found to be seriously lacking in ruscogenin content.

Butcher's broom has excellent vasculotonic properties

French scientists were the first to reveal that butcher's broom extract possessed vasoconstrictive (blood vessel narrowing) and anti-inflammatory properties. Since that time, the extract has become very popular in European medicine as a treatment for venous circulatory disorders (especially for women complaining of a heavy sensation in the legs), as well as hemorrhoidal ailments.

Early research showed that simple alcohol extracts of whole butcher's broom rhizomes were very effective in constricting peripheral blood vessels.[1-4] Concomitant toxicological screenings suggested that the herb was extremely safe to use, much more so than other preparations being used to treat hemorrhoids. Clinical trials with external preparations have been supported down through the years by continued pharmacological investigation of the vasoconstrictive effects.[5-9] Besides the simple vasoconstrictor action, butcher's broom tones up a sluggish venous system and reduces capillary fragility. An enzymatic effect reduces pain and swelling. Insufficient circulation to the extremities is reversed. (This pertains also to circulation problems involving the retina.)

An anti-inflammatory property of butcher's broom has also been established.[10-13] This is not surprising, since butcher's broom has such a potent vasoconstrictive property. (Dilation of blood vessels is a substantial part of the inflammatory process.) At any rate, since a great many vascular problems are associated with inflammation, this finding suggests even more uses for butcher's broom.

Butcher's broom is an effective treatment of hemorrhoids

In Europe, butcher's broom is recognized for its usefulness in treating hemorrhoids and venous problems involving inflammation. European clinical trials of varying quality tend to support the medical claims, as reviewed below.

Both external and internal hemorrhoids yield to repeated application of butcher's broom. Inflammatory states of the anorectal mucosa are quickly reduced in size (reducing pain), and the return of a healthy appearance can be fairly quickly achieved.[14-16]

Tablets, salves and suppositories are used by the medical profession for treating hemorrhoids, as well as related problems in the vicinity around the rectum. Butcher's broom is also used before and after the surgical removal of hemorrhoidal knots. It works by rapidly decreasing inflammation and pain, and by strengthening the capillaries that feed this area.[17,18]

Butcher's broom helps relieve circulation disorders

Butcher's broom preparations have become a primary treatment for phlebitis (inflammation of the veins) resulting from insufficient circulation, and are recommended in the treatment of post-thrombotic syndrome, venous circulatory disturbances such as chilblains (a common vasomotor disorder of the extremities), peripheral circulatory edema, varicophlebitis, pregnancy-related varicose veins (e.g., milk leg), varicose ulcers, postoperative venous disorders, and other disorders of the peripheral hemodynamic. Dramatic improvement in both subjective and objective measures is often observed within days. Thousands of European women use butcher's broom to augment the tone and elasticity of capillary walls in the treatment of the common "heaviness in the legs" syndrome (edema experienced after standing at work all day). More resistant to permanent alteration, but still capable of cure, are varicose veins, varicose ulcers and surface veins.[19-22]

SAFETY DATA

Side effects, outside of occasional nausea or gastritis, are not known to have occurred using therapeutic doses. Studies on toxicity have shown a remarkable lack of such effects, even at high doses.[23]

REFERENCES

1. Caujolle, F., Stanilas, W., Roux, G. and Labrot, P. "Recherches pharmacologiques sur l'intrait de ruscus aculeatus L." *69e Congres Assoc. Fr. Avanc. Sci.*, Toulouse, 1950.

2. Caujolle, F., et al. "Sur la valeur du fragon en medication antihemorroidaire." *Therapie*, 7, 428, 1952.

3. Caujolle, F., et al. "Sur les proprietes pharmacologiques de ruscus aculeatus L. *Ann. Pharm. Franc.*, 11, 109, 1953.

4. Moscarella, C. "Contribution a l'etude pharmacologique du ruscus aculeatus L. (fragon epineux)." *These de pharmacie*, Toulouse, 1953.

5. Capra, C. "Studio farmacologico e tossicologico di componenti del ruscus aculeatus L." *Fitoterapia*, 43, 99, 1972.

6. Tarayre, J.P. and Lauressergues, H. "Etude de quelques proprietes pharmacologiques d'une association vasculotrope." *Ann. Pharm. Franc.* 34, 375, 1976.

7. Tarayre, J.P. and Lauressergues, H. "Action anti-oedemateuse d'une association enzymes proteolytiques, flavonoides, heterosides de ruscus aculeatus et acide ascorbique." *Ann. Pharm. Franc.*, 37, 191, 1979.

8. Marcelon, G., et al. "Effect of ruscus aculeatus on isolated canine cutaneous veins." *Pharmacology*, 14, 103, 1983.

9. Rubanyi, G. et al. "Effect of temperature on the responsiveness of cutaneous veins to the extract of ruscus aculeatus." *Gen. Pharmac.*, in press.

10. Chevillard, L. et al. "Activite anti-inflammatoire d'extraits de fragon epineux (ruscus aculeatus L.)." *Med. Pharmacol. Exp.*, 12, 109–114, 1964.

11. Cahn, J., et al. "Antiphlogistic and anti-inflammatory activity of F191." *Int. Symp. Non Steroidal Anti-inflammatory Drugs*, Milano, 1964.

12, 13. Capra, C. op. cit., 1972.

14. Lemozy, J., et al. "Interet du proctolog dans le traitement des hemorroides et des fissures anales." *Mediterranee Med.*, 92, 87, 1976.

15. Chabanon, R. "Experimentation du proctolog dans les hemor-

roides et les fissures anales." *Gaz. Med. de France*, 83, 3013, 1976.

16. Pris, J. "Proctolog: utilisation dans un service d'hematologie." *Gaz. Med France*, 84, 2423, 1977.

17. Caujolle, F., et al, op. cit., 1952.

18. Moscarella, C. op. cit., 1953.

19. Cohen, J. "Traitment par le ruscus des incidences veineuses de la contraception orale." *Vie Medicale*, X, 1305, 1977.

20. Sterboul, K. "Etude clinique d'un vasomoteur veineux. Extrait de fragon epineux." *Gaz. Hop. Civils et Militaires*, 134, 375, 1962.

21. Verne, J.M., et al. *Ann. de Chirurgie*, 14, 1221–51, 1960.

22. Sicard, P. "Resultats obtenus avec Cyclo 3 dans le traitement des ulceres variquex." *Phlebologie*, (1), 117–121, 1971.

23. Capra, C. op. cit., 1972.

KELP
(Laminaria spp.)

Kelp is today an important general nutritive tonic in essentially every land in which it grows. Until recent years, however, it was eaten almost exclusively and universally by the Japanese. Studies have shown that the Japanese intake of kelp is significantly responsible for that country's dramatically lower breast cancer rates, as well as the presence of less obesity, heart disease, respiratory disease, rheumatism and arthritis, high blood pressure, thyroid deficiency, infectious disease, constipation and other gastrointestinal ailments. The Japanese consume between 5 and 7.5 grams of kelp per capita per day. It is used in almost every meal, as garnish, vegetable, in soups, cakes, jellies, sauces, salads and flour. The most common Japanese food is noodles made from kelp. Among heavily Westernized Japanese social-economic groups, kelp consumption is decreasing and all of the above diseases are increasing. Among the poor and the rural populations, kelp consumption is increasing and disease rates are decreasing.

Three of the major effects of kelp are nutritive, antibiotic and hypotensive. A preparation called *kombu*, which is the blades of various *Laminaria* species, has been employed as a hypotensive agent in Japan for many years. Recent studies have verified its efficacy. The active principles appear to be laminine and histamine. Brown kelp is the primary source of algin, a kind of fiber that has shown considerable cholesterol-lowering activity. Kelp has cardiotonic action. It has been found to increase the contractile force in the atria, and to stimulate the hearts of frogs.

Kelp has hypotensive properties

Research on kombu from Japan has found that human hypertensive patients who drank kombu experienced significant improvement in blood pressure readings, subjective well-being and cardiac efficiency, without any side effects. Other studies have obtained the same results, in humans and in rabbits, rats and other animals. The active principles are believed to include histamine, laminine, and other cardiotonic principles that find their way into the kombu medication. Studies on independent species of *Laminaria* have also found laminine to be hypotensive.[7-13]

Kelp has cardiotonic activity

Several components of kelp, including laminine, have been shown to have good cardiotonic action. Two cardiac principles were isolated from nekombu (the basal part of the blade of a laminariaceous seaweed). Fatty acids found in kelp stimulated heart muscle, while a histamine compound accelerated contractions of the atrium. Histamine and iodine content of nekombu were 501 milligrams per kilogram and 3200 mg/kg respectively, indicating that 36 percent of the total iodine present in nekombu is in the salt form of histamine. In another test, extract from *Undaria pinnatifida* was found to increase contractile force in the atria.

Another fraction of the same seaweed also increased contractile force in the atria; the fraction had no effect on the rate of spontaneously beating right atrium, but had a positive inotropic action in the left atrium.[12, 13]

SAFETY DATA

Kelp has no known toxicity. The degraded carrageenan, derived from two red seaweeds (Irish moss), has been implicated in causing colonic lesions in rats, but none of the brown seaweeds or their derivatives have been found to be carcinogenic. Even Irish moss, if ingested in whole (i.e., nondegraded) form is perfectly safe, since it is nonabsorbable.[1-3]

Some kelp species are known for their relatively high arsenic content; however, extensive testing has found that the arsenic, although certainly present, is in a biologically unavailable form. Recently, four men were fed different kinds of seaweed in order to monitor the urinary excretion of aresenic. For kelp, 100 percent of the ingested arsenic was excreted in the urine within 60 hours, providing further evidence for the biological inertness of arsenic in seaweed. Thus brown seaweeds appear to be neither carcinogenic nor toxic.[4-6]

REFERENCES

1. Watt, J. "Effect of degraded and undegraded alginates on the colon of guinea pigs." *Proc. Nutr. Society*, 30, 81A, 1971.
2. Nilson, H. and Wagner, J.A. "Feeding tests with some algin products." *Proceedings of the Society for Experimental Biology and Medicine*, 76(4), 630–635, 1951.
3. Ershoff, B.H. and Marshall, W.E. "Protective effects of dietary fiber in rats fed toxic doses of sodium cyclamate and polyoxyethelene sorbitanmonstearate (Tween 60)." *Journal of Food Science*, 40, 357, 1975.
4. Shimokawa, K., Horibe, N., Teramachi, M. and Mori, H. "Arsenic content of inedible seaweeds on the market." *Shokuhin Eiseigaku Zasshi*, 12(4), 330–332, 1971.

5. Watanabe, T., Hirayama, T., Takahashi, T., Kokubo, T. and Ikeda, M. "Toxicological evaluation of arsenic in edible seaweed hizikia species." *Toxicology*, 14, 1–22, 1979.

6. Fukui, S., Hirayama, T., Nohara, M. and Sakagami, Y. "The chemical forms of arsenic in some seafoods and in urine after ingestion of these foods." *Shokuhin Eiseigaku Zasshi*, 22(6), 513–519, 1981.

7. Funayama, S. and Hikino, H. "Hypotensive principle of laminaria and allied seaweeds." *Planta Medica*, 41, 29–33, 1981.

8. Takemoto, T., Daigo, K. and Takagi, N. "Studies on the hypotensive constituents of marine algae. I. "A new basic amino acid 'laminine' and other basic constituents isolated from laminaria angustata." *Yakugaku Zasshi*, 84(12), 1176–1179, 1964.

9. Kameda, J. "Medical studies on seaweeds, I." *Fukushima Igaku Zasshi*, 11, 289–309, 1961.

10. Ozawa, H., Gomi, Y. and Otsuki, I. "Pharmacological studies on lamininemonocitrate." *Yakugaku Zasshi*, 87(8), 935–939, 1967.

11. Kameda, J. "Medical studies on seaweeds, II." *Fukushima Igaku Zasshi*, 10, 251, 1960.

12. Kosuge, T., Nukaya, H., Yamamoto, T. and Tsuji, K. "Isolation and identification of cardiac principles from laminaria." *Yakugaku Zasshi*, 103(6), 683–685, 1983.

13. Searl, P.B., Norton, T.R., and Lum, B.K.B. "Study of a cardiotonic fraction from an extract of the seaweed, undaria pinnatifida." *Proceedings of the Western Pharmacology Society*, 24, 63–65, 1981.

TURMERIC
(Curcuma longa)

This common spice has been the subject of considerable research and much is known about its medicinal value.

There are many species of turmeric, but *Curcuma longa* is most important because it is highest in content of curcumin, the major active constituent. Guaranteed potency extracts of turmeric should contain a 95 percent standardized concentration of curcumin.

Turmeric is the primary ingredient in many varieties of curry powders and sauces. It provides the typical yellowish color of curry and a lot of the flavor. Curries contain other herbs, among them coriander, cumin, garlic, cayenne, fennel, fenugreek, anise, nutmeg, mace, cinnamon, cloves, black pepper, cardamon, ginger and onion. Different combinations of these are used by different cultures for different foods. The curry herbs contribute significantly to the digestion process, to the health of the liver, and to the elimination of wastes from the body.

Curry herbs exhibit cardiotonic activity

Almost all of the curry herbs, including turmeric, exhibit the following important vascular activities:

• *Inhibition of platelet aggregation.* The incidence of thrombosis in countries using curry is much less than that in countries not using these spices.
• *Anticholesterol action.* Most of the curry herbs have been shown to prevent rises in serum cholesterol that would occur from eating fatty foods.
• *Fibrinolytic activity.* This action also helps keep the blood flowing correctly. While fibrin is necessary for proper blood clotting when an injury occurs, an excess of this substance can be dangerous. Sometimes the fibrinolytic system of the body (the system that normally removes excess fibrin) malfunctions, particularly when other aspects of the body's health are being threatened. Many of the curry herbs give the fibrinolytic system a boost.

The interesting thing about these effects is that they are all fairly short-term in nature. Your body requires the aid provided by these herbs only as long as dietary toxins, harmful fatty acids, etc., are floating around in the blood. The herbs negate the action of the harmful chemicals and boost the ability of the liver to filter them out, and help regenerate any cells killed by toxic substances. After the digestive and assimilative war is over, the activity of the herbs ceases. (The overactivity of any of these mechanisms could be just as bad as underactivity—for example, a constant state of thinning in the blood could lead to just as severe complications as blood that is in danger of clotting.) The obvious inference is that anybody could benefit from the frequent and proper use of various combinations of the curry herbs.

Turmeric has specific cardiovascular activity

Much research has sought to determine the influence of turmeric on characteristics of the blood. For example, curcumin has been found to lower blood cholesterol levels.[1]

A recent article reviewed some of that research and looked specifically at the effects of curcumin on platelet aggregation inhibition and synthesis of prostacyclin (anti-inflammatory principle). The herb was very effective, so much so that the researchers recommended that it be used as a treatment of choice in patients prone to vascular thrombosis and those requiring antiarthritic therapy.[2]

The potent anti-inflammatory activity (in the essential oil and in curcumin) of turmeric has also been substantiated. Like other nonsteroidal anti-inflammatory agents (e.g., licorice root), curcumin appears to act through some sort of adrenal mechanism (when the adrenals are removed, turmeric has no effect).[3–7]

SAFETY DATA

Turmeric is perfectly safe to use in reasonable amounts. It has no known toxicity. However, in large quantities it can produce such strong activity in the common bile duct that it might aggravate the passage of gallstones in people currently suffering from the condition. In normal amounts, used for tonic purposes, the likelihood of that effect is remote.

REFERENCES

1. Leung, A. *Encyclopedia of Common Natural Ingredients in Food, Drugs, and Cosmetics*, John Wiley & Sons, New York, 1980, pp. 313–314.

2. Srivastava, R., et al. "Effect of curcumin on platelet aggregation and vascular prostacyclin synthesis." *Arzneimittel-Forschung*, 36(4), 715–717, 1986.

3. Srimal, R.C. and Dhaman, B.N. "Pharmacology of diferuloyl methane (curcumin), a non-steroidal anti-inflammatory agent." *J. Pharm. Pharmacol.*, 25, 447–452, 1973.

4. Mukhodapadhyay, A., et al. "Anti-inflammatory and irritant activities of curcumin analogues in rats." *Agents Actions*, 12, 508–515, 1982.

5. Chandra, D. and Gupta, S. "Anti-inflammatory and anti-arthritic activity of volatile oil of curcumin longa." *Indian J. Med. Res.*, 60, 138–142, 1972.

6. Arora, R. et. al. "Anti-inflammatory studies on curcuma longa (turmeric)." *Indian J. Exp. Biol.*, 56, 1289–95, 1971.

7. Ghatak, N. and Basu, N. "Sodium curcuminate as an effective anti-inflammatory agent." *Indian J. Exp. Biol.*, 10, 235–36, 1972.

MOTHERWORT
(Leonurus cardiaca)

Notice that the common name and Latin name refer to the two most common uses of this herb: the female system and the heart. Motherwort is primarily hypotensive in the cardiovascular system, but is a tonic in that it does not depress activity under normal conditions. Motherwort is often compared to valerian root (discussed in the chapter on the nervous system) because it seems to exhibit several of the same properties; namely, it is used as a hypotensive and sedative.

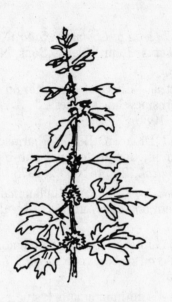

MOTHERWORT

In women it is used to promote menstruation, though its actions on the female reproductive system are not tonic in nature.

Several experimental studies have confirmed these actions, but none agree that the effects of this herb and those of valerian match up exactly. Older studies concluded that motherwort was not as effective as valerian root. But more recent studies have reached the opposite conclusion, rating motherwort's hypotensive action as up to three times that of valerian root. The observed experimental properties of motherwort in general support its use as a remedy for nervous heart conditions.

Motherwort has a hypotensive action

Different investigators at different times, with slightly different preparations, have reached conflicting conclusions regarding the efficacy of motherwort as a potential cardiac tonic and hypotensive substance. This suggests that the herb contains constituents with opposing properties, in keeping with the definition of a tonic.

The modern era of motherwort research opened in 1930 when Manchurian researchers investigated the pharmacological properties of *Leonurus sibiricus*, L., an ancient Chinese species of motherwort closely related to *L. cardiacus*. As the following brief review of their research indicates, these researchers appeared to be stumbling across different aspects of the tonic action; it did not appear that they knew what was happening. They isolated an alkaloid which they called leonurin. Leonurin was found to cause central nervous system paralysis in frogs. When injected into mice it caused irritation followed by cramp and finally respiratory paralysis. Injected into the vein of cat it caused a temporary fall in blood pressure, sometimes followed by a slight rise; this seemed to be a peripheral action. As far as the heart was concerned, a certain amount of leonurin was apparently not toxic. In excised frog heart, small doses were slightly stimulating, while large doses were paralyzing. In perfusion experiments on toads and rabbits, a contraction of the blood vessels was observed in several organs. A small amount of leonurin injected into cats acted as a stimulant on respiration, quickening the frequency and magnifying the amplitude, but an excessive dose caused, after a temporary stimulation, a paralysis, the respiration becoming weaker and irregular; this effect was attributed to effects on the respiratory center.[1,2]

In 1948 an Italian study reported similar kinds of opposing forces at work in motherwort, depending on how it was prepared and administered. The whole plant was used to prepare either ethanol or aqeuous extracts. These extracts exhibited mild sedative effects, which were attributed to both organic and inorganic components, practically insoluble in ethanol. The ethanol extracts had a fleeting depressor effect and a still less marked stimulating effect on respiration. Large doses depressed the heart muscle, perhaps mainly because of the potassium content.[3]

Other research has reported one action or the other. For example, extracts of motherwort have been obtained that exhibited good antispasmodic and hypotensive properties. These preparations had sedative effects three times stronger than those obtained from valerian root. Clinical studies showed antiepileptic activity. Similar effects were obtained in other studies. In one study the sedative action of motherwort was one-and-a-half times that of valerian. A mixture of motherwort and valerian produced a persistent sedative action. Another study reported using liquid extracts of motherwort to obtain paralysis of the central nervous system and contraction of vessels by fairly high doses of the concentrated extract. Low doses had no effect on the heart, but high doses decreased the amplitude of contraction. Intravenous injection of the extract sharply decreased blood pressure. Most pertinently, lasting hypotension was observed in dogs with experimentally induced hypertension.[4-6]

Recently, motherwort was shown to improve metabolism in the heart, reduce heart rate, increase coronary perfusion and inhibit blood platelet aggregation. In another study both motherwort and its alcohol extract, K substance, exhibited direct inhibitory action on normal beating myocardial cells. K substance was more potent than the whole herb.[7,8]

SAFETY DATA

No toxicity has been observed from the ingestion of motherwort, but sensitive individuals may incur allergic contact dermatitis from prolonged contact with the plant.

REFERENCES

1. Kubota, S. and Nakashima, S. "The study of leonurus sibiricus L. I. Chemical study of the alkaloid (leonurin) isolated from leon-

urus sibiricus, L." *Nippon Yakugaku Zasshi*, 11(2), 153–158, 1930.

2. Kubota, S. and Nakashima, S. "The study of leonurus sibericus L. II. Pharmacological study of the alkaloid leonurin isolated from leonurus sibericus L." *Nippon Yakugaku Zasshi*, 11(2), 159–167, 1930.

3. Erspammer, V. "Ricerche farmacologiche sul leonurus cardiaca L. and leonurus marrubiastrum L." *Archiv. Intern. Pharmacodynamie*, 76, 132–152, 1948.

4. Isaev, I., and Bojadzieva, M. "Obtaining galenic and neogalenic preparations and experiments for the isolation of an active substance from leonurus cardiaca." *Nauchney Trudy Visshiia Meditsinski Institu (Sofia)*, 37(5), 145–52, 1960.

5. Polyakov, N.G. "A study of the biological activity of infusions of valerian and motherwort and their mixtures." In: *Information on the First All-Russian Session of Pharmacists*, 1962, Meditsina: Moscow, pp. 319–324, 1964.

6. Arustamova, F.A. "Hypotensive effect of leonurus cardiaca on animals in experimental chronic hypertension." *Izvestiya Akademii Nauk Armyanski SSR, Biologicheski Nauki*, 16(7), 47–52, 1963.

7. Yanxing, Xia. "The inhibitory effect of motherwort extract on pulsating myocardial cells in vitro." *J. Traditional Chinese Medicine*, 3(3), 185–188, 1983.

8. Zhang, C. et al. "Studies on actions of extract of motherwort." *Journal of Traditional Chinese Medicine*, 2(4), 267, 1982.

ROSEMARY
(Rosmarinus officinalis)

Rosemary, an herb of ancient origin and use, contains good concentrations of minerals, such as calcium, magnesium, phosphorus, sodium and potassium, all of which are involved in the electrolytic balance of fluids surrounding nerves and cardiac tissues. One of the primary uses of rosemary is to lower blood pressure. The leaf also decreases capillary permeability and fragility, thereby contributing even further to cardiovascular health.

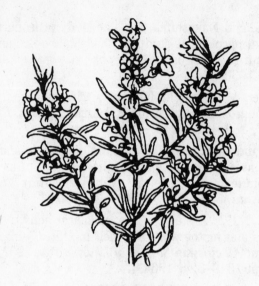

ROSEMARY

Rosemary leaf has certain cardiovascular effects

Rosemary leaf contains several potent aromatic oils, including borneol, camphor, cineol and many terpenes. In addition, it contains the active rosemaricine, and the flavonoid pigment diosmin, both of which contribute to cardiovascular health. Diosmin decreases capillary permeability and fragility. Hypotensive activity has also been observed in rosemary leaf extracts. In Germany, rosemary is generally recognized by physicians still using natural medicines as an agent to use during convalescence and during old age for quickening and quieting circulation, for rheumatism and for neuralgia.[1,3,5]

SAFETY DATA

Rosemary is nontoxic and perfectly safe when used in therapeutic amounts. Care should be taken, however, to avoid the ingestion of extremely large amounts, which can be toxic.[1,2]

REFERENCES

1. Pahlow, M. *Das Grosse Buch der Heilplanzen*. Graefe und Unzer GmbH. Munich, 1979, pp. 124–126.
2. List, P.H. and Hoerhammer, L.H. *Hagers Handbuch Der Pharmazeutischen Praxis*, six volumes, Springer-Verlag, Berlin 1968–1979. Citation for Rosemarinus.
3. *British Herbal Pharmacopoeia*, British Herbal Medicine Association, 1983, pp. 180–181.
4. Boido, A., Sparatore, F. and Biniecka, M. "N-substituted derivatives of rosmaricine." *Studi. Sassar. Sez.* 2, 53(5–6); 383–393, 1975.
5. Von Haler, A. "Kraeuter-Heilkraefte der natur." *Krakenpflege*, 29(3), 96–97, 1975.

SIBERIAN GINSENG, ELEUTHERO
(Eleutherococcus senticosis)

Eleuthero is one of the better tonics for the heart and vascular system. Athletes love this plant because it increases the flow of blood to the heart and lowers blood pressure (but without any tendency to lower pressure when it is normal). In addition, eleuthero increases the amount of time muscle cells can remain in aerobic respiration during exercise; thus, one can work out longer without the buildup of lactic acid, muscle soreness or exhaustion. The reader is referred to the section on Siberian ginseng in the chapter on the nervous system for a complete discussion of this important tonic herb.

VALERIAN ROOT
(Valeriana officinalis)

Valerian has become a popular constituent of European cardiovascular compounds in the last few years. This popularity may be attributed to the herb's ability to reduce blood pressure, relax and calm the heart, and generally remove much of the tension that is created by our modern hectic pace. Tension is one of the leading stressors of modern life; by reducing the severity of this stressor, valerian contributes meaningfully to the continued health of the heart and vascular system. For a complete discussion of valerian root the reader is referred to the section on this herb in the chapter on the nervous system.

CENTELLA, GOTU KOLA
(Centella asiatica, Hydrocotyle a.)

Centella and gotu kola are two very closely related plants growing in India and Madagascar respectively. They differ mainly in their native content of the active constituents asiaticosides and other triterpenes. Centella is the more concentrated of the two, and new guaranteed potency extracts of centella exert powerful effects on the vascular system. Gotu kola, on the other hand, is still a significant source of these active materials, but has found application primarily as a topical agent to help in the repair of infected tissue. Both gotu kola and centella are considered tonic in action, especially in terms of their effects on the cardiovascular system and the nervous system.

Whole centella, or a standardized extract of whole plant sprayed back onto original plant material, is preferable to simple extracts, or to any one of the individual constituents. Research suggests that the combination of triterpenes is most effective.[1] Centella does not contain caffeine or any of its analogues.

Centella and gotu kola enjoy a rich heritage of folklore use.

Asian medicine has relied upon this plant for hundreds of years for the treatment of skin sores and infections. The ethnobotanist K. Heyne remarked that the plant was equivalent to an entire drug store.[2] It is used extensively in the Ayurvedic system where it is called *Brahmi*. Centella and gotu kola are used routinely to treat problems of the skin, blood and nerves, including leprosy and syphilis.[3]

In both Western and Eastern traditions, these plants have gained a solid reputation as nerve tonics. They are used to increase the ability to remember and learn, probably by increasing the integrity of the flow of blood to the brain.[31,32]

The therapeutic use of centella in the treatment of skin and blood disorders probably depends to some degree on a proven bacteriostatic property.[5] In China, centella is said to be a "cooling" herb, and is used to reduce fever and detoxify the blood. In actual practice that means using it for acute infections and inflammations of the skin externally and internally, as well as drinking a tea to help clear the upper respiratory tract during infection (whooping cough, tightness in chest). This practice is shared by several Southeast Asian countries.

Centella and gotu kola are also said to increase longevity. The first "case history" of such an effect was that of the ancient Chinese herbalist, Li Ching Yun, who purportedly lived for 256 years. Since then, many are the tales coming from obscure regions of India, Pakistan and Madagascar, of people living beyond 100 years, while still laboring in the fields. Sri Lankans purportedly accept centella as a longevity plant on the basis that elephants eat it—and look how old they get!

Asiaticosides enhance the reticuloendothelial system (RES)

Asiaticosides, injected directly into leprosy nodules, perforated ulcers and lesions on fingers and eyes, are thought by Indian doctors to break down these structures, dissolving the waxy covering of the leprosy bacillus so that it becomes fragile and vulnerable, leading the way to subsequent healing.[4] Apparently, asiaticoside works by selectively stimulating the reticuloendothelial system (RES). The RES is a vast network of cells and tissues, found throughout the body, that are concerned with the formation and destruction of blood cells, the storage of fatty materials, the metabolism of iron and pigment, and the course of inflammation and immune responses. The RES is concentrated in the blood, but can be found also in connective tissue, spleen, liver, lungs, bone marrow and lymph nodes. Some of these cells move freely through the system, responding to "distress calls" from distant points. Many RES cells are phagocytic, that is, their primary mission is to ingest and destroy unwanted foreign material. Spleen RES cells can destroy disintegrated or used-up red blood cells, liberating the hemoglobin, which can then be transformed into bile pigments by other RES cells located in the blood cavities of the liver, the connective tissue, and bone marrow. Centella and to a lesser extent, gotu kola, asiaticosides exert a tonic effect on this system.[6-9]

Since about 1979, medicinal preparations containing the triterpenes of centella have been in widespread use (but not in the United States). They are primarily targeted at cellulitis and related conditions involving severe infection and acute inflammation of the skin.

Centella extract is used effectively in the treatment of sclerosis

In one of the earliest clinical trials, scientists administered a purified extract of centella to subjects every day for three months. They found that tissues taken from the thigh bone and the deltoid muscle of these subjects exhibited a significantly reduced tendency to hardening as a result of inflammation (sclerosis) when compared to tissues taken from placebo control subjects.[10]

Centella and gotu kola help in the healing of skin ulcers

Clinically, centella triterpenes are used whenever it is desirable to promote or accelerate the healing of the skin. As far back as

1958, positive research along these lines was being performed.[12] In many studies, all patients with ulcers of the lower limbs were successfully treated. Several of these cases were caused by some kind of alteration in venous circulation, as would typically occur in patients confined to bed for long periods.[11, 13–17] Such problems usually involve more or less severe bed sores and ulcerations, conditions euphemistically known as "traumatic and varicose ulcerative lesions of the limbs." The application of centella triterpenes often results in the rapid shedding of damaged tissues, the intense formation of new epithelial and connective tissues, and a greatly shortened hospital stay. An example of such research: In 1982, researchers reported a series of trials comprising 27 patients with lesions of various types, such as varicose and arterial ulcers, bedsores, burns and wounds. All cases experienced rapid and definite improvement with complete cleansing of the lesion and formation of healthy new tissue.[17]

Asiaticosides are effective in accelerating healing following gynecological procedures

Various lesions and ulcerative problems, involving bleeding, and associated with pregnancy and delivery have been successfully treated with centella. Cervical lesions of several types, some of up to 50 days duration, were treated in one study. The result was the rapid generation of a uniform, normal-looking mucosa in all cases.[18]

Centella extract was subjected to a vigorous series of trials on its properties relative to perineal lesions occurring during delivery and obstetric manipulations. The investigators concluded that by applying the substance early, they could significantly improve the chances of rapid healing.[19–22] Administering the extract later always accelerated the healing of tears that failed to heal on their own. In all cases, healing was usually complete in four to six days, and follow-ups, one or two months later, revealed uniformly good healing.[20]

Episiotomy, an incision of the vulva done during the second

stage of delivery to avoid later tearing, often results in a very uncomfortable healing process. Mercurochrome and novocaine ointments are traditionally used to lessen pain and chances of infection. Compared to these standard treatments, purified extracts of centella yield consistently better results. Almost all women receiving the centella treatment report less pain and more rapid healing than women subjected to standard measures.[23]

Centella helps reverse venous insufficiency and phlebitis

Centella triterpenes have been examined for their effect on venous insufficiency, a decrease in blood flow through the veins, a condition underlying several common ailments. The results have been uniformly positive, in the sense that significant improvement is observed in most cases. A wide range of individual manifestations of symptoms can be exhibited by people suffering from chronic venous insufficiency.

Using phlebitis as a model of venous insufficiency, investigators have attempted to pinpoint the action of centella more exactly in the hope of not only learning more about centella, but of discovering more about the body's healing processes. For example, in one study centella was compared to two commonly used therapeutic agents considered to possess first, the ability to protect capillary stability and second, a capacity for stimulating capillary dynamic activity without inducing active expansion and contraction of the veins. Since centella triterpenes act at the level of connective tissue, the researchers were hoping to elucidate the role of connective tissue in microscopic circulatory dynamics. Patients suffering from phlebitis (inflammation of the veins), due to prolonged confinement to bed, were used as subjects. Such confinement produces complicated changes in the relationship of veins to bones and joints that are thought to produce the inflammation. The centella extract produced the best results on all parameters, leading the authors to conclude not only that centella triterpenes were ideally suited for the treatment of manifestations of venous insufficiency that arise due to prolonged confinement, but to propose the revolutionary hypothesis that metabolic and biochemical factors contribute as much or more to the correction of confinement problems as do tensional and postural factors.[11]

Phlebitis, or inflammation of a vein, is a relatively common condition, especially in the veins of the lower limbs. If the inflammation occurs in a deep vein, the condition may have serious consequences. Phlebitis occurs most frequently where there is poor circulation due to some other condition, such as blood disorders, obesity, other infections, or prolonged confinement without exercise or frequent changes of position. It is also known to occur in about 1 percent of women following childbirth.

Because of its selective effects on connective tissue, centella has been highly successful in studies on its action relative to phlebitis and other examples of venous insufficiency. In one study, 72 percent of 125 patients suffering from varices, phlebitis, capillary fragility and paraphlebitis were successfully treated.[24] The success rate of other studies has ranged from 70 to 90 percent.[25-30] In addition to the symptoms cited above, the following conditions have responded well to centella treatment: heaviness of the legs, tingling, and nocturnal cramps.[25] All of these may require repair of vascular tissue.

The most recent studies have focused on the use of centella to treat persons with long-standing or chronic venous insufficiency. In one study, a purified extract of centella, in tablet form, was administered to 26 female patients over a period of 30 days. Several indices were used to evaluate effectiveness: postural edema, alterations in observable health of skin, induced pain, nocturnal cramps, numbness and sensation of weight. The treatment induced a statistically significant remission of all symptoms, except the numbness and appearance of the skin.[26] In another study, tablets were given to 40 men and women with chronic venous insufficiency, for a period of 30 days. The symptoms chosen for observation were swelling or edema of the lower limbs, dilation of the blood vessels, health of skin, and ulcerative conditions. Centella's effects were significant on all parameters.[27]

SUMMARY

The most general conclusion we can make is that centella triterpenes, as present in a purified centella extract, and to a lesser extent in all species of gotu kola, have a clear and consistent healing effect on most, if not all, solid tissues of the body, including the skin, connective tissues, lymph tissues, blood vessels and mucous membranes. This product has found its most successful applications in the treatment of conditions involving, or based on, venous insufficiency, tissue inflammation and infection, and postsurgical healing. It stimulates and accelerates the normal cellular repair processes, rather than instituting some artificial process.

Whenever circulation is poor, whether due to inactivity or disease, one runs the risk of coming down with additional problems. Purified centella extracts have been shown to strengthen the veins in several ways: by strengthening and repairing the connective tissues around the veins; by decreasing capillary fragility; by nutritively supporting the cells of the vein. Part of this process is indirect; it involves the nourishment of efferent (motor) neurons, whose task it is to stimulate growth and metabolism in peripheral organs and tissues. The tonic action of centella involves the stabilization of cell membranes and the revitalization of connective tissue.

SAFETY DATA

Centella and gotu kola species, asiaticosides and other triterpenes, appear to be completely nontoxic. Both whole plant and active constituents are generally regarded as safe in countries throughout the world.

REFERENCES.

1. Lythgoe, B. and Tripett, S. "Derivatives of centella asiatica used against leprosy. Centelloside." *Nature*, 163, 259–260, 1949, and Boiteau, P., Buzas, A., Lederer, E., and Polonsky, J. "De-

rivatives of centella asiatica used against leprosy. Chemical constitution of asiaticoside." *Nature*, 163, 258–60, 1949.

2. Heyne, K. *De Nuttige Planten van Indonesie*, 3rd Ed. Part I., p. 1211, Wageningen, 1950.

3. Lepine, J. "De l'hydrocotlyle asiatica Linne." *Journal Pharm. Chim.*, III, 28, 47–59.

4. Boiteau. P., Buzas, A., Lederer, E. and Polonsky, J. "Sur la constitution chimique de l'asiaticoside, 'heteroside' naturel contre la lepre." *Bull. Soc. Chim. Biol.*, 31; 46–51, 1949.

5. Boiteau, P. and Saracino, R. "Premiere essais au sujet de l'action de l'asiaticoside sur les lupus erythemateux et sur certains lesions produites par les bacilles de Hansen et Koch." *Medecin Francais*, 8, 251, 1948.

6. Boiteau, P. and Ratsimamanga, A.R., "L'asiaticoside extrait de 'centella asiatica' et ses emplois therapeutiques dans la cicatrisation des plaies experimentales et rebelles (lepre, tuberculose et lupus)." *Therapie*, 11, 125–149, 1956.

7. Lawrence, J.C. "The morphological and pharmacological effects of asiaticoside upon skin in vitro and in vivo." *Europ. J. Pharmacol.*, 1, 414–24, 1967.

8. Del Vecchio, A., Senni, I., Cossu, G. and Molinaro, M. "Effetti della centella asiatica sull'attivita biosintetica di fibroblasti in coltura." *Farmaco, Ed. Prague*, 39, 355–64, 1984.

9. Tincani, G. P. and Traldi, A. "Effect of asiaticoside on the plasma level and urinary elimination of amino acids." *Minerva Med.*, 53, 1587–1588, 1962.

10. Hachen, A. and Bourgoin, J.Y. "Etude anatomo-clinique des effets de l'extrait titre de centella asiatic dans la lipodystrophie localisee." *Med. Prat.* #738–Suppl., 7, 1979.

11. Allegra, C. "Studio capillaroscopico comparativo tra alcuni bioflavonoidi e frazione totale triterpenica di centella asiatica nell' insufficienza venosa." *Clin Ter.*, 110, 555–559, 1984.

12. Boely, C. and Ratsimamanga, A.R. "Traitment des ulceres de jambe par l'extrait de 'centella madagascariensis'." *Presse Med.*, 66, 1933–35, 1958.

13. Farris, G. "L'azione terapeutica dell'asiaticoside in campo dermatologico." *Minerva Med.*, 51, 2244, 1960.

14. Fincato, M. "Sul trattamento di lesioni cutanee con estratto di 'centella asiatica'." *Minerva Med.*, 15, 1235–1238, 1960.

15. Ugo, A. "L'asiaticoside in alcune affezioni della cute." *Boll. Soc. Med. Chir., Varese.*, 15, 145, 1960.

15a. Borsalino, G. "L'asiaticoside nella terapia di lesioni ulcerative traumatiche e varicose degli arti." *Romana Med.*, 14, 335, 1962.

16. Maleville, J. "Etude clinique d'un nouveau tulle gras." *Gaz. Med. It.* 86, 593, 1979.

17. Apperti, M., Senneca, H., Sito, G., Grasso, C. and Izzo, A. "Sperimentazione dell'estratto di centella asiatica nelle ulcere trofiche e nei procesi riparativi tissutalli." *Quad. Chir. Prat.*, 3, 115, 1982.

18. Remotti, G. and Colombo, P.A. "L'asiaticoside nella terapia delle lesioni cervicali di natura non neoplastica." *Riv. Ost. Ginec. Prat.*, 44, 572, 1962.

19. Baudon-Glanddier, Brivady. "Lesion perineales et asiaticoside." *Gaz. Med. France* 70, 2463–2464, 1963.

20. Torre, Ph., Dannadieu, J.M. and Braditch, J.L. "Activite cicatrisante de l'asiaticoside dans les plaies obstetricales du perinee." *Clinique*, 58 (681), 203–206, 1963.

21. Chisal, E., Serra, G.E. and Rapallo, G.B. "L'azione terapeutica dell'asiaticoside su ectopie colposcopicamente diagnosticate." *Min., Ginec.*, 13, 799, 1961.

22. Heller, L. "Madecassol en gynecologie." *Gaz. Med. France,* 32, 6626, 1968.

23. Castellani, L., Gillet, J.Y., Lavernhe, G. and Dellenbach, P. "Asiaticoside et cicatrisation des episiotomies." *Bull. Ped. Soc. Gynec. Obstet. Franc.*, 18, 184–186, 1966.

24. Frileux, C. and Cope, R. "Etude d'une nouvelle medication du tissue conjonctif veineux: l'extrait titre de centella asiatica." *Gaz. Med. France*, 78, 50–52, 1971.

25. Boely, C. "Indications therapeutiques de l'extrait titre de centella asiatica en phlebologie." *Gaz. Med. France*, 82, 741–44, 1975.

26. Pastore, A., and Zorzoli, C. "Terapia medica della I.V.C.: la centella asiatica (sperimentazione in doppio cieco vs/placebo." *Clin. Europ.*, 20, 910, 1981.

27. Mazzola, M. and Gini, M.M. "La centella asiatica nella terapia della insufficienza venos cronica. Ricerca clinica controllata a cecita doppia vs placebo." *Clin. Europ.*, 21, 160–166, 1982.

28. Cappelli, R. "Studio farmacologico clinico sull'effetto dell'estratto titolato di centella asiatica nell' insufficienza venosa cronica degli arti inferori." *Giorn. It. Angiol.*, 3, 44–48, 1983.

29. Mariani, G. and Patuzzo, E. "Il trattamento dell'insufficienza venosa con estratto di centella asiatica." *Clin. Europ.*, 22, 154–158, 1983.

30. Allegra, C. "Studio capillaroscopico comparativo tra alcuni bioflavonoidi e frazione totale treterpenica di centella asiatica nell' insufficienza venosa." *Clin. Ter.*, 99(5), 507–513, 1981.

31. Mowrey, D.B. "Capsicum, ginseng and gotu kola in combination." *The Herbalist*, Premier Issue, 22–28, 1975.

32. Ramaswamy, A.S., Periyasamy, S.M. and Basu, N. *Journal of Research in Indian Medicine*, 4, 160–175, 1970.

BILBERRY
(Vacinium myrtillus)

In Europe, bilberry has been used for several decades to help repair the vascular supply to the eye and to help correct eye problems. The development of a guaranteed potency form of this plant has made its application very attractive for the American market.

The standardized constituents in guaranteed potency bilberry are anthocyanosides. Whole bilberry fruit is preferable to isolated anthocyanosides. The standardized level of active principle should be no less than 15 percent. Compared to traditional dry bilberry extract with a maximum anthocyaniden content of 1 to 2 percent, the concentrate is appreciably more cost-effective, and much more easily matched to individual needs on a dosage basis.

Bilberry fruit has been a popular source of fresh jam for hundreds of years. The berry is a native of northern Europe and Asia. The nearest American counterpart is the blueberry. However, the blueberry is probably unsuitable for standardized medical uses. During World War II, Royal Air Force pilots ate bilberry jam to improve visual acuity during night missions. Over the course of several years, reports were published that associated bilberry fruit extract with the effective treatment of a variety of visual problems including night blindness (nyctalopia), visual fatigue from prolonged reading and working in dim light, severe nearsightedness (myopia), and various vascular disturbances of the retina.[1-3] From there, research expanded to demonstrate the effectiveness of bilberry in a wide variety of vascular disorders.

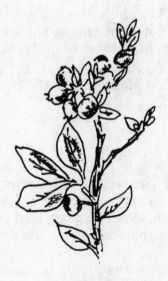

BILBERRY

Bilberry improves visual acuity by improving blood supply

In early studies, airline pilots, air traffic controllers, car and truck drivers, students, computer terminal operators, navigators, watchmakers and sports enthusiasts of various kinds were treated, with promising results.[4-6] The findings of the first real controlled experiment, carried out by a team of French scientists, confirmed the anecdotes: dark adaptation, following prolonged exposure to bright light, was significantly accelerated, and some improvement in visual acuity in dim light was observed in experimental subjects.[7] Other studies showed that bilberry was a quick-acting substance with practically no residual or long-term habituating action on the body[8-9]

In patients with pigmentary retinitis, bilberry produced an enlargement of the range of vision as well as a more responsive adaptation to darkness.[10-11] In yet other studies, bilberry has been effective in improving day and night visual acuity, eye strain of almost any kind (studying, driving, using computer terminals, etc.) and in aiding hemeralopia (day blindness, the opposite of nyctalopia).[12,13] Additionally, many specific diseases of the visual apparatus may be effectively treated with bilberry extract, particularly vascular retinal disturbances, cataracts, diabetic-induced glaucoma, and myopia.

Bilberry is helpful in a great variety of vascular disorders

Bilberry's effectiveness in treating visual problems is due to a complex network of supportive actions that strengthen capillary integrity and promote a healthy interplay of important enzymes. Bilberry anthocyanosides favorably affect the operation of crucial enzymes in retinal cellular metabolism and function, such as glucose-6-phosphatase and phosphoglucomutase.[14]

Hyperpermeable, or leaky, capillaries underlie many disorders, such as inflammatory responses, allergic reactions, hypertension, and venous and arterial insufficiency. Bilberry is a very powerful agent, even more effective than the bioflavonoids.[15] in its ability to stabilize capillary membranes and reduce their permeability.[16]

People with evidence of purpuras (bleeding under the skin, frequent and easy bruising, and abundant red patches) and people exhibiting various problems with blood supply to the central nervous system, as well as people suffering from coagulation problems and varicose veins, have all been successfully treated with bilberry.[17]

Bilberry has been successfully used in cases where fragile capillaries are accompanied by increased permeability.[18] This double whammy produces leaky, stiff, sclerotic capillaries that tend to break easily, thus leading to various arterial and venous problems.

An in-depth investigation of the effects of bilberry on patients suffering from marked hyperpermeability of the capillaries found that the treatment effectively restored health to these structures.[19] Even fragile capillaries caused by advanced diabetes returned to a healthy state following the administration of bilberry extract.[20]

Pregnant women suffering from varices and various blood disorders have been treated with anthocyanosides. A combination of bilberry anthocyanosides and vitamin E has proved very effective and seems to be well tolerated with no side effects occurring in either the mother or the infant.[21]

Other findings include the following:

• Stimulation of peripheral circulation.[22]
• Therapeutic benefits on disorders of the vessels in the conjunctiva of diabetic and pre-diabetic patients with tendencies toward glaucoma.[23]
• Antispasmodic and CNS sedative action.[24]
• Inhibition of platelet aggregation; implicated in the prevention of thromboses.[25]
• Control and prevention of retinal hemorrhaging during long-term anticoagulant therapy.[26]

In summary, bilberry extracts can be used effectively to treat varicose veins and related conditions, coagulation problems such as thrombosis, varices of assorted origin, capillary rigidity and permeability-related ailments of many kinds, including: hypertension; advanced diabetes; arteriosclerosis; purpuras or hemorrhages of the skin, mucous membranes, internal organs and other tissues; brain circulation disorders; kidney hematuria; and bleeding gums.

The tonic action of bilberry is evidenced by its lack of

physiological action in normal conditions. It does not stimulate the over production of rhodopsin; nor does it result in *hypo*permeability or flaccidity of capillaries.

SAFETY DATA

Anthocyanosides have been shown to be completely non-toxic when administered orally. In toxicity tests on mice and rats, no toxicity was observed when the anthocyanosides were administered orally. Intraperitoneal and intravenous administration produce LD50's of very high values, again validating the low toxicity of the product. Since the preferred route of administration is oral, no toxicity should be expected.[27]

REFERENCES

1. Bailliart, J.P. "Tentative d'amelioration de la vision nocturne." *Le Medicin de Reserve*, 121, 1969.

2. Ala El Din Barradah, M., Shourkry, I. and Hegazy, M. "Difrarel 100 in the treatment of retinal vascular disorders and high myopia." *Bull. Ophth. Soc. Egypt*, 60, 251, 1967.

3. Gil Del Rio, E. "Los antocianosidos del vaccinium myrtillus en oftalmologia." *Arch. Soc. Oftal. Hisp.-Amer.*, 26, 969, 1966.

4. Chevaleraud, J. and Perdriel, G. "Peut-on ameliorer la vision nocturne des aviateurs." *Gaz. Med. de France*, 18, 25 June 1968.

5. Rouher, F. and Sole, P. "Peut-on ameliorer la vision nocturne des conducteurs automobiles." *Ann. Med. Accidents Traffic*, 3–4, 1965.

6. Belleoud, L., Leluan, D. and Boyer, Y. "Etude des effets des glucosides d'anthocyanes sur la vision nocturne du personnel navigant." *Rev. Med. Aero. Spat.*, 6, 5, 1967.

7. Jayle, G.E. and Aubert, L. "Action des glucosides d'anthocyanes sur la vision scotopique et mesopique du sujet normal." *Therapie*, 19, 171, 1964.

8. Volpi, U. and Bertoni, G. "L'azione del 'pourpranyl' sulfa sinsibilita luminosa retinica del soggetto normale." *Ann. Ottal. Clin. Ocul.*, 90, 492, 1964.

9. Mercier, A., Perdriel, G. and Carves, H. "Note concernant l'activite des glucosides d'anthocyanes sur la vision scotopique et l'acuite visuelle mesopique des sujets normaux." *Rev. Med. Aero.*, 13, 57, 1965.

10. Mercier, A., Perdriel, G., Rozier, J. and Chevaleraud, J. "Note concernant l'action des glucosides d'anthocyanes sur l'electroretinogramme humain." *J. Bull. Soc. Ophtalm. Fr.*, 65, 1049, 1965.

11. Scialdone, D. "L'azione delle antocianine sul senso luminoso." *Ann. Ottal. Clin. Ocul.*, 92, 43, 1966.

12. Zavarisse, G. "Sull'effetto del trattamento prolungato con antocianosidi sul senso luminoso." *Ann. Ottal. Clin. Ocul.*, 94, 209, 1968.

13. Jueneman, G. "Ueber die wirkung der anthozyanoside auf die hemeralopie nach chininintoxikation." *Augenheilkunde*, 151, 891, 1968.

14. Cluzel, C., Bastide, P., Wegman, R. and Tronche, P. "Activities enzymatiques de la retine et anthocyanosides extraits de vaccinium myrtillus." *Biochem. Pharm.*, 19, 2295, 1970.

15. Demure, G. "Etude experimentale et clinique d'un nouveau facteur vitaminique P: les anthocyanosides." *These Medecine Clermont*, 1964.

16. Pourrat, H., Bastide, P., Dorier, P., Pourrat, A. and Tronche, P. "Preparation et activite therapeutique de quelques glucosides d'anthrocyanes." *Chim. Therap.*, 2, 33, 1967.

17. Terrasse, J. and Moinade, S. "Premiers resultats obtenus avec un nouveau facteur vitaminique P 'Les anthocyanosides' extraits du vaccinum myrtillus." *Presse Med.*, 72, 397, 1964.

18. Demure, G. op. cit.

19. Cuvelier, R., Terrasse, J., Derycke, Ch., Andraud, G. and Aublet-Cuvelier, J.L. "Essai d'appreciation par le test de landis de l'action sur les capillaries d'un complexe anthocianique." *Clermont Med.*, 63, 61, 1966.

20. Thomas, Ch. and Barisain, P. "L'action des anthocyanosides

sur al fagilite des capillaries oculaire dans le diabete et l'hypertension arterielle." *Bull. Soc. Ophthalm. Fran.*, 65, 212, 1965.

21. Baudon, J., Bruhat, M., Plane, C. and Hermabessiere, J. "Utilisation d'une association d'angio-protecteur et de vitamine E." *Lyon Medit. Medical*, 46, Oct. 1969.

22. Terrasse, J., Aubiet-Cuvelier, J.L. and Marcheix, J.C. "Action des anthocyanosides sur la circulation peripherique et le test de Landis." *Vie Medicale, Dic.,* 1969.

23. Romani, J.D. "Action des anthocyanosides sur l'angiopathie conjonctivale au cours du diabete et du prediabete." *Vie Medicale, Dic.,* 1969.

24. Canivet, J. and Passa, Ph. "Interet therapeutique d'une association d'anthocyanosides, d'antispasmodiques et de neuro- sedatif central." *G.M. de France*, 78, 682, 1971.

25. Rasmussen, Ch. "Anthocyanosides. Adhesivite plaquettaire et prevention des thromboses." *Therapeutique*, 48, 399, 1972.

26. Neumann, L. "Erfahrungen mit anthocyanosid-behandlung von netzhautblutungen unter antikoagulantien-dauertherapia." *Augenheilkunde*, 163, 96, 1973.

27. Pourrat H., et al., 1967, op. cit.

CHAPTER THREE

The Nervous System

❧ The nervous system is the central processing unit of the body. Nothing happens without input from this system. The heart doesn't beat, the muscles don't move, the stomach doesn't digest, the eyes don't see, the glands don't secrete, the blood doesn't move, nothing at all happens. Therefore, a great deal of attention must be paid to keeping the nervous system as healthy as possible; overstimulation is almost as bad as understimulation.

The human nervous system is generally divided into three major parts, though there are numerous ways to subdivide it after that. The first part is the central nervous system (CNS), which consists of brain and spinal cord and is really the central processing unit; the second is the peripheral nervous system, which comprises the nerves leading from the spinal cord to all parts of the body and innervates mainly the skeletal muscles and their appendages; the third is the autonomic nervous system (ANS), which is composed of the nerves that innervate organs, glands, blood vessels, smooth muscle and the heart and control these vital functions.

The basic working unit of the nervous system is the nerve

cell, or neuron. Some understanding of the structure of the nerve cell is essential to understanding the rest of the nervous system. Like most cells, nerve cells have a centrally located cell body in which can be found cytoplasm and the nucleus. But similarity to most other cells ceases there. From the cell body emanate filaments or fibers that can be as short as a few millimeters to as long as several feet. The longest of these fibers is called the axon; it carries signals away from the cell body. The shorter fibers, of which there may be as few as one, or as many as 200, are called dendrites. They carry impulses toward the cell body.

Many neuron fibers are covered by a fatty sheath known as myelin. At intervals along the myelin are uncovered or thinly covered spots known as nodes. Neural transmission can jump from node to node; internodal distance can therefore affect the speed of transmission. Some neuron fibers do not have myelin sheath. Neural transmission in these fibers is slowest of all.

Neurons are generally classified by their function, and this gives us a clear understanding of how the nervous system works. Some neurons carry messages to the brain and/or spinal cord. They are called afferent or sensory neurons. Efferent or motor neurons, on the other hand, relay messages from the brain or spinal cord to distant places in the body. Afferent neurons are stimulated by data coming in from receptors, which can be specialized neurons—as are the olfactory sensors in the nose—or specialized organs. A stimulus is anything that activates a receptor. Finally, there are neurons that sometimes occur between the afferents and efferents. These are called associative neurons, or interneurons. The brain and spinal cord are made up mostly of interneurons; these are what make our lives so rich, complex, and interesting.

The picture we have built so far of neural functioning, then, goes like this. A stimulus acts upon a receptor, which undergoes some change, the result of which creates an electrochemical signal in an afferent neuron. This signal travels to the spinal cord or brain where it interacts with one or many interneurons which can take that signal, modify it and carry it to other places in the nervous system where it can further interact and associate. Eventually, you may decide to act on the stimulus, or maybe it simply elicits a reflex. In either event an outgoing signal is generated which travels along efferents, perhaps interacting with interneurons along the way until it reaches some muscle fiber, gland or organ in which it stimulates activity.

A nerve must be distinguished from a nerve cell. A nerve is a bundle of nerve fibers bound together by a sheath of connective tissue. Nerves are primarily axons. Sometimes cell bodies are gathered together in a bundle; these groups of cell bodies are called ganglia (plural of ganglion) if they occur outside of the central nervous system. In the CNS they are called nuclei (although some nuclei are called ganglia, e.g., the basal ganglia).

The nerve impulse

Once impulses are generated in a neuron, they speed along like a chain reaction of electrochemical events that cannot be stopped until they reach the end of the neuron. These events depend upon minute differences in electric potential between the inside and the outside of the cell, and they occur very rapidly; a nerve impulse can travel over 100 meters per second—that's the length of three football fields in one second. There are many ways that the initial nerve impulse, or "action potential," is created in the first sensory neuron: pressure, heat, chemical changes, etc., arising in the specialized sensory receptors. But how does the impulse get transmitted to the next neuron along the way? How does it get across the gap between the first neuron's axon and the second neuron's dendrites? The gap is called a synapse; communication across the gap is called synaptic transmission. It requires the presence of special hormones called neurotransmitters. These are stored in the ends of the axons, and when an impulse reaches that point, it causes the neurotransmitters to spill out into the synapse. The transmitter substances set up an action potential in special receptor sites on the dendrites of the next neuron which is then carried along the dendrites, through the cell body and down the axon to the next synapse.

Great modification of neural signals can take place at the synapse as different kinds of transmitters interact to either increase or inhibit the intensity of the original signal, send it off in different directions, create memory traces, initiate reflexive motor responses, and so forth.

Reflexes are the simplest kind of neural circuit. Let's say you step on a sharp object. The pressure receptors in the skin of your foot would send a signal through sensory neurons directly to the spinal cord, where the signal would be relayed directly to motor neurons which would activate an appropriate escape response in the muscles controlling your legs and feet. That action requires no input from "you." It is a reflex. Meanwhile, signals from pain receptors in your foot are being relayed through three or four more neurons to your brain. When the messages reach the brain, you experience the sensation of pain. If these neurons are cut, you don't feel pain. Pain, therefore, requires the brain. The fact that you feel the pain in your foot and not in your brain is one of the wonders of life.

Some say that behavioral habits, actions we engage in without thinking are like cerebral equivalents of the lower order reflex—reflexes we have allowed to occur and which take great effort to regain control of.

The central nervous system

Just be glad we are not requiring you to memorize the structures of the CNS. Try to remember that the brain is here, and that it is the organ of control, thought, speech and emotion. You might also be aware that the cerebellum, brain stem and spinal cord are all part of the CNS.

The peripheral nervous system

Ditto here.

The autonomic nervous system

You're not so lucky here. Because so many essential body functions require input from the ANS, we should know something about how it works and how we can maintain the wellness of this system. Also, it will be seen that the manner of function of the ANS underlies many of the effects of tonic herbs.

The ANS consists of two parts, the sympathetic division (SNS) and the parasympathetic division (PNS). Both systems innervate the same organs: the brain, the heart, intestines, bladder, blood vessels, kidneys and other organs. Much of the work of one system is counteracted by the work of the other system. Each functions in its own due time, and left to themselves, they will generally coordinate the health of the body in an efficient manner. Unfortunately, the stresses imposed on our body by daily living, diet and genetics tend throw off the balance between the SNS and PNS, resulting in sickness. Generally, the SNS heightens activity in the body, while the PNS slows things down.

The primary neurotransmitter of the SNS is norepinephrine (NE)(or noradrenalin). This chemical causes certain muscle cells to relax and others to contract. Stimulation of the PNS is under the control of acetylcholine (ACh). This chemical has exactly the opposite effect to that of NE. The muscle that contracted with NE will relax under the influence of ACh, and vice versa.

Here are some other examples. When blood pressure is too high, a message is sent to the brain that stimulates a message in the PNS which will tend to slow the heart rate and decrease blood pressure. The SNS constricts the pupils, inhibits salivation, dilates the bronchi, accelerates the heart, increases adrenocortical secretions, constricts blood vessels in the skin and abdominal organs, increases blood flow to muscles, inhibits peristalsis in the stomach and gastric juice production, relaxes the bladder, inhibits activity in the colon and rectum, produces contractions in the male urethra by which sperm are ejaculated, and causes you to sweat. PNS stimulation has the opposite effect on each of those systems. Interestingly, the PNS is responsible for producing and maintaining erection of the penis.

Stimulation of the SNS also has a specialized effect on the conversion of fat calories into heat.

Usually, both the SNS and the PNS are operating at the same time, with one dominating the other to one degree or another. Seldom, if ever, does one side shut down altogether. In case of severe fright, the SNS assumes almost total control. And while you are asleep, the PNS takes over most control to help you recover from the day's stresses. Most of the time, however, the two systems are working closely together to maintain homeostasis in the body's structures whose function they control.

DISORDERS OF THE NERVOUS SYSTEM

Congenital defects

Babies can be born with a number of different nervous system dysfunctions: Down's syndrome, Tay-Sachs disease, cri cu chat, microcephaly, anencephaly and hydrocephaly, to name a few. Most of these are not correctable; some are correctable; others can be dealt with through patient and intensive care from parents and medical personnel.

Infection

Infections can attack the brain, the spinal cord or any peripheral nerve. Encephalitis and meningitis are examples. Viruses and bacteria are mostly responsible. The rabies and herpes simplex viruses are responsible for a great many cases of meningitis. Simple ear infections can spread to the brain and create life-threatening abscesses.

Injury

Most critical parts of the nervous system, such as the brain and spinal cord, are fairly well protected, yet serious injuries do occur. Damage can range from barely perceptible to total dysfunction. Neurons of the central nervous system cannot generally regenerate, but they can often take over the functions of other severely damaged neurons.

Impaired blood and oxygen supply.

Since brain cells cannot survive more than a few minutes without oxygen, it is imperative that the flow of blood to the brain not be interrupted. One of the causes of cerebral palsy is temporary asphyxiation during the birth process. Later in life, progressive cerebrovascular disease produces increasingly large impairments to blood supply with resultant loss of neurons throughout the brain. Senility of various kinds may result, or even a stroke.

Degeneration

The most well known degenerative disease of the nervous system is multiple sclerosis, characterized by the gradual destruction of the myelin sheath along the nerves. Alzheimer's disease and Parkinson's disease are receiving a lot of attention today as scientists are beginning to understand more about these forms of dementia. Destruction and interference by free radicals are thought to be leading causes of neural degenerative diseases.

Miscellaneous conditions

There are many disorders of the nervous system that are little understood. Usually, these are characterized more by certain symptoms than by any observable defect. Examples are migraines, narcolepsy, epilepsy, mental illness, schizophrenia and organic brain syndromes. Epilepsy is becoming better understood all the time. Certain kinds have been traced to underlying causes, such as tumor and infections, but most are still inexplicable.

Organic brain syndromes are disturbances of conscious thought and reasoning ability that are thought to have physical substrates rather than psychiatric. They could be due to metabolic disturbances, vitamin deficiencies, mineral imbalances, infections, medication, drug abuse, tumors, strokes, toxins, and so forth. Symptoms can range from mild confusion to stupor or coma and may involve memory impairment, delusions, disorientation and even hallucinations.

Aphasia

Aphasia is the name given to loss of the ability to speak. Many of us joke about creeping aphasia as we find ourselves groping for the right word, stumbling through sentences and forgetting names and dates. Though this progressive deterioration of thought processes is not truly aphasia, it seems to characterize the aging process, and may be a mild form of organic brain syndrome.

Autonomic control disorders

Sometimes imbalances occur in the relationship between the SNS and the PNS. When that happens, any of the functions governed by the two systems could run out of control. Childhood hyperactivity, bed wetting, hypochondria, insomnia, headaches, attention deficits and even some forms of obesity may be the result of autonomic imbalance.

Nervous breakdown

When your life goes all to pieces, your nervous system simply cannot cope with the amount of stress you are subjecting it to. Severe anxiety makes tremendous demands on the ANS. Tension, episodes of emotional distress marked by shouting, crying, screaming, social withdrawal, and constant worry all exact their toll on the nervous system. What is needed is a period of rest, a time to get away from it all. Or maybe just a stronger nervous system.

Neuropathy

Neuropathy is a term that is gaining widespread acceptance in recent years. It is replacing older terms such as neurasthenia and neuritis. It refers to disease, inflammation or damage to the peripheral nerves. Symptoms include numbness, tingling sensations, pain and muscle weakness. The myelin sheath of axons is the common victim of the damage or inflammation. It may thin, become patchy, or suffer complete loss; this causes slowing or blocking of nerve impulses. Alcoholism and diabetes are two common causes of the most painful neuropathies, but in most cases there is no detectable cause. Dietary deficiencies (especially of the B vitamins) may be responsible for some cases; intoxication by environmental pollutants may be a cause. Infections are probable factors, as are autoimmune disorders. In arthritis, lupus and other diseases, there is often damage to blood vessels that supply the nerves. Both sensory and motor fibers can be affected. If the autonomic system is involved, symptoms such as blurred vision, impaired sweating, fainting, low blood pressure, impaired sexual ability, loss of bladder control, and poor digestion might be experienced.

Insomnia

A general term for any kind of sleeping disorder. Surveys show that as many as one-third of all adults in the United States have trouble sleeping. This may involve trouble falling asleep, trouble staying asleep, or trouble with the quality or depth of sleep. The problem is further compounded by the usual treatment, hypnotic drugs. Thus other common complaints of insomniacs, such as daytime fatigue, irritability, nausea, anxiety, etc., may be as much the fault of the sleeping aids as they are intrinsic to insomnia itself.

Insomnia is often caused by an inability to let go of the day's worries. It can be aggravated by sleep apnea (a breathing problem that causes snoring), restless leg syndrome, noise, light, caffeine, sugar, lack of exercise and drug abuse.

🌿 HERBAL TONICS FOR THE NERVOUS SYSTEM

The preceding discussion, especially of the ANS, may have alerted the reader to the important role tonic herbs might play in regulating the health of all the internal organs and glands of the body, in addition to the heart and blood vessels. Virtually every system we have discussed so far in this book depends upon input from the ANS. Because the health and wellness of all of these structures depends on the ability of the opposing forces of the ANS to maintain homeostasis, the support provided by herbal materials with constituents that act on both halves could have an enormous influence on overall health. And this is exactly what so many tonic herbs do; they provide materials the body can draw from to tone either the PNS or SNS, whichever needs it at the time.

These herbs also affect the other divisions of the nervous system in a tonic manner. It is surprising to some people to find out, for example, that the use of valerian root can help you sleep better and the next day can be used to help you concentrate better.

VALERIAN ROOT
(Valeriana officinalis)

Valerian root has been used for centuries to calm upset nerves, treat mood problems, pain and headache. In medieval times, valerian was so popular it became known as "all-heal." It is currently one of the most popular orthodox antispasmodic medications in Russia and Germany. Other parts of the world, including China and Asia and North America, have incorporated valerian root in their pharmacopoeias.

The root is used to treat insomnia, nervous tension, anxiety, muscle cramps and spasm, muscle pain, headache, stress, menstrual pain and discomfort, hysteria, epilepsy (as an anticonvulsant), autonomic nervous disorders of all kinds (including hypochondria), hypertension, a wide variety of gastrointestinal disorders, and others.

In herbal terms, valerian is antispasmodic (muscle relaxant), calmative (sedative, depressant), a nervine (tranquilizing), carminative (good for upset stomach and digestion), and anodyne (pain reliever). One old folk tradition depicts married couples hanging valerian in their houses to help bring peace and prevent contention in the home.

Stress, muscle spasms, nervous exhaustion, headaches with nervous components, heart problems involving nervous tension, insomnia, and even whooping cough are the kind of disorders for which valerian is best suited. During the First World War, valerian was used to prevent shell shock in front-line troops, and in the Second World War it was used during air raids to reduce strain and anxiety among the civilians.

Valerian is used medically in much the same manner as the popular drug Valium, though the two are totally unrelated. One of the major differences in action between valerian and Valium is the characteristic lack of side effects experienced by persons using valerian root.

In a remarkable series of animal studies in the 1960s, the herb was proven to be sedative, to improve coordination, and to antagonize the hypnotic effects of alcohol.[1] At the same time, clinical evidence in humans was showing that valerian root constituents were strongly sedative, though large doses were not any more effective than small or moderate doses, except to extend the duration of the effect. The root also had a marked tendency to increase concentration ability and energy levels.[2]

More recent research has shown that valerian sedates and regulates the autonomic nervous system in patients and children with control disorders, to help regulate psychosomatic disorders, and to relieve tension and restlessness.[3] Valerian root preparations have neurotropic effects directly on higher centers of the central nervous system. Childhood behavior disorders and learning disabilities are particularly susceptible to the positive effects of valerian root. Valerian root is a primary sedative for use when sleep disorders are the result of anxiety, nervousness and exhaustion, headache and hysteria. In addition, it has been effective in treating tachycardia that just precedes going to sleep.[4]

Valerian root contains at least three major groups of active constituents: volatile oil, esters, and alkaloids. But there are probably still other active constituents remaining to be discovered in other fractions of the plant, which substances probably modify or augment the action of the three major groups. The most obviously active components of valerian root are found in the volatile oil group. Among them are the valepotriates, valerianic acid, valeranone and valernal.

Central nervous system sedative effects

The main effect of valerian root on the central nervous system is depressant,[6] although certain species appear to be mildly stimulating in a minority of people. Until the critical variables in valerian production and processing have been identified, the occasional stimulant effect must be expected. It is probable that the tonic nature of valerian root is being exhibited; therefore, it would be expected to depress or stimulate where necessary, depending on the current needs of the nervous system. Since most people only turn to valerian when they are obviously overstimulated, the sedative effect would be most often observed. This is indeed the case.

Numerous studies have published clinical observations of the effect in humans of all ages, and these are supported by research on lower organisms.[7-11] In one of the best studies to date, using a rat brain preparation, researchers were able to demonstrate definite EEG changes; loosely speaking, they found significant sedative activity, recorded as a reduction in waking brain wave activity and an increase in relaxing and sleeping brain waves.[5]

In most clinical studies, valerian acts to level upset nervous disorders, including both physical and psychological symptoms. That is, it acts as both sedative and tranquilizer. In one clinical study, a tincture of valerian root was given to 23 hypertensive males. The preparation produced a general tranquilizing effect, and had an elective neurotropic action on higher brain centers as measured by a depression of the third order waves on the digital plethysmogram in 18 men on the following day.[12]

Effects on locomotor activity

One of the paradoxes of valerian effects, at least as viewed from the perspective of orthodox medicine, is its ability to maintain, even improve, motor coordination and mental acuity while simultaneously depressing overall motor activity.[13–15] But such results are in perfect agreement with the concept of a tonic. In one of the best controlled studies to date, valerian constituents significantly inhibited locomotor activity in mice.[16] Interestingly, higher doses did not produce catalepsy (a kind of rigidity induced by high doses of standard sedative drugs), but instead seemed to simply prolong the sedative effect. Other animal studies have also reported this depressant effect. These findings accord well with clinical observations in human.[17,18] Some research has shown that valerian extracts increase the length of time hyperactive subjects are able to concentrate on some given task.[19]

Insomnia

One of the strongest areas of application of valerian root has been in the treatment of insomnia. Although not all insomniacs respond to valerian root, the majority do quite well objectively and subjectively, in taking the herb just a few minutes before retiring.

In one study, a group of 8 volunteers suffering from mild insomnia received a placebo, 450 mg or 900 mg of an aqueous extract of valerian root (in a double-blind, repeated measures, random-order design).[20] Subjective sleep ratings were assessed by questionnaire and movements were recorded throughout the night with wrist-worn activity meters. The study found a significant decrease in sleep latency (the amount of time taken before falling asleep) with valerian compared to placebo. Higher doses produced no further improvement in sleep latency. These results were similar to those of a study involving 128 volunteers in which an aqueous extract of valerian root improved subjective ratings for sleep quality and sleep latency but left no "hangover" the next morning, as is often observed with traditional sleeping aids.[21] The improvements in the quality of sleep were especially marked in people who considered themselves habitually poor sleepers. In neither of the above studies was a carryover from one night to the next observed.

It appears from these studies, 1) that the effects of the valerian preparation are confined to the early part of the night; 2) that the herb is quickly metabolized; 3) that the effects are gone by morning (and may not be exerting any effect after as few as 2–3 hours after sleep begins); and 4) that there are no side effects, no morning hangover, no need to grab a cup of coffee or pep pill to get going again.[22]

Experimental results indicate that valerian root is at least as effective as small doses of barbiturates and benzodiazepines, without the side effects of the latter substances.[23]

Numerous other clinical studies have demonstrated the sedative action of valerian root and its derivatives in insomnia and other sleep disorders. Valerian root is contained in dozens of popular over-the-counter European sleeping aids, many of which have been proven to be effective. In America, only the enlightened use valerian root for insomnia.

Control disorders of the autonomic nervous system

In Europe, for about the last 20 years, valerian root has been used in the treatment of childhood behavior disorders including hyperactivity and learning disabilities. Experimentally, valerian root has been shown to increase coordination ability in mice. In cats, it decreases unrest, anxiety and aggressiveness without decreasing reaction time at all. In fact, valerian actually has been found to improve reaction times. In human patients with poor concentration ability, valerian has been able to significantly increase performance on several psychological variables. On the other hand, in patients with strong concentration abilities, the substance produces a mild decrease in some variables. In one study, valerian extract was given to 120 children with a variety of behavioral disorders, including gross nervous restlessness, sleep disorders, headaches, migraines, learning disorders, enuresis, anxiety, and pathological habits such as nail biting and thumb-sucking. Length of study was at least 3 weeks in each case. All of the children tolerated the drug very well; there were no allergic reactions or other side effects. Significant deviations from normal in blood and urine tests were not observed. In 74.4 percent of the cases very good or good results were obtained on the experimental variables. These results are extraordinary, given the lack of toxicity observed. Valerian root would make a very good addition to the therapy of childhood behavior problems.[24]

Clinical observations of the last couple of decades have almost uniformly shown that valerian root preparations appear to stabilize the autonomic nervous system in psychosomatic patients and those with disorders of the autonomic nervous system. These kinds of disorders are rarely diagnosed in the United States. In Germany, however, clinicians are more sensitive to subtle dysfunctions of the autonomic nervous system, and recognize these as the basis for a great many cases of functional insufficiency including anxiety, insomnia, hysteria, ulcers, exaggerated nervousness, PMS, postmenopausal depression, etc. Valerian root products produce a clear increase in performance coupled with moderate sedation; therefore, patients' motor coordination, concentration ability, and reasoning skills increase, but without any hypnotic or depressive symptoms.[25–27] These effects may be summarized as stress reduction.[28] In one German study with 70 hospitalized patients diagnosed as having dysregulation of the autonomic nervous system due to various etiologies, valerian extract suppressed and regulated all the symptoms, and produced a mildly relaxing sedative effect; it was especially effective in relieving symptoms of restlessness and tension.[29]

Coronary dilatory and hypotensive properties

As far back as Roman times, valerian was used to treat certain heart conditions, especially palpitations and arrhythmias. The hypotensive effect of valerian root has been regularly observed in modern clinical and experimental settings. In one study, the coronary flow of rabbit heart was found to increase by more than 50 percent following valerian root extract administration. This effect has also been observed in living cats and dogs.

Valerian root is included in one German heart tonic to provide inhibition of reflex hypersensitivity and to help maintain neuro-coronary equilibrium. Hypotensive, anticonvulsant and antiarrhythmic properties have been observed in several studies. Also, valerian has been found to prevent the appearance of acute coronary insufficiency in experimental animals. Moderately positive inotropic (increases cardiac contractility) and negative chronotropic (slows heartbeat) effects have also been observed.[30–36]

SAFETY DATA

Perhaps one of the most remarkable aspects of valerian root preparations is the almost total lack of toxicity they exhibit, even with prolonged use. Considering that many thousands of people have been using these preparations, surprisingly few reports of heartburn, upset stomach, diarrhea, and allergic reactions have come forth.[37] Blood pressure, blood and liver parameters are not influenced.[38] Furthermore, in cats and dogs the oral lethal dose has not been determined because it is so high that that much substance cannot be administered.[39]

One of the main advantages of using valerian is that it has no synergy with alcohol; if alcohol is ingested with conventional tranquilizers, the effects combine to produce potentially very dangerous effects. Valerian is free of that danger. Valerian also lacks other commonly experienced side effects of prescriptions sedatives: depressed coordination, groggy drugged feelings, dependence.

As with all substances, however, there is always the chance of overdose. Overdosing with whole valerian root is extremely difficult to do, but concentrated valerian extracts pose a somewhat larger risk. Signs of overdose might include headaches, illusions, spasms, and either profound depression or profound anxiety. These symptoms disappear completely after a short while.

REFERENCES

1. von Eickstedt, K.S., et al. "Psychopharmacologic effects of valepotriates." *Arzneimittel-Forschung,* 19, 316–319, 1969, and 19, 993, 1969.

2. Schaette, R. *Dissertation* Muenchen, 1971. and Schaette, R. "Stable valerian preparations." *Ger. Offen.,* 2,230,626, 10 Jan. 1974.

3. Boeters, U. "Behandlung vegetativer regulationsstoerungen mit volepotriaten (valmane)." *Muenchener Medizinische Wochenschrift,* 37, 1873–1876, 1969.

4. Straube, C. "The meaning of valerian root in therapy." *Therapie der Gegenwart,* 107, 555–562, 1968. (In German.)

5. Fink, C., Hoelzl, J., et al. "Wirkungen vonvaltrat auf das EEG des isoliert perfundierten ratenhirns." *Arzneimittel-Forschung,* 34(2), 170–174, 1984.

6. Wagner, H. "Comparative studies on the sedative action of Valeriana extracts, valepotriates and their degradation products." *Planta Medica,* 38, 358–365, 1980.

7. Stoll, A., et al. "New investigations on valerian." *Schweizerische Apotheker Zeitung,* 95, 115–120, 1957.

8. Hendricks, H., et al. "Pharmacological screening of valeranal and some other components of the essential oil of valeriana officinalis." *Planta Medica,* 42, 62–68, 1981.

9. Hendriks, H., et. al. "Central nervous system depressant activity of valerenic acid in the mouse." *Planta Medica,* 49, 28–31, 1985.

10. Riedel, et al. "Inhibition of GABA breakdown by valerenic acid." *Planta Medica,* 46, 219–220, 1982.

11. Hazelhoff, et al. "Antispasmodic effects of valerian compounds: an in vivo and in vitro study on guinea pig ileum." *Archives Internat. de Pharmacoidyn.,* 257, 274–287, 1982.

12. Kempinskas, V. "On the action of valerian." *Farmakologiia i Toksikologiia,* 4(3), 305–309, 1964. (In Russian.)

13. Buehring, M. "The effect of valerian-hops preparation on the reaction time of clinic patients." *Der Kassenartz,* 16, 1976.

14. Stoll, A., et al., op.cit.

15. von Eickstedt, K., et al., op.cit.

16. Hoelzl, J. and Fink, C. "Untersuchungen zur wirkung der valep-otriate auf die spontanmotilitaet von maeusen." *Arzneimittel-Forschung,* 34(1), 44–47, 1984.

17. Mayer, B. and Springer, E. *Arzneimittel-Forschung,* 24, 2066, 1974.

18. Kempinskas, op.cit.

19. Broeren, W. *Pharmakopsychiatr. Neuropharmakol.,* 2, 1, 1969.

20. Leathwood, P.D. and Chauffard, F. "Aqueous extract of vale-rian reduces latency to fall asleep in man." *Planta Medica,* 2, 144–148, 1985.

21. Leathwood, P.D., Chauffard, F., et. al. "Aqueous extract of valerian root (Valeriana officinalis L.) improves sleep quality in man." *Pharmacol. Biochem. and Behav.,* 17, 65–71, 1982.

22. Chauffard, F., et. al "Detection of mild sedative effects: valerian and sleep in man." *Experientia,* 37, 622, 1982.

23. Leathwood, P.D. and Chauffard, F., op.cit.

24. Klich, R. and Gladbach, B. "Verhaltensstoerungen im kinde-salter und deren therapie." *Mendizinische Welt,* 26(25), 1252–1254, 1975.

25. Broeren, op.cit

26. Straube, C., op.cit.

27. Buchtala, M. *Hippokrates, 12,* 466–468, 1969.

28. Moser, L. "Medicine for stress behind the wheel?" *Deutsche Apotheker Zeitung,* 121, 2651–2654, 1981.

29. Boeters, U., op.cit.

30. Petkov, V. and Manolov, P. "Pharmacological studies on sub-stances of plant origin with coronary dilating and anti-arrhythmic action." *Comparative Medicine East and West,* 6(2), 123–130, 1978.

31. Mrnov, V.N. "Blood coagulation changes under the effect of valerian officinalis." *Farmakologiia i Toksikologiia,* 29, 187–188, 1966. (In Russian.)

32. Hanak, T. "Phytotherapie in der kardiologischen alltagspr-axis." *Zhurnal der Allgemein Medizin,* 56, 276–283, 1980.

33. Kempiunskas, V. op.cit.

34. Zburzhinsky, V.K. "An investigation into the sedative effect of

valerian." *Farmakologiia i Toksikologiia*, 27(3), 301–305, 1964. (In Russian.)

35. Manolova, P. and Petkov, V. "Screening studies on valepotriatic fractions from valerian officinalis roots." *Farmazia*, 26(2), 29–34, 1976. (In Russian.)

36. Petkov, V.D., et al. "Pharmacological studies of a mixture of valepotriates isolated from valerian officinalis." *Dokl. Bolg. Akad. Nauk*, 27, 1007–1010, 1973.

37. List, P.H. and Hoerhammer, L. *Hagers Handbuch der Pharmazeutischen Praxis*. Berlin, Springer-Verlag, 1968–1979, citation for Valeriana.

38. Dziuba, K. *Medizinische Welt*, 1866–1868, 1968.

39. Reported in Klich, R. and Gladbach, B. "Verhaltensstoerungen im kindesalter und deren therapie." *Medizinische Welt*, 26(25), 1252–1254, 1975.

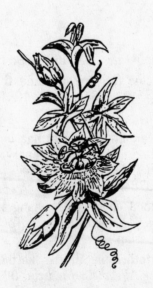

PASSION FLOWER

PASSION FLOWER
(Passiflora incarnata)

Passion flower, like valerian root, has a long, colorful history of use as a sedative. Passion flower usually takes the back seat to valerian, but in a recent survey of popular herbal sedatives in Great Britain, passion flower narrowly outscored valerian root for top honors.[1]

Passion flower is used primarily as a sedative or nervine to combat excess nervousness and anxiety, to tranquilize, and to induce sleep; as an anodyne, anti-spasmodic and anti-convulsant to treat dysmenorrhea and muscle cramps.

Passion flower was first discovered, in Peru, by the Spanish doctor Monardes in 1569. According to his reports, the herb was treasured highly by the mountain people of Peru, and by tribes throughout Brazil. Monardes, and other explorers after him, took the herb back to the Old World where it quickly became a favorite herb tea. Many years later, the herb returned to America with the early settlers as a part of their standard pharmacopoeia. In the United States *Passiflora incarnata* is commonly found in Florida, Texas, Virginia and in the southern part of Oklahoma, Missouri and North Carolina.

Primarily, passion flower is used world wide as a mild sedative or nervine that reduces anxiety, nervous tension, high blood pressure, and encourages sleep. It has also been employed as an antispasmodic (or spasmolytic) in the treatment of muscle cramps, convulsions, premenstrual tension, and even epilepsy. Passion flower preparations have been observed to overcome nervous symptoms and cramps that inhibit sleep, and to produce a restful and deep sleep free from frequent awakenings and disturbances. The antispasmodic action is also successfully used in the treatment of bronchial asthma.

Passion flower is well known for its analgesic or anodyne action. Topically it has been used in Europe and America on burns and in compresses and has a marked effect against inflammations, especially hemorrhoids. It is used in South America as a diuretic and for hemorrhoidal inflammations. In Brazil it is used as an antispasmodic and sedative. The Brazilians even have a favorite passion flower drink, called *maracuja grande*, that is frequently used to treat asthma, whooping cough, bronchitis and other tough coughs.[2] North American applications include use as an analgesic and anticonvulsant, with some success noticed in cases of tetanus. Italian physicians have placed great emphasis on passion flower in the treatment of asthma, and in Poland it is used in a proprietary drug for treating neurasthenia, hysteria and abnormal sexual excitability. Throughout Europe, passion flower is used to treat nervous conditions and pain that accompany female complaints ranging from dysmenorrhea to PMS to disturbances of menopause.

Other uses of passion flower, several of which have received some support in the experimental literature, include the treatment of nervous, high-strung, and easily excited children, cardiovascular neuroses, coronary sickness, circulation weakness, and concentration problems in school children.

Passion flower is a good sedative

Since passion flower is such a good sedative, most of the research has dealt with this action.[3-8] In keeping with the concept of a tonic, however, it should be noted that this herb does not produce sedation in healthy, conscious individuals who need to remain active and awake. Rather, in humans, it removes the anxiety and tension that prevents a person from relaxing or going to sleep.

The sedative action is intrinsically bound to all other actions, one way or another. It sedates the central nervous system, thus helping to overcome anxiety, nervousness and more serious conditions such as convulsions and hysteria. This also helps prepare the way for better sleeping habits. It relaxes the smooth muscles, and thereby is useful in the treatment of asthma, dysmenorrhea and other conditions that benefit from smooth muscle relaxation. The sedative action also increases the usefulness of the anticonvulsant property.

Experiments conducted in the last century showed that the

herb was effective under varying conditions, from simple nervous exhaustion to radical hysteria, and seemed to be particularly effective on sleeplessness that occurred during convalescence from the flu, in sleep disorders resulting from mental turmoil, overexcitement and irritability. It was also found to have a beneficial effect in cases of chorea, meningitis and strychnine poisoning, where it reduced the incidence and severity of muscular spasms.

In this century, more tightly controlled research has found substantially the same thing. In a typical animal trial, passion flower added to the diet, or injected directly into the stomach or bloodstream, significantly decreases motor activity as measured by such tests as the time required to negotiate a simple maze, or the amount of observable exploratory activity in a novel environment, compared to control animals. In one report, the researchers concluded that passion fruit, due to the presence of small amounts of harmala alkaloids, was an ideal substance for use by people caught up in the hectic pace of the modern world, a substance that not only possessed considerable nutritive value, but also possessed extraordinary potential as a tranquilizer.[9]

Passion flower and insomnia

Passion flower is a common remedy for insomnia, especially when it is caused by nervousness, irritability, anxiety and restlessness. The herb induces normal, peaceful, undisturbed sleep. Experimental observations the day following administration reveal no depression of body or mind, in contrast to the "morning after" usually experienced with narcotic drugs. Combinations of valerian root and passion flower are among the most popular sleeping aids throughout all of Europe, including the former Soviet Union.

The role that passion flower plays in the treatment of insomnia and other sleep disorders is very intriguing. It involves the action of certain constituents on the normal metabolic fate of the brain neurotransmitter serotonin. Serotonin, otherwise known as 5-hydroxytryptamine or 5-HT, is involved in sleep regulation. It is synthesized in the body from tryptophan. One way to increase serotonin levels in the brain is by ingesting tryptophan. For this reason, tryptophan is often included in sleeping aids in order to help provide the body with a pool of precursor from which serotonin can be made. The idea is that the more serotonin occurring in brain cells, the easier it is to fall asleep. (At this writing, the fate of tryptophan as a dietary supplement is uncertain. Reported cases of toxicity, probably as the result of contamination, have jeopardized the future availability of this amino acid to the general public.)

However, there is another way of increasing the stores of serotonin in nerve cells. This involves inhibiting the breakdown or metabolism of the serotonin already present. Serotonin is converted to 5-hydroxyindolacetic acid by enzyme monoamine oxidase (MAO). Substances that inhibit the action of this enzyme prevent the degradation of serotonin. Such substances are called monoamine oxidase inhibitors, or simply MAO inhibitors; the strongest of these substances comprise an important class of orthodox drugs known as antidepressants.

Passion flower constituents also inhibit monoamine oxidase, but only mildly. Nevertheless, this appears to be one of the ways in which passion flower affects the regulation and quality of sleep. It should be noted that only a small fraction of dietary tryptophan is utilized for serotonin synthesis, whereas MAO inhibitors can double the serotonin content of the brain in less than an hour. Even a mild MAO inhibitor such as passion flower would therefore be expected to have measurable effect on serotonin levels. Tryptophan supplementation, on the other hand, could have only minimal effects.

Paradoxically, serotonin is often referred to as a stimulant. This has led some writers to suppose that passion flower is also a stimulant, since it increases serotonin levels. The usual effects of ingesting passion flower, however, are clearly sedative. This may simply reflect the fact that people usually ingest passion flower only when the body needs to utilize the sedative constituents. At other times the stimulant constituents may be desirable. But there is another resolution to this particular contradiction. It requires that we clearly understand the difference between exogenous and endogenous serotonin.

Exogenous serotonin is that which is administered from the outside, for example, in the diet or by injection. Endogenous means it is produced by the body itself. Reports of stimulant action invariably involve exogenous 5-HT. Injected into the body, 5-HT stimulates the gastrointestinal and bronchial smooth muscles, afferent nerve endings, ganglion cells, and adrenal medullary cells. Exogenous 5-HT does not cross the blood-brain barrier, and hence is incapable of affecting brain cells in the same manner as endogenous 5-HT, which is undoubtedly an important neurotransmitter of the central nervous system.

Endogenous 5-HT is depressant. It has been conclusively demonstrated to play an important role in sleep regulation. But, in addition, due to its CNS action, it probably modulates the excitatory action of exogenous serotonin in the gastrointestinal tract and everywhere else the substance occurs in the body.

Observations of the action of exogenous serotonin, therefore, lack critical input from endogenous 5-HT. That input is undoubtedly depressant. This probably explains why much serotonin research is equivocal and contradictory.

On the surface, then, it would appear that passion flower, being an exogenous substance, should be stimulating. However, passion flower does not contain serotonin itself. Rather, it affects endogenous levels of 5-HT by inhibiting the enzyme that normally destroys the neurotransmitter. Passion flower therefore raises levels of endogenous serotonin and thereby produces a net depressant effect on the CNS.

It should also be mentioned that alkaloids of passion flower can cross the blood-brain barrier if administered in high enough doses, and can have psychotomimetic effects, i.e., they can cause hallucinations and so forth. However, in the quantities that occur in passion flower, these alkaloids are incapable of psychostimulation.

Passion flower has analgesic and antispasmodic actions

The analgesic, sedative, sleep-inducing and spasmolytic effects of passion flower are closely related and seldom occur in isolation. The analgesic and antispasmodic properties of this herb are observed simultaneously, and doctors have had the most success treating sleeplessness experienced by neurasthenic and hysteric patients, that is, by persons experiencing either physical or emotional pain, sometimes accompanied by organic or psychogenic convulsions.

Early investigators sometimes noticed that the herb worked especially well in those cases where sleeplessness could be traced to inflammation of the brain—it appeared to act as an analgesic and anticonvulsant. Neuralgia is commonly treated with passion flower. The analgesic or anodyne action of passion flower is regularly cited in noted codexes around the world.

Passion flower is frequently used in the treatment of dysmenorrhea, PMS, pelvic atony and for allaying the general nervousness that sometimes accompanies the menstrual cycle. Neuralgic pains associated with menstruation as well as various pains incurred during pregnancy and menopause have been successfully treated with passion flower.

SAFETY DATA

The use of passion flower appears to be completely free of toxicity and side effects, and has been approved by the FDA for food use. No known contraindications for passion flower exist, but it is wise to use whole plant and to avoid isolated alkaloids, which could be hallucinogenic. Also, it is probably wise to avoid the use of sympathomimetic agents when using passion flower to treat dysmenorrhea.

REFERENCES

1. Ross, M.S.F. and Anderson, L.A. "Selection of plants for phytopharmacological study based on modern herbal practice." *International Journal of Crude Drug Research,* 24(1) 1–6, 1986.

(Valerian and passion flower were most popular; valerian was listed first, but passion flower had the greater point total, so it is questionable which is truly the greater.)

2. Guertzenstein, B. "Aerztlicher fuehrer durch die brasilianische pflanzenmedizin." Sao Paulo o. J. *Deutsche Ausgabe*, 218, 238 (reported in Schindler, H., *Arzneimittel-Forschung*, 5, 491–492, 1955.)

3. *Planta Medica*, 54(6), 488–491, 1988.

4. Lutomski, J., Segiet, E., Szpunar, K. and Grisse, K. "Die bedeutung der passionsblume in der heilkunde." *Pharmazie in Unserer Zeit*, 10(2), 45–49, 1981.

5. Phillipson, J.D. and Anderson, L.A. *Pharmaceutical Journal*, 2, 80, 1984 (review article).

6. Aoyagi, N., Kimura, R. and Murata, T. *Chemical & Pharmaceutical Bulletin*, 22, 1008–1013, 1974.

7. Gagiu, F, Budiu, T, Lavu, P. and Bidiu, O. Romanian patent #59,589; (*Chem. Abstracts* 89, 48897n, 1978).

8. Lutomski, J. and Wrocinski, T. "Pharmacodynamic properties of passiflora incarnata preparations. The effect of alkaloid and flavonoid components on pharmacodynamic properties of the raw material." *Biul. Inst. Roslin Leczniczych*, 6, 176–184, 1960.

9. Lutomski, J., Malek, B. and Rybacka, L. "Pharmacochemical investigation of the raw materials from passiflora genus. 2. The pharmacochemical estimation of juices from the fruits of passiflora edulis and passiflora edulis forma flavicarpa." *Planta Medica*, 27, 112–121, 1975.

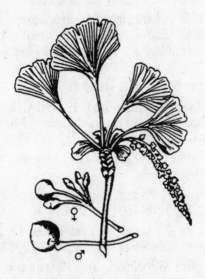

GINKGO BILOBA

GINKGO
(Ginkgo biloba)

The ginkgo biloba tree has been called "the doyen of trees," because of its antiquity.[1] It is believed to predate the last Ice Age. Individual trees are believed capable of living 2000 to 4000 years, and some extant are dated to over 1000 years. The tree is basically native to China and Japan (though there is evidence it was native to Europe at some ancient date), but has been extensively cultivated throughout the world due to its hardy nature. Ginkgo biloba is remarkably resistant to all kinds of pollution, viruses and fungi, possessed of a unique history, unique life cycle, and unique biochemistry.

The active constituents in ginkgo leaves are flavoglycosides (heterosides), and quercetin, as found in the leaf. These constituents should not be isolated, but should be present in a concentrated extract. Such an extract would be expected to contain about 24 percent flavoglycosides and 10 percent quercetin (which is itself a flavonoid). The use of regular whole leaf is of little efficacy. The product is only effective when extracted and concentrated. In addition to the guaranteed potency constituents, a substantial amount of pharmacologically active terpene derivatives (ginkgolides and bilobalides) should also be present.

Ginkgo has a tonic action on several aspects of neural functioning, including the stabilization of neural and muscular membranes, removal of toxic metabolites, normalization of transmitter concentrations, and maintenance of appropriate levels of important electrolytes.

Ginkgo has cerebral vascular effects

In a typical preclinical study using standard pharmacological procedures, microscopic particles are injected into the carotid artery of rats to mimic arterial blockage which normally leads to a decrease in the blood and oxygen supply to the brain. The administration of ginkgo biloba successfully protects the animals against the destructive effects of this procedure. Under the influence of ginkgo, increased levels of glucose and ATP occur, which help to maintain energy levels within individual cells of the brain.[2-5]

In the above procedures, following the injection of microspheres, there is usually a period of several hours characterized by a hypertensive burst, during which time considerable damage is done to the blood-brain barrier (that physiological system that prevents toxic substances from entering the brain mass from the surrounding blood vessels). The damage begins with just small molecules passing the barrier, but progresses until increasingly larger substances cross over. In later stages, considerable swelling (edema) of cerebral tissues becomes evident. The administration of ginkgo during the initial stages prevents the later stages by stabilizing the membranes involved in the blood-brain barrier. The result is a diminution of cerebral edema and essentially complete restoration of function.[6,7]

Since cerebral edema is one of the commonest complications of advancing age, it is profoundly important, then, that ginkgo biloba is able to inhibit its occurrence and the negative neurological consequences.[9]

Ginkgo inhibits platelet aggregation

Ginkgo has an inhibitory effect on blood platelet aggregation, meaning that it effectively reduces the tendency of blood components to stick together; therefore, it reduces the tendency for dangerous clots or thrombi to form in veins and arteries. The ability to inhibit blood clotting implies, of course, that ginkgo is probably an effective agent in the prevention of coronary thrombosis and in recovery from strokes and heart attacks, etc.[9]

Ginkgo is a free-radical inhibitor

Ginkgo demonstrates an ability to neutralize free radicals. That free radicals are directly implicated in the aging process, as well as in many other debilitating conditions, is a reason why medical science is always in search of new and better ways to neutralize or destroy these pathological agents. Since oxygen is the major source of free radicals, oxygen scavengers are among the best substances used to prevent the formation of free radicals. The flavonoids of ginkgo, including quercetin, are extremely potent oxygen scavengers. Possessing a particular affinity for the central nervous system as well as for the adrenal and thyroid glands, ginkgo is ideally suited for use in protecting the heart, blood vessels and brain against the destructive influence of free radicals.[10]

Free radical inhibition by ginkgo has been reported in a number of Petri dish models. Ginkgo not only destroys existing free radicals, but also inactivates their formation, and inhibits membrane lipid peroxidation (a destructive effect for which free radicals are partly responsible). Finally, through its antiradical activity, ginkgo exerts a stimulant effect on the biosynthesis of prostanoids (substances that, among other things, are capable of dilating blood vessels, thereby contributing to the prevention of high blood pressure).[11]

Ginkgo affects important brain neurotransmitters

Treatment with ginkgo significantly increases blood flow to the brain, and, perhaps more critically, it also produces a significant rise in dopamine synthesis, a neurotransmitter that is critical to the transfer of information and electrochemical impulses between nerves and other nerves, and between nerves and muscles, glands, organs, blood vessels and other structures of the body.[15]

Studies on the contractile action of ginkgo on isolated rabbit aorta have found that this action is probably due to the ability of the substance to stimulate the release of still other neurotransmitters: the catecholamines, namely epinephrine and norepinephrine. Because of its capacity to release catecholamines, ginkgo could affect the functioning of the entire network of catecholaminergic, glandular, cardiovascular and nervous systems of the body (perhaps the most extensive network, upon which depend the most important functions of life).[16]

Ginkgo exerts a specific effect on the beta receptors of the noradrenergic nervous system (this is basically a part of the sympathetic division of the autonomic nervous system). Beta receptor sites on muscles and organs, when activated, produce among other things dilation of airways in the lung, and dilation of peripheral blood vessels—i.e., those going to muscles, etc. The best word to describe the effect of ginkgo is "reactivation." In the aging process, the noradrenergic nervous system, especially in the brain, begins to lose vigor; associated symptoms of memory loss, speech defects, and decrease in alertness appear. By reactivating the brain cells of the cerebral cortex, ginkgo promsies to be an important substance in the prevention of premature aging.[17]

Ginkgo also affects the cholinergic aspect of the nervous system. The decline in function of this system is also implicated in the aging process and the onset of dementia. Using rats as a model of this condition, researchers have found that the oral administration of ginkgo significantly increases the population of appropriate cholinergic receptor sites in the brain. So, rather than having a direct effect on transmitter substances, in this case the compound works by proliferating sites that can be activated by cholinergic neurotransmitters. The end result is the same: revitalization of decreasingly effective cerebral tissue.[18]

Ginkgo had important vascular effects in humans

Ginkgo exerts considerable antispasmodic or sedative effects, and has excellent restorative effects on the nervous system.[19] Over one hundred patients with organic and neurological angiopathy, as well as ten healthy volunteers, were observed for changes in several physiological parameters resulting from exercise, after using ginkgo. It was concluded that ginkgo treatment should be considered in any case of central and peripheral vascular disease.

Ginkgo has been found to affect the microcirculation of the conjunctiva in elderly patients suffering from disturbances in cerebral blood supply. These studies have found a consistent increase in capillary and venous blood flow to the head resulting from decreased resistance to flow. The reduction in flow was not accompanied by hypotension or any appreciable variations in blood pressure.[20-21]

It has also been found that the use of ginkgo avoids another common complication caused by the more orthodox hypotensive medications: It increases peripheral blood flow without sacrificing cerebral circulation. A common side effect of standard peripheral vasodilators is that blood tends to accumulate in the expanded vessels rather than circulate to the vessels that feed the central nervous system, whose supporting vascular microstructure is not affected by the drug. Ginkgo avoids this complication by simultaneously increasing blood flow to the periphery and to the brain.

With 20 patients between the ages of 62 and 86 years serving as subjects, a 1977 study attempted to discover the effect of very low doses of ginkgo, administered over a two-week period. All subjects were experiencing a lack of adequate blood supply to the brain (cerebral circulatory insufficiency), due to age and arterio-sclerosis. The expectation of the investigators was that the combination of age, health of subjects, and the low dosage, would preclude any kind of spectacular results. Yet, of 20 subjects, 15 responded dramatically with much improved cerebral hemodynamics.[23]

Administered to patients with Parkinson's disease secondary to cerebral arteriosclerosis, ginkgo increased blood supply to the brain and improved its nutritional status. The latter finding has not been investigated thoroughly. But it crops up now and again, usually as a byproduct of a study, rather than its subject proper.[25]

Many other studies of improved vascular flow could be reviewed here. Instead, we will summarize some of the more important results as follows (over 95 percent of the following studies were double-blind placebo controlled trials):

- 65 percent successful treatment of 30 patients with focal or diffuse cerebral vascular disease.[26]
- 80 percent successful treatment of 47 patients with cerebral circulatory insufficiency, measured as improvement in mental functioning, EEG parameters, and cerebral angiogram. This study was a good demonstration of the potential benefit of ginkgo in the treatment of disease with both neural and circulatory components.[27]
- 80 percent success rate in 60 patients with chronic cerebral insufficiencies measured by improvement in functional symptoms such as vertigo, headache, etc.[28]
- Successful treatment of 60 patients with cerebral insufficiency as measured by ECG, EEG, computed tomography of the skull, and psychological tests.[29]
- 92 percent success rate in patients with cerebrovascular insufficiency in which all pathological findings disappeared after 18 days of treatment.[30]
- 80 percent success in treating headache and lesser percent success in cases of migraine, though still highly significant considering subjects had complained of migraine for a long time and had already received other treatments—the

authors conclude that ginkgo should be considered as one of the most effective drugs against migraine.[31]

- 40 percent success in the treatment of 49 elderly patients with peripheral arteriopathy (arterial insufficiency of lower limbs), some with angiopathy complicating senile diabetes mellitus, as measured by improvement in general psychophysical performance and in capacity to adapt to the environment.[33]

Ginkgo is used to treat vascular disturbances of the inner ear

Both structural and functional disturbances of the inner ear have been successfully treated with ginkgo. These problems all stem from some underlying vascular defect. In one study ginkgo was given to patients suffering from hearing loss due to old age (presbyacusia), patients with persistent ringing in the ears, and patients with vertigo. Improved hearing was experienced by 40 percent of the presbyacusia patients; those who didn't respond were assumed to have irreversible lesions of the sensory structures of the inner ear. Most of those patients with ringing in the ear experienced significant improvement within 10 to 20 days. The action of ginkgo on cerebral circulation resulted in swift and complete disappearance of vertigo. The researcher concludes his study with the admonition to use ginkgo not only for treatment, but also for prevention of otorhinolaryngeal problems.[38]

Similar results were obtained by various other investigators. An 88 percent success rate was obtained in one study involving 49 patients suffering variously from hearing loss, ringing, vertigo and labyrinthine syndrome. The consensus of such studies is that ginkgo is highly recommended in neurosensory diseases of the inner ear of vascular origin which manifest themselves by ringing in the ear, vertigo and headache.[27, 39, 40]

That severe cochleovestibular disturbances with a vascular component are subject to amelioration by ginkgo is reported in a recent study. In deafness of long standing, the results were poor, but even then in about half of such cases definite improvement was seen. Such results are truly remarkable. In recent deafness, following head injuries or sonic damage, the results were very good in more than 60 percent of the cases. Ringing in the ear improved significantly even in very severe cases at a rate of 74 percent. Almost all patients with vertigo reported significant improvement.[29]

In one study devoted explicitly to vertigo, 70 patients were given ginkgo or placebo over a three-month period. The effectiveness of the ginkgo on the intensity, frequency and duration of the disorder was statistically significant. At the end of the trial, 47 percent of the patients receiving ginkgo were completely free of their symptoms (18 percent of the placebo group recovered).[17] Other studies have essentially replicated the findings of this one.[42–44]

Ginkgo has mental and behavioral effects

In a twelve-week study, elderly patients expressing no particular complaint were selected to receive ginkgo (120 milligrams) or placebo on a daily basis. The ginkgo produced definite improvements in alertness measures in persons in whom there was room for improvement, but induced no change in the persons whose initial performance was already at a high level. In comparison to controls, the experimental subjects showed a substantial increase in vigilance as measured by simple reaction time tests and multiple-choice reaction tests. These results contrasted somewhat with results obtained in an early trial in which healthy young girls improved significantly on a memory test after ingesting 600 mg of ginkgo. The general implication of these studies is that ginkgo increases the rate of information processing at neuronal levels, not only in geriatric persons with deteriorating mental function but perhaps also in healthy young individuals.[45, 46]

In another study, eighty healthy female volunteers were administered variable doses of ginkgo one hour before being subjected to a battery of psychological and physiological tests, the results of which tended to differentiate ginkgo from sedative and stimulant drugs and suggested a selective effect of ginkgo on the memory process. Keep in mind that these tests took place just one hour following the administration of the compound. This quick-acting effect, when placed in context with the longer periods required for the vascular action, suggest a whole continuum of properties attributable to this herb.[47]

Utilizing the EEG, one study determined the effects of ginkgo in three pathological animal models, in young healthy volunteers and in elderly people with dementia disorders. It was found that the EEG tracings correlated well with the psychometric tests employed. The results confirmed those of other clinical trials and especially highlighted the ability of ginkgo to enhance alertness in the human subjects.[48]

Not many long-term studies have had a chance to be conducted, given the short history of ginkgo research, but one such study was recently reported. Using 166 patients, researchers tracked the effects of ginkgo on a battery of behavioral, clinical and physiological measures (such as those mentioned above) of cerebral disorders due to aging. Differences between control and treatment groups became clearly apparent after just three months. Over the ensuing months, the differences increased—a dramatic demonstration of benefits available from the use of ginkgo extract.[49]

Ginkgo may affect the course of Alzheimer's disease

Research on the possible effects of ginkgo in patients suffering from Alzheimer's disease and other age-related cognitive disorders is currently under way, and preliminary discussions are extremely promising. In reviewing the available research, one scientist concluded that ginkgo extract showed exceptional promise as the drug of choice "in all types of dementia, and even in patients suffering from cognitive disorders secondary to depression, because of its beneficial effects on mood. Of special concern are people who are just beginning to experience deterioration in their cognitive function. Ginkgo biloba extract might delay deterioration and enable these subjects to maintain a normal life and escape institutionalization. In addition, ginkgo biloba extract appears to be a safe drug, being well tolerated, even in doses many times higher than those usually recommended."[50-52]

SAFETY DATA

Before ginkgo was approved for human consumption it had been extensively tested for potential side effects. Virtually none were found. Some people have reported mild gastrointestinal upset, headache or skin rash that are probably allergic in nature, but that's it. Even doses many times in excess of the recommended therapeutic amount have not produced significant toxicity.

One long-term study was carried out to determine if very large doses of ginkgo had any influence on delicate endocrine balances. The results of all hormonal and blood assays were negative.[53]

REFERENCES

1. Drieu, K. "Preparation et definition de l'extrait de ginkgo biloba." *Presse Med.*, 15(31), 1455–1457, 1986.
2. Larsen, R.G., Dupeyron, J.P. and Boulu, R.G. "Modele d'eschemie cerebrale experimentale par microspheres chez le rat. Etude de l'effect de deux extraits de ginkgo biloba et du naftidrofuril." *Therapie*, 33, 651, 1978.
3. Rapin, J.R. and Le Poncin-Lafitte, M. "Modele experimental d'ischemie cerebrale. Action preventive de l'extrait de ginkgo." *Sem. Hop. Paris*, 55, 2047, 1979.
4. Le Poncin-Lafitte, M., Rapin, J. and Rapin, J.R. "Effects of ginkgo biloba on changes induced by quantitative cerebral microembolization in rats." *Arch. Int. Pharmacodyn.*, 243, 236, 1980.
5. Rapin, J.R. and Le Poncin-Lafitte, M. "Consommation cerebrale du glucose. Effet de l'extrait de ginkgo biloba." *Presse Med.*, 15(31), 1494–1497, 1986.

6. Grosdemouge, C, Le Poncin-Lafitte, M. and Rapin, J.R. "Effets protecteurs de l'extrait de ginkgo biloba sur la rupture precoce de la barriere hemoencephalique le rat." *Presse Med.*, 15(31), 1502–1505, 1986.

7. Spinnewyn, B., Blavet, N. and Clostre, F. "Effets de l'extrait de ginkgo biloba sur un modele d'ischemie cerebrale chez la gerbille." *Presse Med.*, 15(31), 1511, 1986.

8. Etienne, A., Hecquet, F. and Clostre, F. "Mecanismes d'action de l'extrait de ginkgo biloba sur l'oedeme cerebral experimental." *Presse Med.*, 15(31), 1506–1510, 1986.

9. Borzeix, M.G., Labos, M. and Hartl, C. "Recherches sur l'action antiagregant de l'extrait de ginkgo biloba. Activite au niveau des arteres et des veines de la pie-mere chez le lapin." *Arch. Int. Pharmacodyn.*, 243, 236, 1980

10. Brunello, N., Racagni, G., Clostre, F., Drieu, K. and Braquet, P. "Effects of an extract of ginkgo biloba on noradrenergic systems of rat cerebral cortex." *Pharm. Res. Commun.*, 17, 1063–1072, 1985.

11. Pincemail, J. and Deby, C. "Proprietes antiradicalaires de l'extrait de ginkgo biloba." *Presse Med.*, 15(31), 1475–1479, 1986.

12. Doly, M., Droy-Lefaix, M.T., Bonhomme, B. and Braquet, P. "Effet de l'extrait de ginkgo biloba sur l'electrophysiologie de la retine isolee de rat diabetique." *Presse Med.*, 15(31), 1480–1483, 1986.

13. Lebuissen, D.A., Leroy, L. and Rigal, G. "Traitement des degenerescences 'maculaires seniles' par l'extrait de ginkgo biloba. Etude preliminaire a double insu face au placebo." *Presse Med.*, 15(31), 1556–1558, 1986.

14. Clairambault, P., Magnier, B., Droy-Lefaix, M.T., Magnier, M. and Pairault, C. "Effet de l'extrait de ginkgo biloba sur les lesions induites par une photocoagulation au laser a l'argon sur la retine de lapin." *Sem. Hop. Paris*, 62, 57, 1986.

15. Le Poncin-Lafitte, M., Martin, P., Lespinasse, P. and Rapin, J.R. "Ischemie cerebrale apres ligature non simultanee des arteres carotides chez le rat: effet de l'extrait de ginkgo biloba." *Sem. Hop. Paris*, 58, 403, 1982.

16. Auguet, M., De Feudis, V., Clostre, F. and Deghenghi, R. "Effects of an extract of ginkgo biloba on rabbit isolated aorta." *Gen. Pharmac.*, 13, 225, 1982.

17. Racagni, G., Brunello, N. and Paoletti, R. "Neuromediator changes during cerebral aging. The effect of ginkgo biloba extract." *Presse Med.*, 15 (31), 1488–1490, 1986.

18. Taylor, J. E. "Liasions des neuromediateurs a leurs recepteurs dans le cerveau de rats. Effet de l'administration chronique de l'extrait de ginkgo biloba." *Presse Med.*, 15(31), 1491–1493, 1986.

19. Trounier, H. "Klinisch-pharmakologische untersuchungen ueber den effect eines extraktes aus ginkgo biloba L. beim post thrombotischen syndrom." *Arzneimittel-Forschung*, 18, 551, 1968.

20. Massoni, G., Piovella, C. and Fratti, L. "Effets microcirculatoieres de la ginkgo biloba chez les personnes agees.' *Giorn. Geront.*, 20, 444, 1972.

21. Piovella, C. "Effetti della ginkgo biloba sui micorovasi della congiuntiva bulbare." *Minerva Med.*, 64, 4179, 1973.

22. Auguet, M. et al., op. cit., 1982.

23. Galley, P. and Safi, N. "Tanakan et cerveau senile. Etude radio-circulographique." *Bordeaux Med.*, 10, 171, 1977.

24. Bauer, U. "6-month double blind randomized clinical trial of ginkgo biloba extract versus placebo in two parallel groups in patients suffering from peripheral arterial insufficiency." *Arzneimittel-Forschung*, 34, 716, 1984.

25. Hemmer, R. and Tzavellas, O. "Zur zerebralen wirksamkeit eines pflanzenpraparates aus ginkgo biloba." *Arzneimittel-Forschung*, 17, 491, 1967.

26. Montanini, R. and Gaspari, G. "Impiego di un estratto di ginkgo biloba (TEBONIN) nella terapia delle vasculopatie cerebrali." *Min. Card.*, 17, 1096, 1969.

27. Boudouresques, G., Vigourous, R. and Boudouresques, J. "Interet et place de l'extrait de ginkgo biloba en pathologie vasculaire cerebrale." *Medicine Praticienne*, 55–75, 1975.

28. Moreau, Ph. "Un nouveau stimulant circulatoiere cerebral." *Nouv. Presse. Med.*, 4, 2401, 1975.

29. Haan, J., Reekermann, V., Welter, F.L., Sabin, G. and Muller, E. "Ginkgo biloba flavonglykoside. Therapiemoglichkeit der zerebralen insuffizienz." *Medizinische Welt*, 33, 1001, 1982.

30. Eckmann, F. and Schlag, H. "Kontrollierte doppelblind-studie

zum wirksamkeitsnachweis von tebonin forte bei patienten mit zerebrovaskularer insuffizienz." *Fortschrifte der Medizin*, 100, 474, 1982.

31. Dalet, R. "Essai du tanankan dans les cephalees et les migraines." *Vie Medicale*, 35, 2971, 1975.

32. Daniel, F. "Les troubles trophiques d'origine veineuse des membres inferieurs, et leur traitement par le ginkor." *Immex*, Janvier 1972, p. 129.

33. Locatelli, G. R. and Sorbini, E. "Effetto del tebonin (estratto delle foglie di ginkgo biloba 1.) nel trattamento dell'arteriopatia periferica senile." *Min. Card.*, 17, 1103, 1969.

34. Sorbini, E. "La ginkgo biloba nella terapia vascolare." *Minerva Med.*, 64, 4201, 1973.

35. Natali, J. and Cristol, L. "Experimentation clinique d'un extrait de ginkgo biloba dans les insuffisances arterielles peripheriques." *Vie Med.*, 16, 1023, 1976.

36. Ambrosi, C. and Bourde, C. "Nouveaute therapeutique medicale dans les arteriopathies des membres inferieurs: tanakan. Essai clinique et etude par les cristaux liquides." *Gaz. Med. France*, 82, 628, 1975.

37. Garzya, G. and Picari, M. "Trattamento delle vasculopatie periferiche con una nuova sostanza estrattiva il tanakan." *Clin. Europ.*, 20, 936, 1981.

38. De Amicis, E. "Attivita della ginkgo biloba nelle otopatie da arteriosclerosi." *Minerva Med.*, 64, 4193, 1973.

39. Artieres, J. "Effets therapeutiques du tanakan sur les hypoacousies et les acouphenes." *Lyon Mediter. Medical*, 14, 2503, 1978.

40. Natalie, R., Rachinel, J. and Pouyat, P.M. "Le tanakan dans les syndromes cochlevestibulaieres relevant d'une etiologie vasculaiere. Traitement de long cours." *Gaz. Med. France*, 86, 1381, 1979.

41. Haguenauer, J.P., Cantenot, F., Koskas, H. and Pierart, H. "Traitement des troubles de l'equilibre par l'extrait de ginkgo biloba. Etude multicentrique a double insu face au placebo." *Presse Med.*, 15(31), 1569–1572, 1986.

42. Claussen, C.F. "Interet diagnostique et pratique de la craniocorpographie dans les syndromes vertigineux." *Presse Med.*, 15(31) 1565–1568, 1986.

43. Meyer, B. "Etude multicentrique randomisee a double insu face au placebo du traitement des acouphenes par l'extrait de ginkgo biloba." *Presse Med.*, 15(31), 1562–1564, 1986.

44. Dubreuil, C. "Essai therapeutique dans les surdites cochleaires aigues. Etude comparative de l'extrait de ginkgo biloba et de la nicergoline." *Presse Med.*, 15(31), 1559–1561, 1986.

45. Gessner, B., Voelp, A. and Klasser, M. "Study of the long-term action of a ginkgo biloba extract on vigilance and mental performance as determined by means of quantitative pharmaco-EEG and psychometric measurements." *Arzneimittel-Forschung*, 35(9), 1459–1465, 1985.

46. Hindmarch, I. and Subhan, Z. *Clin. Pharmacol. Res.*, 4, 89, 1980.

47. Hindmarch, I. "Activate de l'extrait de ginkgo biloba sur la memoire a court terme." *Presse Med.*, 15(31), 1592–1594, 1986.

48. Pidoux, B. "Effets sur l'activite fonctionnelle cerebrale d l'extrait de ginkgo biloba. Bilan d'etudes cliniques et experimientales." *Presse Med.*, 15(31), 1588–1591, 1986.

49. Taillandier, J., Ammar, A., Rabourdin, J.P., Ribeyre, J.P., Pichon, J., Niddam, S. and Pierart, H. "Traitement des troubles du vieillissement cerebral par l'extrait de ginkgo biloba. Etude longitudinale multicentrique a double insu face au placebo." *Presse Med.*, 15(31), 1583–1587, 1986.

50. Dehen, H., Dordain, G. and Allard, M. "Methodologie d'un essai controle dans la maladie d'Alzheimer." *Presse Med.*, 15(31), 1577–1582, 1986.

51. Allard, M. "Traitement des troubles du vieillissement par extrait de ginkgo biloba." *Presse Med.*, 15(31), 1540–1545, 1986.

52. Warburton, D.M. "Psycho-pharmacologie clinique de l'extrait de ginkgo biloba." *Presse Med.*, 15(31), 1595–1604, 1986.

53. Felber, J.P. "Effet de l'extrait de ginkgo biloba sur les parametres biologiques endocrines." *Presse med.*, 15(31), 1573–1574, 1986.

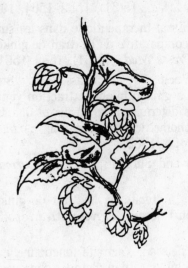

HOPS

HOPS
(Humulus lupulus)

Hops have been used down through the centuries as a mild sedative and sleeping aid. Attempts to discover the active principles, or even to verify the sedative effect experimentally, were frustrated for many years. But finally good experimental procedures produced the expected results, confirmation of sedative action. Apparently, the active principles are extremely labile, and efforts to process the herb during the early stages of the experiments effectively destroyed the active substances. Normally commercial processing undoubtedly also destroys much of the activity of the herb. That's why standardized extracts of hops are becoming the only acceptable form of administration.

Hops have also been shown to have antispasmodic action, which would explain their use as a stomachic. Estrogenic substances are found in hops, as well as good antibiotic activity. As a sleeping aid, hops have been put in pillows and used in teas; this use has also found experimental support.

The primary use is to calm and tone nerves and help induce sleep. For these purposes they are usually combined with other herbal sedatives such as passion flower and valerian root.

Hops have sedative action

The sedative property of hops eluded researchers for many years, suggesting that the active principle may be extremely volatile and short-lived. (One investigator found that after nine months hops retained only 15 percent of its original potency.) Nevertheless, sedative action was eventually found and has since been further substantiated. The sedative action has been shown not to depend on muscle relaxation but instead to be a function of the central nervous system. Generally, a soothing, relaxing calm is experienced within 20 to 40 minutes after ingesting the herb. Lupulin is accepted as the active ingredient, though at least one study found sedative properties in a lupulin-free preparation.[1-7]

An active sedative constituent of hops, 2-methyl-3-buten-2-ol is structurally very similar to a known sedative, methylpentynol. In tests with rats, both chemicals were effective within the same range. Further tests showed that the sedative effect could not be ascribed to a muscle relaxing principle.[1,8]

Hops have antispasmodic principles

In an investigation of hops' antispasmodic effects, it was found that the herb exerted a strong sedative action on smooth muscle preparations obtained from internal organs of various species of animals; it antagonized the spasmogenic effects of acetylcholine, atropine, papaverine, mepoyramine and histamine. This action was produced by a double mechanism, both neurotropic and musculotropic, but the musculotropic element was much the stronger. These findings would seem to justify the use of hops in the treatment of gastric and intestinal spasms.[6]

Hops helps in the treatment of sleep disorders

Hops is found in dozens of proprietary sleeping aids throughout Europe and the United States. For example, it is a constituent (along with valerian, melissa, and passion flower) of a proprietary sleeping aid called Vita-Dor marketed in Germany. This product was submitted to clinical trial, and found to be very effective in a dose-dependent manner. Age was important. Generally, patients over sixty required less. It was impossible to determine how much of the effect was due to the individual components of the drug.[9]

SAFETY DATA

Hops has no known toxicity; however, large doses are not tolerated well by some people.

Hops may also cause contact dermatitis in sensitive individuals.[10]

REFERENCES

1. Wohlfart, R., Haensel, R. and Schmidt, H. "Nachweis sedativ-hypnotischerwirkstoffe im hopfen, 4." *Planta Medica*, 48, 120–123, 1983.

2. Wohlfart, R., Haensed, R. and Schmidt, H. "An investigation of sedative hypnotic principles in hops. Part 3." *Planta Medica*, 45, 224, 1982.

3. Leclerc, H. "La Pharmacologie du houblon (humulus lupulus L.)" *La Presse Medicale*, Samedi (Paris), 42(20 Oct), 1652, 1934.

4. Stocker, H. *Schweizer Brauerei Rundschau*, 78, 80, 1967.

5. Berndt, G. *Deutsche Apotheker Zeitung*, 106, 158–59, 1966.

6. Caujolle, F., et al. "Etude de l'action spasmolytique du houblon (humulus lupulus, C.)." *Agressologie*, 10(5), 405–410, 1969.

7. Haensel, R., Wohlfart, R. and Coper, H. "Narcotic action of 2 methyl-3-butene-2-ol contained in hops. Part 3." *Planta Medica*, 45, 224, 1982.

8. Haensel, R., Wohlfart, R. and Coper, H. "Versuche, sedativ hypnotischewirkstoffe im hopfen nachzuweisen, II." *Zhurnal Naturforschung*, 35c, 1096–1097, 1980.

9. Steyn, D.C. *Onderstepoort J. Vet. Sci.*, O, 107, 111, 573, 1937.

10. List, P.H. and Hoerhammer, L.H. *Hagers Handbuch der Pharmazeutischen Praxis*, six volumes, Springer-Verlag, Berlin, 1968–1979, citation for Humulus.

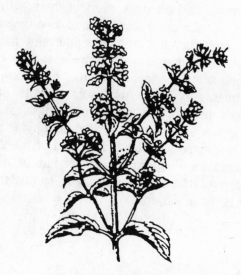

PEPPERMINT

PEPPERMINT
(Mentha piperita)

Peppermint is one of the most popular tonic herbs known to modern man. Its use as a flavoring agent is well known. Medicinally, it is mainly used to aid the various processes of digestion: combatting gas, increasing the flow of bile, healing the stomach and liver, etc. The active constituents are found in the essential oil, mainly menthol and carvone.

The volatile ingredients of peppermint make it an ideal choice for invigorating the mind, for improving the mood and relaxing a tension-filled, anxiety-ridden nervous system. These properties of the oils have been experimentally verified, as have the spasmolytic, antiulcer, anti-inflammatory and antibacterial properties.

Peppermint has spasmolytic properties

Well known to herbalists everywhere are the abilities of peppermint tea to calm upset stomach and tone the gastrointestinal tract. The spasmolytic property of peppermint has been established through comparisons with a wide variety of convulsant drugs, including acetylcholine, histamine, serotonin, anaphylaxotocin. Experiments typically use isolated cuts of rabbit and guinea-pig intestine, isolated guinea pig lungs, cat lungs in situ and whole animals under conditions of anaphylactic shock. The smooth muscle spasmolytic effect is exerted primarily on the neuromuscular junction. Peppermint extract has been found to decrease the tone of the lower esophagus sphincter so that the escape of air is made easier.[1-3]

SAFETY DATA

Peppermint is nontoxic, though some people may be allergic to the leaves, and some hay fever has been associated with fields of peppermint.

It is said that menthol and menthol-containing drugs can be lethal to infants if applied to the nose (as when the infant has a cold). Avoid this practice.[4]

REFERENCES

1. Shipochliev, T. "Pharmacological study of several essential oils. I. Effect on the smooth muscle." *Vet. Med. (Prague)*, 13(8–9), 63–69, 1968.

2. Forster, H. "Spasmolytische wirkung pflanzlicher carminativa." *Zeitschrift der Allgemein Medizin*, 59, 1327–1333, 1983.

3. List, P.H. and Hoerhammer, L.H. *Hagers Handbuch der Pharmazeutischen Praxis*, six volumes, Springer-Verlag, Berlin, 1968–1979, citation for Mentha.

4. Martindale: *The Extra Pharmacopoeia*, The Pharmaceutical Press, London, 1977. Citation for Mentha.

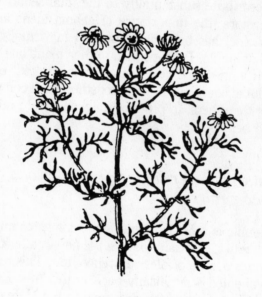

CHAMOMILE

CHAMOMILE
(Matricaria chamomilia)

Since chamomile is one of the most widely used and talked-about herbs, we should try to understand the physiological actions of the plant. Fortunately, scientists have investigated chamomile to some extent, and there is presently substantial evidence we can draw upon to increase our awareness of what chamomile contains and what it does to us.

Chamomile contains a wide variety of active constituents, each of which comes to the fore under certain conditions and plays an important supportive role in other situations. Thus bisabolol is thought to be the major anti-inflammatory constituent, but the total anti-inflammatory effect of whole chamomile depends upon the presence of the flavonoids, such as apiginine and luteoline. Likewise, for years researchers attributed the antispasmodic effect to the flavonoids, but it has recently been demonstrated through numerous trials that other constituents also contribute substantially to the total sedative action.

Furthermore, the importance of chamazulene and its precursor, matricine, has been demonstrated in virtually all of the actions of chamomile. Perhaps in no other plant has the importance of holistic medicine been better demonstrated. Both water- and lipid-soluble components work together, each complementing the action of the others, to produce the wonderful range of activity discussed below.

Chamomile has relaxing properties of a tonic nature

Chamomile is most frequently used for its calming, slightly sedative properties. It is said to calm the nerves after a long day's work, to induce a state of pleasant relaxation. This property was fairly well validated scientifically back in the '50s. Even as long ago as 1914 papers appeared proclaiming the ability of chamomile to block the action of known convulsants, spasmolytic agents, and so forth.[1-4]

In one study, chamomile tea was administered to ventricular catheterized patients in order to determine if the herb affected cardiac function. It didn't. But 10 of the 12 patients fell asleep about 10 minutes after drinking the tea.[5]

High doses of chamomile can have a pronounced depressant effect on normal voluntary activity, if we can generalize from studies involving rats.[6,7] Rats normally perform certain trained tasks very efficiently, intent solely on receiving reinforcement. Large doses of chamomile slow such behavior down. In humans, it is reasonable to expect some inhibition of motor function following the ingestion of, say, a couple of gallons of chamomile tea. So be careful. . . .

Seriously, in some countries both chamomile tea and chamomile medicinal preparations are used primarily for their depressive action on the central nervous system. The behavior of rats after ingesting chamomile tea is instructive. Such animals appear very relaxed; they are certainly not as anxious-acting as control animals. However, when required to perform a task requiring some degree of coordination, they perform as well as the control animals. The tea is therefore not *disrupting* normal performance or function; it appears to be simply reducing anxiety, as would be expected from a nervous system tonic. It is not a primary muscle relaxant, as it does not induce motor incoordination. When rats are introduced to a situation that allows them to stick their noses through holes, most engage in this exploratory kind of behavior with vigor. The chamomile rats don't seem nearly as interested in this opportunity. They won't explore nearly as many holes. So what does that mean? Frankly, who knows? Why do the rats explore the holes in the first place? Curiosity? Hunger? Fear? Sex? No one really knows. About all we can deduce with any certainty is that the behavior is mediated via the central nervous system, and the effect of chamomile is probably somehow involved at that level, too.

Chamomile has a mild calming action on the digestive system

Chamomile is as much used as a carminative as a mild sedative. The carminative action of chamomile depends, of course, on its sedative activity. Drinking warm chamomile tea is recognized among herb users as one of the best ways to calm an upset stomach and ease digestion.[8]

Chamomile has anti-inflammatory action

Much of the effectiveness of chamomile is due to its well-documented anti-inflammatory properties, which involve the nervous system at various levels. In studies, utilizing experimentally-induced gastritis and other mucous membrane inflammations, chamomile consistently demonstrates a quick and prolonged anti-inflammatory effect. Studies have also shown that the individual anti-inflammatory constituents of chamomile, including azuline, chamazuline, bisabolol and matricine, each have their own distinct mode of action. Some are more powerful but perform for a shorter period of time, while others are milder but exhibit activity for a long period of time.[9-13]

One of the most amazing things about chamomile is that, in spite of the fact that the herb was being used throughout Europe and North America for the treatment of acute and chronic gastrointestinal inflammatory conditions, for heartburn, for constipation, for stomachache, and so forth—in spite of all that, it wasn't until 1979 that experimental verification of its protective and healing effect on the mucosa of the GI tract was reported.[14,15] In the first experimental studies, chamomile inhibited the formation of ulcers produced by several conditions, including the administration of drugs and stress. The alcohol-induced model is particularly well suited to the screening of potential antiulcer substances because the pathological/historical picture obtained closely approximates that of typical bleeding ulcerative gastritis. More recent studies have confirmed and extended the ulcer-protective property of chamomile.

Stress-induced ulcers are prevented by chamomile extracts. This effect is probably the result of the herb's antispasmodic property. Though the ultimate role of hydrochloric acid in causing ulcers is the subject of much dispute, it has been shown that chamomile is able to inhibit the formation of ulcers experimentally induced by that substance.

SAFETY DATA

Since the flowering heads of chamomile are used to make teas, washes and poultices, the allergenic potential of this plant must be respected. Hypersensitive reactions have been observed in a small percentage of the population that is allergic to ragweed pollen. If you are sensitive to asters, chrysanthemums and other members of the *Compositae* family, approach the use of chamomile with care at first, until you have established whether you are sensitive to it. This type of sensitivity is extremely rare.[16]

Chamomile is virtually nontoxic to the population at large.

REFERENCES

1. Breinlich, von J., Scharnagel, K. "Pharmakologische eigenschaften des en-in-dicycloaethers aus matricaria chamomilla." *Arzneimittel-Forschung*, 18, 429–431, 1969.

2. Jelicic-Hadzovic, von J. and Stern, P. "Azulene und bradykinin." *Arzneimittel-Forschung*, 22(7), 1210–1211, 1972.

3. Luppold, E. "Matricaria chamomilla." *Pharmazie in Unserer Zeit*, 13(3) 65–70, 1984.

4. Isaac, O. "Die kamillentherapie—erfahrung and bestaetigung." *Zahn Aerztl. Praxis*, 496, 1980.

5. Gould, L., et al. "Cardiac effects of chamomile tea." *Journal of Clin. Pharmacol.*, 13, 475–479, 1973.

6. Della Loggia, R., et al. "Depressive effect of chamomilla recutita (l.) rausch, tubular flowers on central nervous system in mice." *Pharm. Res. Comm.*, 14(2), 153–162, 1982.

7. Fundaro. A. and Cassone, M.C. "Azione degli olii essenziali di camomilla, cannella, assenzio, macis e origano su un comportamento operativo nel ratto." *Boll. della Soc. Ital. Di Biol. Sperimentale*, 56, 2375–2380, 1980.

8. Lind, P. O. and Bruhn, J.G. "Biologiska effekter av kamomill." *Lakartidningen*, 81(51), 4846–4848, 1984.

9. Jakovlev, V. and Von Schlichtergroll, A. "Antiinflammatory activity of (-)-alpha-bisabolol, an essential component of chamomile oil." *Arzneimittel-Forschung.*, 19(4), 615–616, 1969.

10. Verzarne, P.G., et al. "Adatok a kamilla egyes vegyueleteinek hatasahoz." *Acta Pharm. Hung.*, 49, 13–20, 1979.

11. Isaac, O. and Kristen, G. "Alte und neue wege der kemillentherapie." *Med. Welt*, 31, 1145–1148, 1980.

12. Heubner, W. and Grabe, F. "Ueber die entzuendungswidrige wirkung des kamillenoels." *Naunyn-Schmiedebergs Arch. Exp. Pathol. Pharmakol.*, 171, 329–339, 1933.

13. Jakovlev, V., et al. "Pharmakologische undersuchungen von kamillen inhaltsstoffen." *Planta Medica*, 49(2), 67–73, 1983.

14. Szelenyi, I., et al. "Pharmacological experiments with components of chamomile. III. Experimental animal studies of the ulcer-protective effect of chamomile." *Planta Medica*, 35(2), 218–227, 1979.

15. Schimpke, Dr. "Neues ueber pharmakologie und klinische anwendung der kamille und ihrer inhaltsstoffe." *Pharmazie*, 20, 178, 1965.

16. Abramowicz, M., Ed. *Medical Letter on Drugs and Therapeutics*, 21(7), 30, 1979.

LIME/LINDEN FLOWERS
(Tilia cordata, T. platyphyllos)

The inclusion of lime or linden flowers in this book is admittedly a whim of the author. Too many wonderful herbal materials are overlooked because of the lack of a large experimental database. This flower could be one of those. The tea made from these flowers has been used since the Middle Ages to reduce anxiety, to invigorate the mind, and as a general soothing agent for the whole body. It is used to treat headaches, indigestion, hysteria and diarrhea, among others.

THE PHARMACOLOGY OF LIME/LINDEN

Lime-linden contains a number of flavonoid compounds, especially quercetin and derivatives, kaempferol, and coumarins, which are responsible for most of the plant's medicinal activity. Tannic acid and significant quantities of mucilage are also present and add to the plant's activity. A very rich, fragrant and complicated volatile oil is also a part of linden flowers.[1-5]

The reputation of lime or linden flower to calm the nerves and at the same time invigorate the nervous system suggests that it may be one of the best nervous system tonics around. There is little research to support this claim, but a plant with such a consistent reputation deserves closer inspection.

Linden has anti-influenza action

As an interesting sidelight to this discussion, one study may be of interest to the reader. This study says much about herbal medicine in addition to the specific results of the study. A large group of children with influenza were divided into three groups: (1) linden blossom, bed rest, aspirin; (2) as in (1) plus sulphonamides; (3) just antibiotics. The children in group one recovered most quickly with the fewest complications (middle ear infections, etc.). The results were roughly 10:1 in favor of the herbal group.[6]

The British Herbal Pharmacopoeia recognizes linden (lime) tree as a sedative, spasmolytic, diaphoretic, diuretic and mild astringent, for use in the treatment of migraine, hysteria, arteriosclerotic hypertension, and feverish colds; specific for raised arterial pressure associated with arteriosclerosis and nervous tension.[5]

SAFETY DATA

There is some evidence that continued frequent use of linden flower tea can cause heart damage. In therapeutic doses, especially in encapsulated form, linden is nontoxic.[7]

REFERENCES

1. Schauenberg, P. and Paris, F. *Guide to Medicinal Plants*, Keats Publishing, Inc., New Canaan, Connecticut, 1977, p. 257.

2. Braun, H. and Frohne, D. *Heilplanzen-Lexikon fuer Aerzte und Apotheker*. Gustav Fischer Verlag, Stuttgart, New York, 1987, pp. 238–239.

3. Tyler, V. *The New Honest Herbal*, Stickley, Philadelphia, 1987, pp. 148–149.

4. Duke, J.A. *CRC Handbook of Medicinal Herbs*, CRC Press, Inc., Boca Raton, Florida, 1985, pp. 485–486.

5. *British Herbal Pharmacopoeia*, British Herbal Medicine Association, 1983, pp. 213–214.

6. Weiss, R.F. *Herbal Medicine*. Beaconsfield Publishers, Ltd. Beaconsfield, England, 1988, p. 227.

7. Pahlow, M. *Das Grosse Buch der Heilpflanzen*. Graefe and Unzer Publishers, Munich, 1979, pp. 221–223.

SIBERIAN GINSENG, ELEUTHERO ROOT
(Eleutherococcus senticosis)

Siberian ginseng is one of the primary tonic herbs; it finds application in the maintenance of health in almost all body systems. It is the prototypical adaptogenic agent as conceived by Hans Selye (see Introduction). It buffers the body's alarm reaction, and builds up the body's ability to resist stress effects.

But, while eleuthero fits well in the context of the general adaptation syndrome (GAS), it was the Russians who tagged it with the term "adaptogen." However, early Russian efforts to place the adaptogen theory squarely within the context of the GAS met with little success; had the idea caught on, eleuthero might have emerged as the first substance to fulfill all of Selye's criteria for a perfectly safe and effective catatoxic and syntoxic substance.[41, 48] Using the term "adaptogen" in the context of the GAS is an attractive idea; unfortunately, the Russians defined the term strictly according to the properties of Siberian ginseng (so that in a strict sense, in order for an herb to be called an adaptogen, it has to exhibit almost exactly the same effects as Siberian ginseng). To utilize the term to describe the actions of other adaptation-enhancing herbs requires that we loosen the definition a bit. Ironically, that process is already well under way within the area of herbal medicine; many different herbs are being called adaptogens, even though their actions do not meet the strict criteria laid down by the Russians.[1]

Actually, the term "tonic," as well as the idea that it embodied, preceded both the GAS and the adaptogen theories by several centuries. Once medical science achieved the sophistication necessary to reinvent some of the constructs underlying the tonic theory, it had lost touch with the original formulations (which had already been relegated to the status of primitive, worthless humbug), and so viewed the modern concepts as new, fashionable and original.

The author's preference for the term "tonic" reflects both his respect for the rich heritage implied by that term and his dissatisfaction with Selye's awkward terms "catatoxic" and "syntoxic," and his resistance to bastardizing the otherwise attractive and descriptive term "adaptogen."

Selye observed that most of the catatoxic agents he worked with seemed to operate through an action on the pituitary-adrenal axis. It has likewise been theorized that Siberian ginseng operates primarily through the same axis.[2] Hence, the tonic for which the adaptogen theory was developed is actually a classic model for the GAS theory. In this context, it can be theorized that eleuthero increases the body's ability to deal with stress. Studies have shown that eleuthero treatment in animals greatly reduces the typical signs of stress—stomach ulcerations, spleen enlargement, thymus enlargement, blood changes, etc. These reductions are closely correlated with increases in the manufacture of the adrenocortical hormones that mediate the stage of resistance. Furthermore, by reducing the amount of adrenalin-related hormone secretion, administration of the herb also curbs the initial alarm reaction to the stressor.

The tonic nature of this action is manifested in findings that show that the administration of eleuthero (and other kinds of ginseng) in the absence of stress has very little observable effect on the body. A prominent scientist in the area of ginseng research, Stephen Fulder, building on the framework first advanced by the equally astute Russian scientist, O.I. Kirillov,[48] has synthesized pertinent data to show that the locus of action of ginseng is probably the hypothalamus itself.[3] The hypothalamus sends instructions to the pituitary which secretes ACTH (adreno-corticotropic hormone), which in turn stimulates the adrenal glands, and coordinates effects throughout other body systems. The Fulder/Kirillov theory has been supported by a great deal of research. [2, 9–10, 18–19, 26–30, 41.]

The following statements provide a quick summary of the various effects of Siberian ginseng.

1. Helps treat and prevent a wide variety of debilitating conditions, including diabetes, cancer, rheumatic heart disease and other cardiovascular diseases. [3, 16, 17, 21, 24, 25, 44, 47]

2. Possesses a tendency to improve circulation, although the mechanism of action has not been determined, and indeed, the observed results may be completely secondary to other actions. [38,39]

3. Has a nutritive or tonic effect on the adrenal glands, whose secretion of cortisol is critical to the control of several factors that impact on several body systems, including the cardiovascular, nervous, reproductive, digestive and immune systems. [9,10,18]

4. Regulates blood sugar levels in a tonic fashion. [4, 33]

5. Has a tonic effect on blood lipid levels and lipid metabolism. [5,11]

6. Improves thyroid responsiveness to changing body demands. [6]

7. Helps to neutralize the effects of free radicals. [7]

8. Improves the flow of blood to the brain. [8]

9. Improves physical and mental performance; was utilized by the majority of Soviet athletes. [19, 20, 46]

10. Helps the body fight inflammation. [22, 23]

11. Increases the body's nonspecific resistance to disease. [30, 42]

12. Protects against thermal stress. [31]

13. Reduces the stress associated with exercise. [32]

14. Improves endurance. [34, 35, 36]

15. Strengthens and tonifies the immune system. [37]

16. Promotes weight gain and overall health. [12–14, 45]

17. Promotes health in the male reproductive system without any toxic effect on female reproduction system. [15, 40, 45]

SAFETY DATA

Eleuthero is one of the safest and least toxic of all known plants, and may be safely used in reasonable amounts (less than 3 grams) on a daily basis for extended periods of time[42, 43]

REFERENCES

1. Brekhman, I.I. "New medicinal plants of the Araliaceae family—spiny eleutherococcus." *Izvest. Sibir. Otdel. Akad. Nauk S.S.S. R.,* 9, 113, 1960.

2. Fulder, S. "The drug that builds Russians." *The New Scientist,* 21 August 1980, and "Ginseng and the hypothalamic-pituitary control of stress." *Am. J. Chin. Med.,* 9(2), 112–118, 1981.

3. Mischenko, E.D. "Treatment of diabetes mellitus patients with a liquid extract of eleutherococcus roots." *Vladivostok Sb.,* 54, 1962 (C.A., 59, 14483f, 1963).

4. Brekhman, I.I. and Oleinikova, T.P. "Comparative data on the effect of ginseng and eleutherococcus on artificially elevated blood sugar level." *Mater. Isuch. Zhen-shenya Drugikh Lek. Rast. Dal'n Vost.,* 249, 1963 (C.A. 60, 16389b, 1964).

5. Dambeneva, E.A. and Salnik, B.Y. "Effect of extracts of eleutherococcus and leuzea on lipid metabolism during physical stress." *Stimulyatory Tsent. Nerv. Sist.,* 51, 1966 (C.A. 66, 84586u, 1967).

6. Saratikov, A.S. and Cherdyntsev, S.G. "Effects of certain stimulators on the central nervous system on thyroid function." *Stimulvatory Tsent. Nerv. Sist.,* 62, 1966 (C.A. 66, 93853f, 1966).

7. Tkhor, L.F., et al. "The free radical mechanism of the radioprotective action of some natural compounds." *Tr. Mosk. Obshchest. Ispvt. Prir. Otd. Biol.,* 16, 73, 1966.

8. Zyryanova, T.M. "Effect of extracts of panax, eleutherococcus and leuzea on blood supply to the brain." *Stimulytory Tsent. Nerv. Sist.* 37, 1966 (C.A. 66, 114460t, 1966).

9. Kirillov, V.A. and Semaskevich, G.M. "Effect of eleutherococcus extract on the adrenal glands of white rats." *Tr. Bla-*

goveshch. Gos. Med. Inst., 7, 133, 1966 (C.A. 66, 10233a 1967).

10. Barchas, J.D., Mefford, I.N., Roth, K., et al. "Neuroregulators and stress." *Naval Res. Review*, 23(4), 2–12, 1981.

11. Golikov, A.P. "Cholesterol synthesis in the small intestine of rabbits and the effect of eleutherococcus during a five day cholesterol load." *Mater. Izuch. Zhen'shenya Drugikh Lek. Rast. Dal'ne Vost. Akad. Nauk. SSSR, Sib. Otd.*, 7, 63, 1966 (C.A. 67, 41641m, 1967).

12. Dardymov, I.V. and Kirillov, V.A. "On the mechanism of eleutherococcus's property to increase gain in weight in animals." *Eleutherococcus and Other Adaptogens Among Far Eastern Plants*, Vladivostok, USSR, 1966.

13. Saratlkov, A.S. "Adaptogenic action of eleutherococcus and goldenroot preparations." In: *Adaptation and Biologically Active Substances.* The Far Eastern Scientific Center, USSR Academy of Sciences, Vladivostok, 1976.

14. Brekhman, I.I., ed. *Eleutherococcus and other Adaptogens Among the Far Eastern Plants*, Far Eastern Publishing House, Vladivostok, USSR, 1966.

15. Maxisimov, J.L. "Thorny eleutherococcus plant stimulator of the reproductive function of bulls." *Eleuthero. in Livestock Breeding.* 96–102, 1967.

16. Bezdetko, G.N. "Prophylactic and therapeutic effects of eleutherococcus on alloxan diabetes." *Mater. Izuch. Zhensh. Drugikh Lek. Sredstv. Dal'n Vost.*, 17, 81, 1966 (C.A. 67, 80980r, 1967).

17. Yaremenko, K.V. "Effect of eleutherococcus, panax, and dibazol on the inoculability of intravenously introduced tumorous cells." *Mater. Izuch. Zhensh. Drugikh Lek. Sredstv. Dal'n Vost.*, 7, 109, 1966 (C.A. 68, 11557s, 1968).

18. Dardymov, I.V., et al. "Effect of the prolonged intake of eleutherococcus and ascorbic acid on the body of a healthy human being." *Mater. Izuch. Zhensh. Drugikh Lek. Sredstv. Dal'n Vost.*, 7, 133 1966 (C.A. 68, 11649, 1968).

19. Brandis, S.A. and Pilovitskaya, V.N. "Effectiveness of the use of an extract from the roots of the prickly eleutherococcus during prolonged physical work and inhalation of oxygen-enriched gas

mixtures." *Mater. Izuch. Zhensh. Drugikh Lek. Sredstv. Dal'n Vost.*, 7, 141, 1966 (C.A. 68, 11650s, 1968).

20. Brandis, S.A. and Pilovitskaya, V.N. "Effectiveness of the use of an extract from the roots of the prickly eleutherococcus during work in a high temperature environment." *Mater. Izuch. Zhensh. Drugikh Lek. Sredstv. Dal'n Vost.*, 7, 155, 1966 (C.A. 68, 11651t, 1968).

21. Mikumis, R.I., et al. "Effect of eleutherococcus on some biochemical blood indicators in the treatment of patients with rheumatic heart diseases." *Mater. Izuch. Zhensh. Drugikh Lek. Sredstv. Dal'n Vost.*, 7, 227, 1966 (C.A. 68, 11653v, 1968).

22. Golikov, P.P. "Effect of the preventive administration of antiinflammatories on the vascular permeability in rats during various types of inflammation." *Mater. Izuch. Zhensh. Drugikh Lek. Sredstv. Dal'n Vost.*, 7, 295, 1966 (C.A. 68, 20786t, 1968).

23. Fedorov, Yu.V., et al. "Effect of some stimulants of plant origin on the development of antibodies and immunomorphological reactions during acarid-born encephalitis." *Stimulytory Tsent. Nerv. Sist.*, 99, 1966 (C.A. 69, 104731e, 1968).

24. Malingina, L.L. "Effect of eleutherococcus senticosis max. in combined treatment of experimental tumors." *Vop. Onkol.*, 15, 87, 1969.

25. Moskalik, K.G. "Effects of adaptogens on the growth and metastasis of pliss lymphosarcoma in laparatomized animals." *Voprosy Onkol.*, 16, 74, 1970.

26. Krasnozhenov, E.P. "Effect of rodosine, pyridrol and eleutherococcus extract on the nonspecific immunological reactivity of animals." *Izv. Sib. Otd. Akad. Nauk SSSF, Ser. Biol. Nauk*, 139, 1970 (CA 74, 86141j, 1971).

27. Dardymov, I.V. "Effect of ginseng and eleutherococcus preparations on metabolism under physical load conditions." *Sb. Rat. Inst. Tsitol. Akad. Nauk SSSR*, 14, 76, 1971.

28. Brekhman, I.I. and Dardymov, I.V. "Pharmacological investigations of glycosides from ginseng and eleutherococcus." *Lloydia*, 32, 46, 1969.

29. Brekhman, I.E. and Dardymov, I.V. "Mechanism of increasing organism resistance under the effect of ginseng and eleuthero-

coccus senticosis preparations." *Sb. Rat. Inst. Tsitol. Akad. Nauk SSSR.,* 14, 82, 1971.

30. Wagner, H. et al., "Immunostimulating action of polysaccharides (heteroglycans) from higher plants." *Arzneim.-Forsch.,* 35(7), 1069–1075, 1985.

31. Novozhilov, G.N. and Silchenko, K.K. "Mechanism of adaptogenic effect of eleutherococcus on the human body during thermal stress." *Fiziol. Cheloveka,* 11(2), 303–306, 1985.

32. Martinez, B. and Staba, E.J. "The physiological effects of aralia, panax and eleutherococcus on exercised rats." *Jpn. J. Pharmacol.,* 35(2), 79085, 1984.

33. Medon, P.J. et al. "Hypoglycemic effect and toxicity of eleutherococcus senticosis following acute and chronic administration in mice." *Chung Kuo Yao Li Hsueh Pao,* 2(4), 281–285, 1981.

34. Berdyshev, V.V. "Effect of the long-term intake of eleutherococcus on the adaptation of sailors in the tropics." *Voen. med. Zh.,* (5), 57–58, 1981.

35. Batin, V.V. et al. "Experience in using sugar and an eleutherococcus extract with the workers of the hot shops and the night shifts of the Raichikhinsk Glass Plant." *Gig. Tr. Prof. Zabol.,* (5), 36–38, 1981.

36. Berdyshev, V.V. "Effect of eleutherococcus on body functions and the work capacity of sailors on a cruise." *Voen. Med. Zhurnal,* (2), 48–51, 1981.

37. Barkan, A.I. et al. "Effect of eleutherococcus on respiratory viral infectious morbidity in children in organized collectives." *Pediatriia,* (4) 65–66, 1980.

38. Blokhin, B.N. "Effect of extracts from the roots and leaves of eleutherococcus on the working capacity of athletes." In: *Materials of the 3rd Conference on the Central Research Laboratory of the Tomsk Medical Institute.,* Tomsk, 1966.

39. Brekhman, I.I. and Dardymov, I.V. "A stimulating action of individual glycosides of eleutherococcus." In: *3rd Conference of the Central Research Laboratory.* Tomsk, 1966.

40. Dardymov, I.V. "On the gonadotropic effect of eleutherococcus glycosides." *Lek. Sred Dal-nego Vostoka,* 11, 60–65, 1972.

41. Brekhman, I.I. and Kirillov, O.I. "Effect of eleutherococcus on

alarm-phase of stress." *Life Sci. Physiol. Pharmacol.*, 8(3), 113–121. 1969.

42. Dardymov, I.V. et al. "The effect of prolonged intake of an extract of eleutherococcus on human health." *Kharbarovsky Med. Inst., Mat. Nauk Sess.*, 20–23, 1963.

43. Darymov, I.V. et al. "On the absence of toxicity in eleutherococcus glycosides introduced over two months." *Lek. Sred. Dalnego Vostoka*, 11, 66–69, 1971.

44. Dardymov, I.V. et al. "Insulin like action of eleutherosides from the roots of eleutherococcus senticosis." *Rast. Resur.*, 14(1), 86–89, 1978.

45. Darymov, I.V. and Kirillov, O.I. "Weight differences in certain internal rat organs when eleutherococcus and testosterone are administered in doses identically increasing animals' weight gains." *Eleutherococcus and Other Adaptogenic Plants of the Far East*, Far Eastern Publishing House, Vladivostok, 1966, pp. 43–47.

46. Golikov, P.P. "Influence of aqueous extracts of roots, stems and leaves of eleutherococcus and ginseng on mental working humans (correctness test)." *Mater. Izuch. Zhen-shenya Drug. Lek. Dal'n. Vost.*, (5), 233–235, 1963.

47. Golikov, P.P. "Material on treating atherosclerotic patients with eleutherococcus root extract." *Eleuthero and Other Adaptogenic Plants of the Far East*, 7th Ser., 1966, pp. 213–19.

48. Kirillov. O.I. "The effect of fluid extract of eleutherococcus root on the pituitary-adrenocortical system." *Sib. Otd. Acad. Nauk SSSR.*, 23, 3–5, 1964.

BALM
(Melissa officinalis)

Its very name suggests the primary application of balm—a soothing, calming agent for stressed nerves. Balm, like the various members of the mint family, is invigorating and yet relaxing to the nervous system because it is highly aromatic. These effects are felt throughout the body, and have earned balm the reputation of being a mild panacea.

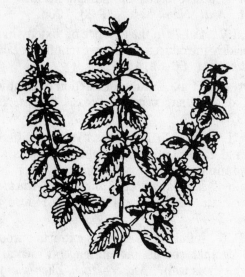

BALM

Balm is a common constituent of relaxants, nervines and sleeping aids throughout the world. Seldom used alone, it seems to interact with and enhance the activity of other beneficial tonics for the nervous system.

In folk medicine, balm is used as a stomachic (to reduce turmoil in the GI tract), antispasmodic (to reduce tension and cramping in both smooth and striated muscle throughout the body), and carminative (to neutralize the effects of gas on the stomach and intestines). Balm is frequently employed in treatments for female discomforts of all kinds, for nervous system problems, for insomnia, cramps, headache, muscle tension and soreness.

Science has yet to investigate the medicinal properties of balm thoroughly, yet what work has been done has established the nervine,[1] antispasmodic,[2,3] antihistamine,[4] carminative,[5] and antimicrobial[6,7] properties of the plant.

SAFETY DATA

Balm is generally regarded as safe by the FDA. It is free of side effects.

REFERENCES

1. Steger, W. "Zur wirksamkeit von vita-dor als einschlaf- und durchschlafmittel." *Fortschr. Med.*, 97(29), 5–8, 1979.
2. Reiter, M. and Brandt, W. "Relaxant effects on tracheal and ileal smooth muscles of the guinea pig." *Arzneim.-Forsch.*, 35(1A), 408–414, 1985.
3. Wagner, H. and Sprinkmetyer, L. *Dtsch. Apoth. Ztg.*, 113, 1159, 1973.
4. Debelmas, A.M. and Rochat, J. *Plant. Med. Phytother.*, 1, 23, 1967.
5. Wichtl, M. *Teedrogen: Ein Handbuch fuer die Praxis auf wissenschaftlicher Grundlage.*, 2nd ed. Wissenschaftliche Verlag., Stuttgart, Germany, 1989, pp. 339–342.
6. Kucera, L.S., Cohen, R.A. and Herrmann, E.C. "Antiviral activities of extracts of the lemon balm plant." *Annals New York Academy of Sciences*, 474–482, 1968.
7. Cohen, R.A., Kucera, L.S. and Herrmann, E.C. "Antiviral activity of melissa officinalis (lemon balm) extract." *Proc. Soc. Expertl. Biol. Med.*, 117, 431–434, 1964.

CHAPTER FOUR

The Digestive System

The digestive system is essentially a tube that runs from one end of your body to the other, with openings at both ends. You put stuff in one end, and as it passes through the body the organs of digestion extract from the stuff what they want and pass the unwanted stuff out the hole on the bottom end. That's admittedly not a very glamorous portrait, but it's one way of looking at the process that occupies a good deal of each day.

Without fuel, the body slows down, runs out of gas and stops. To keep it running, and operating at peak efficiency, we have to pay attention to not only the quantity of stuff we eat, but the quality of the stuff. We also must keep the organs of digestion healthy. Exposed as they are to both the good and bad aspects of anything we happen to put in our mouths, they go through periods of good and bad operating condition. In addition, they respond to the condition of other body systems, including the nervous system, the immune system and the cardiovascular system.

STRUCTURES AND FUNCTION OF
THE DIGESTIVE SYSTEM

The digestive system consists of the mouth, esophagus, stomach, small intestine and large intestine. It relies on secretions from the salivary glands, the pancreas, the liver and gallbladder. It requires the mechanical grinding ability of the teeth and jaws, and the interaction of the tongue.

The ultimate purpose of digestion is to break large pieces of food down into molecules tiny enough to pass unhindered into the bloodstream and from there into individual microscopic cells throughout the body. In addition, many substances need to be altered chemically to become utilizable. Only vitamins, minerals and water can be used by the body just as they are. The tasks of digestion are enormous. Digestion must, and does, begin as soon as food enters the mouth.

THE MOUTH

Many important aspects of digestion occur in the mouth. Mechanical breakdown of food begins with the chewing and grinding action of the teeth. Chemical breakdown begins with addition of saliva secreted by the salivary glands that line the mouth cavity (these include the parotid, sublingual and submandibular glands). These glands are so sensitive that the mere thought of food can get them going. The sight and smell of food are major stimuli: "It's enough to make your mouth water." Saliva is mostly water mixed with mucus and the enzyme amylase. Enzymes throughout the digestive tract stimulate chemical reactions that gradually break apart complex molecules into very simple ones. Amylase works on the starches, or carbohydrates, beginning the process of breaking them down into maltose. Saliva makes the taste of foods possible, since only dissolved substances can be tasted. Saliva contains a variety of other substances not directly related to digestion: sodium, potassium, calcium, chloride, proteins, mucin, urea, white blood cells and debris from the linings of the mouth.

The tongue serves the purpose of mixing things up, pushing food against the roof of the mouth and making small, wet balls of food, called boluses, and pushing these toward the back of the throat in preparation for swallowing. When you get ready to swallow, which for most of us is too soon, a flap of cartilaginous tissue in the throat called the epiglottis moves downward, closing off the trachea, or windpipe, to prevent food from passing into the lungs.

THE ESOPHAGUS

Assuming that your food bypassed the trachea without a hitch, it now enters the esophagus, a muscular tube that connects the mouth to the stomach. Muscular contractions in the esophagus cause the food to move downward. This action is called peristalsis. During the passage through the esophagus, the amylase continues to work on the starches. If you swallow too big a chunk of food it might become lodged in the esophagus, causing discomfort.

THE STOMACH

After food passes through the esophagus, it now empties into the stomach, a saclike organ that connects the esophagus to the duodenum of the small intestine. The stomach is flexible, allowing it to expand when filled with food and collapse when empty. It can hold about 1.5 liters of fluid. The walls of the stomach consist of layers of muscle lined with special glandular cells that secrete gastric juice. The stomach is richly endowed with blood vessels and nerves. A very strong muscle at the lower end of the stomach forms a ring called the pyloric sphincter which controls the passage of food from the stomach to the duodenum. The upper part of the stomach is called the fundus; a section of the lower part is called the antrum.

The stomach has two main functions. The first is to continue the process of digestion begun in the mouth; the second is to store food. Without this storage capacity, you would have to eat much more frequently than the normal two to three times per day.

Like the salivary glands, the gastric glands begin secreting at the mere smell, sight or mention of food. The arrival of food in the stomach initiates even more activity. Gastric juice contains enzymes, hydrochloric acid (HCl) and mucus. The HCl regulates the pH or acidity of the stomach to optimize digestion. It also kills unfriendly bacteria and activates pepsin, one of the main digestive enzymes of gastric juice. Pepsin begins the digestion of proteins. The other main enzyme of gastric juice, lipase, begins the digestion of fats. The mucus is important in protecting the stomach wall from abrasion from food particles and from the caustic action of the HCl.

Gastric juice also contains a substance called intrinsic factor, which facilitates the absorption of vitamin B12 in the small intestine. About the only substances absorbed from the stomach are water and some glucose. The rest must await further breakdown and absorption in the small intestine.

Mechanical action continues in the stomach as the muscles create a churning action that mixes food with gastric juice forming a pastelike mixture called chyme. At regular coordinated intervals the stomach contracts and the pyloric valve relaxes, squirting an amount of chyme into the duodenum. This is a continuation of the peristaltic movement originating in the esophagus.

THE SMALL INTESTINE

The small intestine is a muscular tube about 6.5 meters (21 feet) long and about 35 mm (1.5 inches) in diameter. It comprises three sections: the duodenum (a short, curved, fixed section), the jejunum and ileum (two larger, coiled, mobile segments). Two ducts, one from the gallbladder and one from the pancreas, enter at the duodenum. The walls of the small intestine consist of muscles with an internal lining (the mucosa) and an external lining (the serosa). Peristalsis continues here as food is pushed along the length of the intestine by the contraction of the muscles.

The mucosa consists of thousands of thin, fingerlike projections called villi that are in turn covered with millions of fronds, the microvilli. The result is an incredible total surface area that helps in the absorption of substances into the blood.

When chyme reaches the small intestine it is ready for continued digestion. Secretions from the pancreas, the gallbladder and intestinal glands complete the digestion of food. The fluid from the gallbladder is called bile. It is actually produced by the liver, but it is stored in the gallbladder until stimulated to secrete it down the common bile duct into the duodenum. Bile consists of a variety of waste products from the liver (including bilirubin) as well as cholesterol and bile salts. It is the bile salts that aid in the digestion and absorption of fats (through emulsification). Secretions from the pancreas contain the enzymes trypsin, amylase and lipase. These continue the digestion of proteins and nucleic acids, starch and fats, respectively. Intestinal glands secrete peptidases that complete the last stages in the digestion of proteins, and the enzymes lactase, maltase and sucrase that complete the digestion of carbohydrates.

The end products of digestion are as follows: proteins (polypeptides, peptides and amino acids); starches, complex sugars and simple sugars (glucose, fructose and galactose); fats (glycerol, glycerides, and fatty acids). These materials are absorbed by the villi and pass directly into the bloodstream for distribution throughout the body.

THE LARGE INTESTINE

The large intestine is a muscular tube about 1.8 meters (6 feet) long and 50 mm (2 inches) in diameter. It brackets the small intestine like a picture frame. It is fixed in position, unlike the jejunum and ileum, contains no villi, and has bands of muscle along its length at specific intervals. A small section just past the small intestine is called the cecum. From the cecum hangs the appendix. Past the cecum lies the major part of the large intestine, the colon. The final part of the intestine, just before the anus, is a small section called the rectum. The colon is usually divided into the ascending, transverse, descending and pelvic portions. The pelvic, hanging down into the pelvis, is sometimes called the sigmoid colon.

Unabsorbed material left behind in the small intestine is passed on to the large intestine. It is mostly liquid and fiber. Nutrients, including vitamins and mineral salts, along with most of the remaining water, continue to be absorbed during transit through the large bowel, leaving feces made up of undigested food residue, small amounts of fat, secretions from the stomach, liver, pancreas and bowel wall and a variety of bacteria. The feces are slowly compressed and pass into the rectum. Distention of the rectum normally produces a desire to empty the bowel.

Eventually, the water absorbed from the intestines is eliminated from the body as urine.

THE PANCREAS

The pancreas lies under the stomach, except for its head, which is tucked into the curve of the duodenum. The pancreas consists primarily of exocrine tissue, which in turn consists of "nests" of endocrine cells (the islets of Langerhans) which secrete digestive enzymes into a network of ducts that come together to form the main pancreatic duct. This duct joins the common bile duct. The islets of Langerhans also secrete hormones, such as insulin, directly into the blood.

Pancreatic enzymes are secreted in an inactive form and must be activated by enzymes in the small intestine. The pancreas also secretes bicarbonate, which neutralizes stomach acid entering the duodenum.

THE LIVER

The liver is one of the most important organs of the body. Several of its functions relate directly to digestion. The liver produces bile, a yellowish, bitter mixture, full of pigments and salts. Bile emulsifies fats, which are normally insoluble in water; once emulsified, they are more water-soluble and can be more easily attacked by enzymes. Like pancreatic juice, bile contains a small amount of sodium bicarbonate that helps neutralize gastric acid. Bile also increases the absorption of vitamins A, D, E and K which are insoluble in fats.

ABSORPTION

Food enters the bloodstream and lymph system primarily from the lower portion of the small intestine. This process is called absorption. The mucosa of the small intestine contain millions of villi, presenting an appearance like a soft, thick carpet. The villi contain blood and lymph vessels. Most digested food enters the blood vessels in the villi. Larger fat molecules may pass into the lymph vessels of the villi. It should be noted that absorption occurs partly by diffusion and partly by active transport. The first process occurs due to typical pressure gradients; the second requires the health of special membrane-bound pumps that push substances through against the pressure gradient.

DISORDERS OF THE DIGESTIVE SYSTEM

Indigestion

A general term for several symptoms that follow the ingestion of food, including heartburn, abdominal pain, flatulence (gas) and nausea. The typical burning sensation in the upper abdomen is usually the result of eating too fast or of eating very rich, spicy, fatty foods in which the flow of digestive juices into the small stomach and small intestine is inadequate. Nervous indigestion is often the result of stress which inhibits the flow of gastric juice and slows down peristalsis. Other causes of heartburn can be peptic ulcers, gallstones and esophagitis (see below).

Esophagitis

Inflammation of the esophagus. There are two types, corrosive and reflux. Corrosive occurs following the ingestion of some kind of corrosive chemical or poison such as lye or acid. Reflux esophagitis is a common ailment caused by the regurgitation of stomach contents into the esophagus. It may be the end result of a chain of ailments that begins with a tear in the diaphragm which allows a portion of the stomach to protrude, resulting in hiatal hernia. This weakens the lower segment of the esophagus, which allows the reflux of stomach contents, producing symptoms of heartburn. Overeating, alcohol consumption and smoking all aggravate this condition.

Infection

The hydrochloric acid of the stomach normally kills the harmful bacteria that enter along with the food we eat. When there is insufficient HCl the bacteria can proliferate and spread throughout the digestion system, resulting in a variety of gastrointestinal infections.

Ulcers

Ulcers are single or multiple open sores on the mucous membrane of the gastrointestinal tract lining (peptic ulcer) or the small or large intestine (ulcerative colitis). Peptic ulcers occur where the g.i. tract is bathed in gastric juice (esophagus, stomach or duodenum). They can occur, though rarely, in the jejunum (Zollinger-Ellison syndrome) or ileum (Meckel's diverticulum). Characterized by a gnawing pain, especially when the stomach is empty. Duodenal ulcers occur three times more often than gastric ulcers. No one knows for certain what causes ulcers. Genetic and dietary factors have been implicated. Stress probably does not cause an ulcer, but it may aggravate an existing one.

Ulcerative colitis

Chronic inflammation and ulceration of the lining of the colon and rectum. Characterized by bloody diarrhea and pus-and mucus-containing feces. Diarrhea and bleeding can be mild or severe. Severe cases are usually accompanied by abdominal pain, weakness, tenderness and fever. Complications can be anemia, arthritis and cancer.

Gastritis

Pre-ulcerative inflammation of the gastric lining caused by large amounts of irritative substances such as aspirin or alcohol.

Pernicious anemia

A deficiency in vitamin B12 or folic acid caused by lack of intrinsic factor, a substance produced by the gastric lining that must combine with these nutrients in order to make them absorbable. Lack of intrinsic factor is thought to be an autoimmune disorder in which antibodies are produced that block the production of that critical substance. Because the liver has long-range storage capacity for B12 but not folic acid, most pernicious anemia is probably due to folic acid deficiency.

Intestinal obstruction

Refers to a partial or complete blockage of the small or large intestine. Caused by a variety of conditions including paralytic ileus (loss of peristalsis), strangulated hernia, genetic factors, stenosis (narrowing of the canal), adhesions following operations, twisting and knotting, Crohn's disease, diverticular disease, cancer, impacted food, feces, and gallstones (listed in decreasing order of likelihood).

Congenital disorders of the intestines

Noticeable within the first weeks of life. The intestines may be closed off completely (atresia), be abnormally narrowed (stenosis), be twisted and looped (volvulus), or be blocked by fecal intestinal contents.

Gastroenteritis

A general term for inflammation of the stomach and intestines. May occur for many reasons: from a variety of viruses, bacteria and parasites; from food intolerance, alcohol, antibiotics, and so forth. Symptoms include loss of appetite, nausea, vomiting, cramps and diarrhea, usually of sudden appearance. Symptoms can be mild or severe. Food poisoning, travelers' diarrhea and gastrointestinal flu are forms of gastroenteritis. Typhoid fever and cholera are serious forms of gastroenteritis demanding hospitalization.

Giardiasis

An infection of the small intestine caused by an insidious parasite known as *Giardia lamblia*. Formerly confined to tropical regions, it is now becoming more prevalent in North America and Europe. It contaminates a good portion of mountain rivers and springs. A common cause of giardiasis is the drinking of these waters by campers and hikers. Some reservoirs are also contaminated, causing epidemics of giardiasis. Can be acute or chronic and can reappear. Characterized by attacks of diarrhea and gas, stomach pain, cramps and nausea.

Colitis

Inflammation of the colon causing bloody, mucus-filled diarrhea, abdominal pain and fever. Caused by viruses, parasites (amoebas), and bacteria. The use of antibiotics may cause colitis by killing the normal bacteria in the intestine and allowing other types to grow, especially *Clostridium difficile*.

Crohn's disease

A chronic inflammation of any part of the GI tract from mouth to anus, causing pain, fever, diarrhea and weight loss. Related to colitis. Usually occurs at the end of the ileum (where the small intestine joins the large intestine). Cause unknown; may be a response to infectious organisms or predisposition, perhaps genetic. Many associated complications, including fistulas, ulcers and abscesses.

Diverticular disease

Diverticula are small sacs caused by protrusions at weak points of the inner lining of the intestine. They usually affect the lower part of the colon. Diverticulosis is the term denoting the presence of diverticula. Diverticulitis indicates inflammation in the area of the diverticula, usually caused by obstruction or perforation in one or more diverticula.

Paralytic ileus

The usually temporary failure of intestinal muscles to contract, resulting in the buildup of intestinal contents and bowel obstruction. Commonly follows abdominal surgery, injury or other trauma.

Irritable bowel syndrome

IBS refers to a constellation of diffuse abdominal aches and pains, intermittent nausea and diarrhea alternating with constipation that occurs in the absence of a diagnosis of anything specific. A catch-all for hundreds of difficult-to-diagnose conditions.

Hepatitis

Inflammation of the liver which results in the loss of many liver cells. Usually caused by viruses, but may result from drug abuse or poisoning of various kinds. There are many kinds of hepatitis, differing according to the causative agent and according to whether the condition is acute or chronic. Jaundice is the most common sign. Symptoms include nausea, vomiting, loss of appetite, tenderness in right upper abdomen, aching muscles, joint pain. Type A or infectious hepatitis is transmitted by fecal contamination, e.g. by infected people handling food, and can reach epidemic proportions. Type B or serum hepatitis is present in the blood of infected people and is spread through sexual contact, needle-sharing, etc.

Liver failure

A complication of acute hepatitis in which so much of the liver is destroyed that it is no longer able to carry out normal functions. The most immediate result is dysfunction of other organs, especially the brain, which is quickly poisoned by chemicals normally filtered out by the liver.

Cirrhosis

A chronic liver disease caused by severe damage to its cells that results in fibrosis or scarring of tissue. Gradual loss of liver function results as living cells become surrounded by pockets of fibrosis, thereby shutting off the flow of blood to the healthy tissue.

Cholangitis

Inflammation of the common bile duct. Caused either by bacterial infection following blockage of the duct by gallstones or parasites or by a narrowing of all the bile ducts within and outside the liver for unknown reasons.

Diabetes mellitus

A term for the failure of the pancreas to produce sufficient insulin. Insulin is a hormone that governs the absorption of glucose into cells to meet their energy needs and into the liver and fat cells for storage. Blood levels of glucose become very high. Can lead to serious complications. Symptoms include fatigue, blurred vision, constant thirst, muscle weakness, frequent urination, cystitis, candidiasis, and tingling sensations, followed by numbness in hands and feet.

Cystic fibrosis

An inherited disease in which the pancreas fails to produce enzymes involved in the breakdown of fats and proteins, resulting in their malabsorption from the intestines; this causes malnutrition and excessive fat in the feces. The bronchial tubes produce excessive amounts of thick mucus, which causes constant coughing, breathlessness, pneumonia and bronchitis.

Pancreatitis

Inflammation of the pancreas, resulting in scarring and impaired function. May be a complication of gallstones or alcohol abuse.

Gallstones

Small, smooth, round clumps of cholesterol, bile pigments and other related substances that occur when the chemical composition of the bile is upset. Normally they occur when the liver puts too much cholesterol into the bile, as it does in obesity or in high cholesterol diets.

Biliary colic

A condition characterized by severe pain in the upper right quadrant of the abdomen that is usually caused by gallstones, or, more specifically, by the body's attempt to pass them through the bile ducts.

Cholecystitis

Inflammation of the gallbladder. Causes severe abdominal pain. May be acute or chronic. Acute cholecystitis is usually the result of obstruction of the cystic duct by a gallstone. Repeated mild attacks of acute cholecystitis may lead to a chronic condition marked by thickening of the gallbladder walls which leads to reduced capacity for storing bile.

Cancer

Cancer can, of course, attack virtually any part of the digestive system. Genetic predispositions to certain kinds of cancer, e.g., colon cancer, can be aggravated by bad dietary practices.

HERBAL TONICS FOR THE DIGESTIVE SYSTEM

The purpose of ingesting tonic herbs is to nurture, soothe, stimulate and condition the organs of digestion so that they can operate efficiently at all times. Paying attention to the other systems by nurturing them with tonic herbs also affects gastrointestinal health. There are probably more herbs that act on the digestive system than any other system of the body. Many of these have a rather direct effect on one or another aspect of digestion itself. Others are used in the treatment of specific disorders. The tonic herbs usually combine specific effects on digestion with an overall influence on the health of the organs of digestion. The liver and gallbladder are favorite targets of tonic herbs, as these are perhaps the most critical organs. The nurturing of the stomach lining is another frequent action. While stimulation of the salivary glands and oral hygiene are perhaps the easiest effects to realize from herbal products, the wellness of the pancreas is the most difficult, both in terms of objective measurement and in terms of subjective improvements that can be directly related to that gland. Yet there are tonic herbs that seem to level out blood sugar response curves and fat digestion, thereby suggesting an influence on pancreatic function.

Tonic herbs for the digestive system usually exhibit bidirectionality to one degree or another. Thus ginger root will absorb excess gastric acid, but will stimulate the gastric glands to secrete gastric juice when the digestive process should be under way. Several of these herbs stimulate the production and flow of bile, but they do not do it indiscriminately, only when necessary. Likewise, the secretion of insulin is regulated, not simply increased by the tonic dandelion. Although the herbal sections that follow do not dwell at length on the tonic qualities of each herb, the reader should realize that none of these herbs pushes any components of the body's digestive system in a direction away from homeostasis.

THE ISSUE OF LAXATIVES

While laxatives may not be thought of as tonics in the usual sense of the word, the reader may be surprised to discover that certain herbs do in fact exert a toniclike action on the large bowel. This action is in direct contrast to that exerted by most proprietary laxatives. What, after all, is the laxative habit? It is a dependency on laxatives for promoting bowel movements. When laxatives become a necessary substitute for normal muscular contractions of the large bowel, one is said to have acquired the laxative habit. But how does that happen? It typically happens after months or years of using (abusing?) laxatives. The situation is puzzling to the extent that constipation is usually a temporary phenomenon caused by poor dietary habits, lack of bulk-producing foods or failure to heed the reflexive feelings that signal the need for proper evacuation; under these kinds of conditions, the use of a laxative is typically a short-term proposition. How does it become long-term? Rarely, a person may experience a chronic health problem, such as hypothyroidism or intestinal obstruction, that results in long-term constipation requiring the daily use of a laxative for prolonged periods of time. In this circumstance it is possible for a laxative habit to form. Usually, however, the repeated use of a laxative is the direct result of using the laxative in the first place.

Drug companies (and some herbal companies) learned long ago that certain laxatives have an astringent side effect which tends to reconstipate the system. The person interprets the astringent and constipative action as a continuation of the original problem, and therefore reapplies the laxative. It is easy to see that under these circumstances a person could get caught up in a never ending circle of constipation–laxative use–reconstipation–more laxative–reconstipation, and so forth until a laxative habit was formed. This results in big sales for the drug and herb companies.

Fortunately, there are laxative herbs without astringent side effects. In fact, there are herbs which will actually help to restore tone and normal muscular activity to the lower bowel. Primary among these is cascara sagrada (*Rhamnus purshiana*), buckthorn (*Rhamnus frangula*), and butternut root bark (*Juglans cinera*). These laxative herbs are nonhabituating and gentle when used properly. Six to eight hours after ingesting a few capsules (2–5), one can expect a pleasant bowel movement, without griping. Trying to hurry the process up by overdosing can cause cramps and discomfort. Be patient.

Cascara is the perhaps the best-researched of the laxative

herbs. The Formulary Service of the American Society of Hospital Pharmacists emphasizes the mildness of cascara, and acknowledges that it will not lose its effectiveness with repeated use. It is another characteristic of habituating laxatives that larger and larger doses are required over time; cascara, buckthorn and butternut do not possess this negative property.

Many over-the-counter laxatives contain cascara, but if you look closely, you will see that they also contain other substances, many of which are habituating. Avoid laxatives that contain strychnine (*Nux vomica*), aloin, aloes, baraloin, belladona alkaloids (atropine, scopolamine, hyoscyamine), podophyllum, synthetic drugs and senna.

Cascara, butternut and buckthorn may be viewed, in a liberal sense, as tonics, for they possess the following properties: 1) their cathartic or laxative action is mild; 2) they do not create discomfort in reasonable doses; 3) their action is limited to the large bowel, that is, to the site of action, and therefore does not create problems in the rest of the gastrointestinal tract; 4) their effectiveness is not lost with repeated use; 5) they are not habit-forming; 6) they can be used to restore and maintain tone in the colon; and 7) in *small* doses they can be used on a daily basis to enhance the health of the liver and other organs.

Good herbal laxatives should also contain herbs that are tonic to the organs of digestion, and which soothe and heal an inflamed GI tract, and that help to ameliorate whatever harshness might arise from the laxatives themselves. Among the best adjuncts are licorice root, Irish moss, small amounts of ginger root, turmeric, and slippery elm.

MILK THISTLE
(Silybum marianum L. Gaertn. or Carduus marianus L.)

(This section on milk thistle represents a small fraction of the data currently available on this fascinating herb. For a complete review the reader is referred to the chapter on milk thistle in the author's book, *Guaranteed Potency Herbs: Next Generation Herbal Medicine*, Keats Publishing, 1989.)

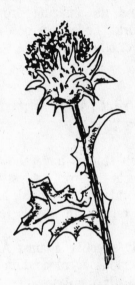

MILK THISTLE

Milk thistle is one of the most ancient known herbal medicines. At some point in time, milk thistle seed has been used in the treatment of gall stones, disorders of the liver, gallbladder and spleen, as a cholagogue to promote the flow of bile, as a tonic for the spleen, gallbladder and liver, as a remedy for jaundice from any cause, for indigestion, dyspepsia, lack of appetite and other stomach and/or digestive disorders, and to treat peritonitis, coughs, bronchitis, uterine congestion and varicose veins. A fine bitter tonic is commonly made from the seeds to aid digestion.

One of the earliest published reports established the ability of milk thistle to stimulate the flow of bile.[1] This action helped to explain why milk thistle appeared to be so effective in the treatment of indigestion and other disorders of the digestive system. However, its cholagogic property is not strong enough to totally explain its many beneficial effects on the digestive system.

Milk thistle contains large amounts of extraordinarily therapeutic substances known as flavonoids. A group of the most potent flavonoids is known collectively as silymarin. Silymarin, at the time of its discovery, was seen to constitute a whole new class of compound, and its amazing properties continue to astound the scientific world. Today, the best milk thistle contains a standardized amount of silymarin.

Milk thistle extract (Mte) protects the liver against toxicity

Numerous research studies have shown that milk thistle seed extract (Mte) protects the liver against the effects of toxins such as carbon tetrachloride, hexobarbital, amanita mushrooms, thioacetamide, salts of rare earth metals (e.g., praseodymium, indium and cerium).[2-8]

Mte is particularly effective against Amanita (death cap) mushroom, a very poisonous agent containing several different kinds of toxins. Mte greatly increases lifespan in poisoned animals. It also significantly inhibits the loss of weight normally observed in poisoned animals. This kind of research has been replicated many times; the outcome is always the same.[9-12]

Another experimental toxin commonly utilized in the study of the hepatoprotective role of Mte is thioacetamide (TAA). When TAA is fed to animals over a period of weeks to months it produces a picture of liver damage that closely resembles that of cirrhosis in man. Eventually death results from chronic administration of TAA. Thus two measures of the effectiveness of Mte are immediately suggested by experiments using TAA. First, it should reduce the amount of liver damage occurring; second, it should increase the lifespan of experimental subjects. Both of these objectives are achieved by Mte administration.[13,14]

Mte strengthens and stabilizes cell membranes

Milk thistle extract appears to protect and heal the liver in three primary ways. First it acts directly on the cell membrane of the liver, and probably most other cells of the body by stabilizing and strengthening that structure.[15,16] In support of this concept is the finding that Mte and some of the toxins actively compete for the same cell membrane receptor sites.[17-19] That toxins are unable to affect cell membranes in the presence of Mte argues for the stabilizing action of these substances. The observable result is the regeneration of liver cells.

One of the major theories offered to explain Mte's action is that it acts as an acceptor of free radicals—that is, it is a free-radical scavenger.[20,21] This idea is supported by the observation that flavonoids in general are good free-radical scavengers.

Mte interferes with enterohepatic circulation

Another mechanism of action is involved in the hepatoprotective action of Mte. Humans develop toxic reactions to certain poisons due to the presence of a continuous enterohepatic circuit. That means the toxins are cycled continuously between the gastrointestinal tract and the liver (with some biliary excretion), increasing the amount of liver damage on each pass.[22] Toxicity produced through an enterohepatic circuit usually takes considerable time to develop. The larger and heavier the organism, the longer it takes to produce toxicity. Once administered, Mte concentrates in the liver and quasi-interrupts the enterohepatic circuit. It first interrupts the primary absorption of toxins, then it helps prevent their reabsorption due to enterohepatic circulation.[23] Cells not yet poisoned are protected from damage from circulating toxins, and act as centers for the generation of new liver cells.[24-26] With time, complete restoration of the liver is possible.

Mte stimulates protein synthesis

One of the ways Mte accelerates the regeneration of destroyed liver tissue is by stimulating cellular protein synthesis. In studies in which the livers of rats were partially removed, the administration of Mte effectively accelerated the regeneration of liver tissue. The mechanism of action is the stimulation of nuclear polymerase A activity which in turn stimulates ribosomal RNA, and subsequent generation of protein from which new cells can be built and nourished.[27,28]

In summary, the effectiveness of Mte is due to an alteration of cell membranes in such a way that only small amounts of toxins may penetrate into the cell, an acceleration of the rate of protein synthesis and thereby the promotion of cellular regeneration, the interruption of the enterohepatic circuit, and the scavenging of membrane-damaging free radicals.

THE USE OF MTE IN CLINICAL SETTINGS

Extensive clinical trials have clearly substantiated the ability of Mte to reverse the symptoms of many liver disorders, both acute and chronic.[29-31] It stimulates liver cells to generate tissue to replace that which has been damaged or destroyed by disease. Although the liver already possesses such ability to a greater extent than perhaps any other organ of the body except the skin, which infected or damaged by alcohol or other drugs, the regenerative capacity slows down or ceases altogether. Hence the need for a medicine like Mte.

Toxic-metabolic liver disease, acute viral hepatitis, chronic persistent hepatitis, chronic-aggressive hepatitis, cirrhosis of the liver, fatty degeneration of the liver, and various liver diseases of unknown etiology are among the conditions that have been significantly affected by Mte. The strongest positive effects have been observed in various forms of toxic-metabolic hepatitis (including alcohol-induced and iatrogenic, drug-induced forms), and in cirrhosis. Although Mte has no antiviral properties, it has been shown to shorten the course of viral hepatitis and to minimize post-hepatitis complications.[32-39]

A typical study involved the participation of 129 patients for a period of about one month. The patients suffered from a number of different conditions, including obvious toxic or toxic-metabolic liver damage, fatty degeneration of the liver for various reasons, and chronic hepatitis. A control group of 56 patients was used for comparison. Mte proved significantly more effective than placebo in modifying subjective and objective symptoms, in stimulating a return to normal enzymatic activities, improvement in digestive disorders (from the very first week); enlarged livers diminished substantially in volume; there was a 50 percent regression in pathological symptoms versus 25 percent in controls; and no cases of intolerance, side effects, or allergic reactions were observed.[40]

The implications of the research heavily favor the idea that regular ingestion of Mte will provide a substantial amount of protection to the sick or healthy liver during the course of normal living. By stabilizing cell membranes and encouraging the regeneration of cells destroyed during the normal detoxification process, Mte should provide the liver and the body with the ability to triumph over the deleterious effects of daily encounters with air-, water- and food-borne toxins.

SAFETY DATA

Original toxicity trials in mice, rats, guinea pigs and dogs, using different routes of administration, in acute, subchronic and chronic regimens, found that even very large doses of Mte were non-toxic and produced no side effects or allergic reactions.[3] Tests in humans also showed that high doses of Mte were well tolerated both subjectively and in view of objective measurement.[37] A few people may report minor gastrointestinal discomfort at first since Mte stimulates a cleansing action.

REFERENCES

1. Westphal, K. *Gallenwegsfunktionen und Gallenleiden*. Springer Verlag, Berlin, 1931, p. 326.

2. Koehler, P. *Zhurnal Ges. Inn. Med.*, 19, 599, 1964.

3. Hahn, G., Lehman, H.D., Kurten, M., Uebel, H. and Vogel, G. "Zur pharmakologie und toxikologie von silymarin, des antihepatotoxishcen wirkprinzipes aus silybum marianum (L.) Gaertn." *Arzneimittel-Forschung*, 18(6), 698–704, 1968.

4. Floersheim, G.L. "Antagonistic effects against single lethal doses of amanita phalloides." *Naunyn-Schmiedeberg's Archives of Pharmacology*, 293, 171–174, 1976.

5. Wieland, Th. "Poisonous principles of mushrooms of the genus amanita." *Science*, 159, 946–952, 1968.

6. Strubelt, O., Siegers, C.P. and Younes, M. "The influence of silybin on the hepatotoxic and hypoglycemic effects of praseodymium and other lanthanides." *Arzneimittel-Forschung*, 30, 1690–1694, 1980.

7. Braatz, R. "The effect of silymarin on acute cadmium toxicity." In: Braatz and Schneider, (eds): *Symposium on the Pharmacodynamics of Silymarin*, Urban & Schwarzenberg, Berlin, 1976, pp. 31–36.

8. Antweiler, H. "Effects of silymarin on intoxication with ethionine and ethanol. In Braatz and Schneider, (Eds): *Symposium on the Pharmacodynamics of Silymarin*, Urban & Schwarzenberg, Berlin, 1976, pp. 80–82.

9. Matschinsky, F., Meyere, U. and Wieland, O. *Biochem. Z.*, 333, 48, 1960.

10. Vogel, G. and Trost, W. "Zur anti-phalloiden-activitat der silymarine silybin und disilybin." *Arzneimittel-Forschung*, 25, 392–393, 1975.

11. Frimmer, M. and Kroker, R. "Phalloidin-antagonisten. 1. Mitteilung. Wirkung von silybin-derivaten an der isoliert perfundierten rattenleber." *Arzneimittel-Forschung*, 25, 394–396, 1975.

12. Petzinger, E., Homann, J. and Frimmer, M. "Phalloiden-antagonisten. 2. Mitteilung. Protektive wirkung von disilybin bei der vergiftung isolierter hepatozten mit phalloidin." *Arzsneimittel-Forschung*, 25, 571–576, 1975.

13. Schriewer, H., Badde, R., Roth, G. and Rauen, H.M. "Die antihepatotoxische wirkung des silymarins bei der leberschaedigung durch thioacetamid." *Arzneimittel-Forschung*, 23, 160, 1973.

14. Schriewer, H.M. and Lohman, J. "Regulationsstoerungen des

phospholipidstoffwechsel der gesamtleber, mitochondrien und mikrosomen bei der akuten intoxikation durch thioacetamid und deren beeinflussung durch silymarin." *Arzneimittel-Forschung*, 26, 65, 1976.

15. Vogel, E., Trost, W., Mengs, U. and Sieck, R. *Abstr. Proc. 7th Int. Congr. Pharmcol.*, Paris, 1978, p. 572, Pergamon Press, Ltd., Oxford.

16. Vogel, G. "Silymarin das antihepatotoxische wirkprinzip aus silybum marianum L. Gaertn., als antagonist der phalloidinwirkung." *Arzneimittel-Forschung*, 18, 1063, 1968.

17. Weil, G. and Frimmer, M. "Die wirkung von silymarin auf die mit phalloidin vergiftete isolierte perfundierte rattenleber." *Arzneimittel-Forschung*, 20, 862–863, 1970.

18. Vogel, G. & Temme, I. "Die curative antagonisierung des durch phalloidin hervorgerufenen leberschadens mit silymarin als modell einer antihepatotoxischen therapie." *Arzneimittel-Forschung*, 19, 613–615, 1969.

19. Vogel, G., Braatz, R. and Mengs, U. "On the nephrotoxicity of alpha-amanitin and the antagonistic effects of silymarin in rats." *Agents Actions*, 9, 221–226, 1979.

20. Rauen, H.M. and Schriewer, H. "Die antihepatotoxische wirkung von silymarin bei experimentellen leberschaiedigungen der ratte durch tetrachlorkohlenstoff, d-galakosamin and allyakohol." *Arzneimittel-Forschung*, 21, 1194, 1971.

21. Rauen, H.M. and Schriewer, H. "Enzymaktivitaetskorrelationen im serum nach experimentellen leberschaedigungen der ratte." *Arzneimittel-Forschung*, 21, 1206, 1971.

22. Fauser, U. and Faustlich, H. "Beobachtungen zur therapie der knollenblaetterpilzvergiftung. Verbesserung der prognose durch unterbrechung des enterohepatischen kreislaufs (choledochusdrainage)." *Deutsche Medizinische Wochenschrift*, 98, 2259, 1973.

23. Faulstich, H., Jahn, W. and Wieland, Th. "Silybin inhibition of amatoxin uptake in the perfused rat liver." *Arzneimittel-Forschung*, 30(3), 452–454, 1980.

24. Flammer, R. "Hinweise auf silymarin bzw. silybin. Therapieempfehlungen bei knollenblaetterpilzvergiftungen." In: Flammer, R. *Differentialdiagnose der Pilzvergiftungen*, G. Fischer, Stuttgart, New York, 1980, pp. 17, 23, 24.

25. Homann, J., Wizemann, V., Matthes, K.J. and Lasch, H.G. Therapie der akuten "Knollenblaetterpilzvergiftungen." *Hepatology*, 12, 1522–1523, 1982.

26. Hruby, K., Lenz, K., Moser, C.D., Bachner, J. and Korninger, C. "Knollenblaetterpilzvergiftungen in Oesterreich." *Wien. Med. Wschr.*, 91, 509–513, 1970.

27. Magliulo, E., Carosi, P.G., Minoli, L. and Gorini, S. "Studies on the regenerative capacity of the liver in rats subjected to partial hepatectomy and treated with silymarin." *Arzneimittel-Forschung*, 23, 161–167, 1973.

28. Sonnenbichler, J., Mattersberger, J. and Machicao, F. "Stimulierung der RNA-polymerase A und der RNA-synthese in vivo und in vitro durch ein flavonderivat." *Hoppe-Seylers Z. Physiol. Chem.*, 357, 337, 1976.

29. Holzgartner, H. "L'impiego della silimarina in medcina interna." *Therapiewoche*, 20, 698, 1968.

30. Muescher, C.H. "Silymarin bei chronischen erkrankungen der leber." *Therapie der Gegenwart*, 11, 1768, 1973.

31. Poser, G. "Erfahrungen mit silymarin bei der behandlung chronischer lebererkankungen." *Arzsneimittel-Forschung*, 21, 1207–1209, 1971.

32. Martiis, M.D., Fontana, M., Assogna, G., D'Ottavi, R. and D'Ottavi, O. "I derivati del cardo mariano nella terapia delle epatopatie chroniche." *Cl. Terap.*, 94(3), 283–315, 1980.

33. Floersheim, G.L., Eberhard, M., Tschumi, P. and Duckert, F. "Effects of penicillin and silymarin on liver enzymes and blood clotting factors in dogs given a boiled preparation of amanita phalloides." *Toxicology and Applied Pharmacology*, 46, 455–462, 1978.

34. Morelli, I. "Costituenti del 'silybum marianum' e loro impiego in terapia." *Boll. Chim. Farm.*, 117(11), 258–267, 1978.

35. Saba, P., Galeone, F., Salvadorini, F., Guarguaglini, M. and Troyer, C. "Therapeutische wirkung von silymarin bei durch psychopharmaka verursachten chronischen hepatopathien." *Gass. Med. Ital.*, 135, 236–251, 1976.

36. Benda, L., Dittrich, H., Ferenzi, P., Frank, H. and Wewelka, F. "Zur wirksamkeit von silymarin auf die ueberlebensrate von patieten mit leberzirrhose." *Wien. Klin. Wochenschrift*, 92, 678–683, 1980.

37. Benda, L. and Zenz, W. "Ambulante langzeitbehandlung der leberzirrhose mit silymarin." *Therapiewoche*, 24, 3598–3608, 1974.

38. Fintelmann, V. and Albert, A. "Nachweis der therapeutischen wirksamkeit von legalon bei toxischen lebererkrankungen im doppelblindversuch." *Therapiewoche*, 30, 5589–5594, 1980.

39. Schilder, M. "Silymarin in der klinischen pruefung. Ein bericht ueber 36 faelle von verschiedenen leberkrankheiten in laengsschnittuntersuchungen." *Therapiewoche*, 20, 3444, 1970.

40. Schopen, R.D., Lange, O.K., Panne, C. and Kirnberger, E.J. "Auf der suche nach einem neuen therapeutischen prinzip." *Med. Welt*, 15, 888, 1969.

ARTICHOKE
(Cynara scolymus)

Anyone who has made a comparative study of the approaches different cultures take to health care will have noted that some cultures, such as the European, are much more interested than others, especially the American, in the effects of a healthy digestive system on overall health. Europeans have typically emphasized the importance of maintaining the wellness of organs, glands and muscles. For this purpose, they choose tonics.

Good health, according to that view, is a reflection of properly functioning body systems. Keeping a healthy liver and gallbladder is very important. Hence, the sophistication achieved by Europeans in this area is extraordinary.

The concern for digestive health is nowhere better typified than in ideas surrounding the value of agents that affect the production, storage and secretion of bile. One of the best of these agents over the past half-century has been the artichoke.

Artichoke is a thistlelike plant that belongs to the daisy family, as does milk thistle. (The milk thistle is sometimes called wild artichoke.)

Artichoke contains a bitter principle, cynaropicrin, with a bitter index of 11,500, which means that the bitter taste is still present in a dilution of 1:11,500; therefore, artichoke should exert considerable beneficial effect on digestion. It also contains cynarin (a crystalline phenolic substance that appears to be an ester of di-caffeic acid of quinic acid; often designated as 1,4-dicaffeylquinic acid, or 1,5-dicaffeylquinic acid—in case you're interested). Other constituents of artichoke include apigenin, luteolin, cynaroside, cyanidine, scolimoside, cosmoside, quercetin, rutin, chlorogenic acid, caffeic acid, isochlorogenic acid, hesperitin, hesperiodoside, maritimein, mucilage, pectins, tannins, sugars, salts, inulin and enzymes.[2,3,19,23,35,37,38,44,45,48]

Before we can discuss the actions of artichoke, we must understand some basic terms. Fine distinctions in terminology are made in Europe that are largely ignored in America. Thus, a cholagogue must be distinguished from a choleretic, which must be distinguished from a cholekinetic.

A *cholagogue* is an agent that produces an increase in the production of bile by the liver.

A *choleretic* is an agent that increases the flow of bile from the gallbladder.

The term *cholekinetic* refers to the ability to increase the contractive power of the bile duct.

To the European, even these distinctions are not sufficient. It has become important, for example, to distinguish between choleretics that increase the volume of bile without producing a corresponding increase in the concentration of biliary solids in the bile, and agents that increase the volume of both the liquid and solid phases. This distinction is important, since a simple increase in volume of liquid would lead to a reduction in the concentration of important solids such as the bile salts, with a corresponding reduction in digestive power. The fact that artichoke is one of the few agents that increases both the solid and liquid phases helps to account for its popularity among European physicians.[59,49]

The above distinctions are presented because research on artichoke has emphasized their importance relative to increasing our understanding of the importance of those processes to digestive health. The reader may find it useful to refer back to the above definitions while reading the following sections.

Artichoke extract and/or cynarin, the main active constituent, has cholagogue/choleretic/choliokinetic action.

Research has shown that caffeic acid, a component of cynarin, is almost as effective as pure cynarin, suggesting that caffeic acid is the substance responsible for the *choleretic* action.[48-51] Artichoke has been shown to increase the production and volume of bile flow by as much as four times normal in a 12-hour period.[6,11-13,28,43,46,59,63] Not all chologogues and choleretics have a choliokinetic action. Artichoke does; in this regard, the action of artichoke closely resembles that of curcumin in turmeric.[30]

Artichoke has hepatotonic and hepatoprotective action

Artichoke protects liver from poisonous effects of toxins in a manner similar to silymarin from milk thistle.[1,4,21,20,27,58] Artichoke extract has many of the same properties as milk thistle extract. It is able to prevent liver damage from the same wide range of poisons as milk thistle.[39,40,42,55] Artichoke extract is also able to stimulate the regeneration of liver cells in much the same manner as does silymarin.[1,27,31,33,34] The usefulness of artichoke for preventing blood and liver cholesterol elevation in the presence of toxins such as alcohol is also of note.[69-71] Application in today's world would also include the prevention of liver damage due to air-, water- and food-borne toxins. A French patent describes an artichoke extract for treating liver disease, high cholesterol levels and kidney insufficiency.[39] Cynarin, and not pure caffeic acid, appears to be the component most responsible for this action. The basic research paradigm for investigating this action in animals is to administer cynarin either prior to, or simultaneously with, the administration of some toxic substance such as carbon tetrachloride, alcohol or arsenic and observe the results. Like milk thistle, artichoke is able to completely protect the liver and the animal against poisoning and death from normally morbid doses of the poisons. Physiological studies reveal that the probable protective action results from the ability of the extract to interrupt the enterohepatic circuit that would otherwise recirculate the toxins between the

GI tract and the liver over and over again until cumulative liver damage became extensive.

The hepatotonic action arises from the ability of cynarin to restore healthy growth and reproduction to liver cells.[31,33,39] Over a period of several weeks of administration of artichoke extract, significant repair and restoration to a severely damaged liver may occur. Mechanisms of action include a stimulation of cellular division, or mitosis, and an increase of binucleated cells with enhanced capacity for division.

Artichoke has lipid-reducing and anticholesterolemic action

Artichoke reduces blood fats. It reduces cholesterol and cholinesterase levels. These effects were first observed in the 1930s during observations that artichoke reversed fatty degeneration of the liver in patients with biliary disease.[64,65] Subsequent research has revealed that the action of cynarin is fairly complex. In simplest terms, the net effect of artichoke extract appears to be the result of both an activation of and an interference with cholesterol metabolism. That is, it mobilizes fat stores from the liver and other tissues such as white adipose tissue, and these fats pour into the blood from which they are subsequently excreted from the body.[14–18,22,28] Along the way, artichoke may produce higher or lower blood cholesterol levels, depending on the method and timing of measurement. The interference mechanism comes into play with regard to the destructive effects of cholesterol on the liver. Cynarin decreases the rate of cholesterol synthesis in the liver, enchances biliary excretion of cholesterol, and increases conversion towards the bile acids.[69,70.]

As far back as the 1930s it was observed that artichoke extract produced a temporary increase in blood cholesterol levels, followed by an elimination and decrease in the blood levels. The initial rise was astutely observed to be due to a mobilization of cholesterol in the tissue.[66]

It should be noted that not all research has found a positive therapeutic effect of cynarin on high levels of lipoproteins in the blood, but the vast majority have.[47,73]

One effect that appears to be fairly consistent from trial to trial is the ability of artichoke extract to prevent rises in blood and liver cholesterol that would otherwise be induced by agents such as ethyl alcohol.[69,71] Not only cholesterol but other blood fats such as triglycerides can be reduced through the use of artichoke.

Artichoke is a useful agent in the maintenance of efficient bile production and composition

Artichoke and other cholagogues not only increase the availability of bile but significantly alter its composition. While the American medical establishment does not recognize bile deficiency as a sign of disease or as a cause for alarm, physicians throughout Europe report seeing and treating patients on a daily basis with this problem. Treatment results in the elimination of many common complaints: epigastric discomfort, biliary tract dysfunction, dyspepsia, pain, nausea, retching and so forth.[4,9,13,29,30,38,39,53,62,66,67]

Artichoke protects against high cholesterol levels

In one human trial, cynarin was clinically evaluated for use in the treatment of hyperlipidemia (high fat levels). In a controlled trial, two groups of 30 patients were treated for 50 days with cynarin (500 mg) or placebo. Cynarin was observed to produce a significant reduction in blood cholesterol levels, in lipoprotein levels, and in body weight.[41,52]

Other studies carried out in the last 20 years have substantiated these findings in humans and animals. Basically, the daily ingestion of artichoke extract would help prevent the absorption of dietary cholesterol, and would help inhibit excess cholesterol production by the liver.[28,39,49,64]

Arising from the research on cholesterol were several studies that related the use of artichoke extract to the prevention and treatment of atherosclerosis and arteriosclerosis.[8,14,16,18,22,60,74] In one animal trial, for example, artichoke extract prevented the formation of atherosclerotic changes, prevented serum cholesterol increase, caused a decrease in lipid phosphorus, increased the level of glycoproteins in the blood, prevented serum beta-globulin increase, decreased albumin, glycoproteins and liver cholesterol, and increased alpha- and gamma-globulin.[56,57]

OTHER APPLICATIONS

Combining the three methods of action listed above, new areas of application are suggested. For example, while most cholagogues are not suitable for the treatment of gallstones, artichoke may be useful because it lowers cholesterol. For over a hundred years, French physicians have believed in a clinical syndrome that is a composite of gallstones, obesity and rheumatism. An underlying common denominator of these three conditions may be high cholesterol and triglycerides, or hyperlipidemia. Since artichoke extract is a common treatment for the syndrome in France, it may be that it works primarily through the depression of serum cholesterol. The connection between cholesterol and gallstones would thereby be strengthened. A mild diuretic action of artichoke may also play a minor role in the reduction of obesity.

Another property mentioned in the literature but largely unexplored is the effect of artichoke extract on blood platelet aggregation. In one study, conducted in a Polish industrial setting, dozens of men exposed to the toxic fumes of carbcn disulfide were treated with a commercial artichoke extract preparation for two years, during which time the typical hyperaggregation of blood platelets and resulting blood disorder was not seen.[74] This result suggests a possible action of artichoke extract in the prevention of heart disease.

A FEW HISTORICAL PERSPECTIVES

Artichoke use for the treatment of jaundice was documented as early as the 18th century, but it wasn't until the early decades of this century that systematic experimental and clinical research was carried out. Throughout the 1930s French and German physicians and researchers documented the various actions of artichoke extract. The French were particularly active, publishing intensive and extensive observations in clinical settings, which remained the standard for the next three decades. The French have always been fascinated by the liver and its function, so it is not surprising that they would pioneer the work on artichoke. Every pertinent action of artichoke was documented by the French, and decades worth of subsequent research would only serve to tease apart the intricacies of the plant's method of action. But clinical applications have remained basically unchanged since the mid '30s. That means that we have accumulated 60 years' worth of valuable observations about the value of artichoke.

Following a hiatus during the war years, work again resumed on artichoke during the 1950s. Again the French and Germans were prominent, but the Italians produced the most extensive, valuable and accurate work from 1950 to 1970. In 1958, Italian scientists published an extensive summary of prize-winning Italian research on artichoke. During the '60s Italian and French researchers continued to publish findings on artichoke; they were joined in the '70s by Polish, Spanish, Russian, Swiss and South American scientists. The findings continued to support the basic modes of action, whether in animals or in humans.

So methodical and extensive was the work during these decades that use of artichoke throughout the European community became firmly established. During the '80s work on the choleretic, hepatoprotective and anticholesterol actions of artichoke declined—almost all skeptics had been silenced or satisfied; the use of artichoke to prevent and treat liver dysfunction held the day.

SAFETY DATA

Artichoke is generally recognized as safe by the FDA. It has no known toxicology. As with all cholagogues, persons with acute gallstones should exercise extreme care in using such agents.

REFERENCES

1. Adzet, T., Camarasa, J. and Laguna, J.C. "Hepatoprotective activity of polyphenolic compounds from cynara scolymus against CC14 toxicity in isolated rat hepatocytes." *Journal of Natural Products*, 50(4), 612–617, 1987.

2. Atherinos, A.E. "Chemical investigation of cynara scolymus. The steroids of the receptacle leaves." *J. Chem. Soc.* 1962, 1700, 1962.

3. Benard, P. and Laalemand, A. *Bull. Soc. Pharm. Marseille*, 15, 1953.

4. Bernet. G. "Antitoxic, diuretic, laxative." *Fr. Demande*, patent no. 2,336,922, 29 July 1977.

5. Bertolani, F., Dardari, M. and Massa, L. *La Radiol. Med.* 45, 8, 1958.

6. Boehm, K. "Untersuchungern ueber choleretische Wirkungen einiger Arzneipflanzen." *Arzneimittel-Forschung*, 9, 376, 1959.

7. Brel, *Bull. Soc. Therap.*, 1929.

8. Caruzzo, C., Carnaghi, R., Enrico-Bena, L. and De Marco, G. "Considerazioni sull'attivita dell'acido 1,4-dicaffeilchinico sulle frzioni lipidiche del siero nell'aterosclerosi." *Minerva Med.*, 60, 4514, 1969.

9. Cavanno, D. and Rocchietta, S. "Old drugs and modern therapy. Cynara scolymus. Pharmacological properties and therapeutic effects." *Minerva Med.*, 55(94), 1644–1648, 1964.

10. Cela, A.B. "Nota acera de la accion bacteriostatica de cynara scolymus L." *Farmacognosia* (Madrid), 19(52), 165, 1959.

11. Chabrol, E., et al. "L'action choleretique du cynara scolymus." *C.R. Soc. de Biologie,* 108, 5 December, 1931, 1020–1022.

12. Chabrol, E., et al. "L'action choleretique des composees." *C.R. Soc. de Biologie*, 108, 5 December, 1931, 1100.

13. Chabrol, E. and Charonnat, R. "Les agents therapeutiques de la secretion biliare." *Annuales de Medicine*, 37(1), 131–142, 1935.

14. Eberhardt, G. "Untersuchungen ueber die wirkung von cynarin bei leberzellverfettung." *Z. Gastroenterol*, 11, 183, 1973.

15. Eck, M. and Desbordes, J. "Exogenous and endogenous hypercholesterolemia in rabbits. Effect of hepatic stimulation." *Compt. Rend. Soc. Biol.*, 117, 681–683, 1934. (also p. 428)

16. Eggstein, M. and Kreutz, K.H. "Eine neue bestimmung der neutralfette im blutserum und gewebe, I. Mitteilung (prinzip, durchfuehrung und besprechung der methode)." *Klinische Wochenschrift*, 44, 262, 1966.

17. Dierl, H. *Wiener Medizinische Wochenschrift*, 122, 188, 1972.

18. Greten, H., Seidel, D., Walters, B. and Kolbe, J. "Die lipoproteinelektrophorese zur diagnose von hyperlipoproteinaemian." *Deutsche Medizinische Wochenschrift*, 95, 1716, 1970.

19. Fujimoto, M. and Matsuki, K. *Japan. Kokai 76,118*, 814, 19 Oct 1976.

20. Fumaneri, A.B. "Biliary hepatic protective preparation composed of fluid extracts." *Boll. Chim. Farm.*, 97, 24–27, 1958.

21. Gaudin, O. "The influence of artichoke extract on the antitoxic action of the liver in the guinea pig." *Bull Sci. Pharmacol*, 46, 167–178, 1939.

22. Hammerl, H., Kindler, K., Kraenzl, Ch., et al. "Ueber den einfluss von cynarin auf hyperlipidaemien unter besonderer beruecksichtingung des typs II (hypercholesterinaemie)." *Wiener Medizinische Wochenschrift*, 41, 601, 1973.

23. Hinou, J., Harvala, C. and Philianos, S. "Substances polyphenoliques des feuilles de cynara scolymus L." *Ann. Pharm. Fr.*, 47(2), 95–98, 1989.

24. Jain, S.R. and Sharma, S.N. "Hypoglycemic drugs of Indian indigenous origin." *Plant. Medica.*, 15, 439–442, 1967.

25. Kalk, H. and Nissen, K. "Untersuchungen ueber die wirkung der curcuma auf die funktion der leber und der gallenwege." *Deutsche Medizinishe Wochenschrift*, 38, 1613, 1931.

26. Kalk, H. and Nissen, K. *Dtch. Med. Woch.* 44, 1423–1426, 1932.

27. Kiso, Y., Tonkin, M. and Hikino, H. "Assay method for anti-hepatotoxic activity using galactosamine-induced cytotoxicity in primary-cultured hepatocytes." *Journal of Natural Products*, 46(6), 841–847, 1983.

28. Lietti, A. "Choleretic and cholesterol lowering properties of two artichoke extracts." *Fitoterapia*, 48(4), 153–158, 1977.

29. Loeper, M. and Lemaire, A. "General action of bitter substances." *Presse Med.*, 39, 433–435, 1931.

30. Maiwald, L. "Pflanzliche Cholagoga." *Zeitschrift fuer Allgemeinmedizin*, 24, 1304–1308, 1983.

31. Maros, T., Racz, G. et al. "The effects of cynara scolymus extracts on the regeneration of rat liver." *Arzneimittel-Forschung*, 25, 1311–1314, 1975.

32. Mansilla, S. "Accion Farmacologica de la cynara scolimus (alcachofa) sobre colesterolemia de hepatopatas." *Rev. Fac. Farm. Bioquim.* (Lima) 26(96), 100, 1964.

33. Maros, T., Racz, G., Katonai, B. and Kovacs, V.V. "The effects of cynara scolymus extracts on the regeneration of rat liver." *Arzneimittel-Forschung*, 16(2), 127–129, 1966. (In German.).

34. Maros, T., et al. *Arzneimittel-Forschung*, 8(18), 884, 1968.

35. Masquelier, J. and Michaud, J. "Glycosides de l'artichaut." *Bull. Soc. Pharm. Bordeaux*, 95, 65–67, 1958; and 96, 103; and 97, 77.

36. Massacci, P. "Pharmacologic properties of artichoke." *Corriere Farm.*, 22(3), 69–71, 1967.

37. Michaud, J. "Contribution a l'etude chimque et analytique de l'artichaut." *These*, Bordeaux, 1964.

38. Michaud, J. "A new artichoke extract." *Bull. Soc. Pharm. Bordeaux*, 106(4), 181–190, 1967.

39. Michaud, J. "Water soluble artichoke extract for treating hepatic ailments, hypocholesterolemia, and renal incapacity." *Fr. M.*, 6613, 24 Feb 1969.

40. Monville, *Thèse*, Paris, 1933 (title of thesis unavailable).

41. Montini, M., et. al. "Kontrolierte anwendung von cynarin in der behandlung hyperlipamischer syndrome." *Arzneimittel-Forschung*, 25, 1311–1314, 1975.

42. Nichiforescu, E.A. and Velescu, G. "Cynara scolymus extract

for pharmaceutical use in liver disease." Romanian Patent 51, 326, 25 Oct. 1968.

43. Nussbaumer, P.A., Buri, P. and Genecand, M. "Cholagogues et choleratiques." *Schw. Ap. Ztg.*, 106(22), 798–803; (25), 900-906; (26) 930–934, 1968.

44. Panizzi, L. "Caffeic esters of quinic acid and quinide." *German Patent* 1,030,514, May 22, 1958.

45. Panizzi, L. and Scarpati, M.L. "Constitution of cynarine, the active principle of the artichoke." *Nature*, 74, 1062, 1954.

46. Pirtkien, R., Surke, E. and Seybold, G. "Vergleichende untersuchungen uber die choleretische wirkung verschiedener artzneimittel bei der ratte." *Med. Welt*, 1, 1417, 1960.

47. Pommeranze, J. and Cressin, M. "Decholesterolizing agents." *Amer. Heart J.*, 49, 262, 1955.

48. Preziosi, P. "1,4-dicaffeylquinic acid from cynara scolymus." *Farmaco (Pavia), Ed. Sci.*, 17, 701–745, 1962.

49. Preziosi, P. and Loscalzo, B. "L'azione sulla coloresi, sul colesterolo ematico e sulla lipoidosi colesterolica del principio attivo del carciofo e di sostanze ad esso correlate (parte prima)." *Fitoterapia*, 27, 666–690, 1956. Part two appeared in *Fitoterapia*, 27, 690–698, 1956.

50. Preziosi, P. and Loscalzo, B. "Experimental (pharmacological) evaluation of 1,4-bis-(3,4-dihydroxycinnamoyl)quinic acid, the active principle of artichoke." *Arch. It. Scien. Farmacol.*, 23, 4, 249–296, 1957.

51. Preziosi, P., Loscalzo, B., Marmo, E. and Miele, E. "Effects of single or repeated treatment with several anticholesterolemic compounds on biliary excretion of cholesterol." *Biochem. Pharmacol.*, 5, 251–262, 1960.

52. Pristautz, H. "Cynarin in the modern treatment of hyperlipemias." *Wiener Medizinische Wochenschrift*, 223, 705–709, 1975.

53. Ravina, A. "The therapeutic value of artichoke leaves and their crystallized principle." *Presse Med.*, 42, 1307, 1934.

54. Risi, A. "Hypoglycemic action of an oxidase extract of cynara scolymus." *Arch. Intern. Pharmacodynami*, 61, 428–446, 1939.

55. Rosa, G.E. "Pharmacodynamics of the active principle of cynara scolymus and its application in liver and kidney diseases." *Semana Med.* (Buenos Aires), I. 1249–1254, 1968.

56. Samochowiec, L. "Antiatherosclerotic activity of cynara scolymus and cynara cardunculus." *The 8th Congress of the Polish Physiological Society*, Poznan, Dec 7–10, 1960, pp. 879–881.

57. Samochowiec, L. "Antiatherosclerotic activity of cynara scolymus and cynara cardunculus." *Farm. Polska*, 16(13), 257, 1961.

58. Samochowiec, L., Szysyka, K. and Szolomicki, F. "Effect of chronic poisoning with carbon disulfide on certain biochemical changes in serum of white rats." *Med. Pracy*, 20(6), 572–578, 1969. (In Polish.)

59. Schindel, L. "Ueber pflanzliche choleretica." *Archiv fuer Exp. Path. u. Pharmakol*, 175, 313–321, 1934.

60. Schoenholzer, G. "Ueber die beeinflussung des cholesterinstoffwechsels durch das aktive prinzip der artischokke und sein anwendung in der therapie der arteriosklerose." *Schweiz. Med. Wschr.*, 69, 1288, 1939.

61. Sokolova V.E., Lyoubaartseva, L.A. and Vasiltchenko, E.A. "L'influence de l'artichaut (cynara scolymus) sur certains aspects du metabolisme azote chez les animaux." *Farmakologya i Toksikologiya*, 33(3), 340–343, 1970.

62. Steinegger, E. and Haensel, E. *Lehrbuch der allgemeinen Pharmakognosie*. Berlin, Heidelberg, New York, 1972, citation for Cynara.

63. Struppler, A. and Roessler. "Choleretic action of artichoke extract." *Med. Monatsschrift*, 11, 221–223, 1957.

64. Tixier, L., de Seze, S. and Eck, M. "Therapy of diseases caused by excess of cholesterol." *Rev. Med.*, 54, 204–222, 1937. (In French.)

65. Tixier, L., *Presse Med.*, 44, 880, 1939.

66. Tixier, L. "Les actions physiologiques et therapeutiques de cynara scolymus (artichaut), *Presse Med.*, 47, 880, 1939.

67. Tixier, L. "Les indications de la cynaratherapie consacrees par plus de 30 annees d'experimentation et de clinique." *La Semaine des Hopitaux*, 37(8), 704–710, 1961.

68. Tremoliere, Thiery and Fauchet. *Rev. de Med.*, Oct., 1933.

69. Wojcicki. J. "Effect of 1,5-dicaffeoylquinic acid on ethanol-induced hypertriglyceridemia." *Arzneimittel-Forschung*, 26(11), 2047–2048, 1976. (In German.)

70. Wojcicki, J. and Szwed, G. "Action and application of 1,5-dicaffeylquinic acid." *Przegl. Lek.*, 34(12), 865–867, 1977. (In Polish.)

71. Wojcicki, J. "Effect of 1,5-dicaffeylquinic acid (cynarine) on cholesterol levels in serum and liver of acute ethanol-treated rats." *Drug Alchol Depend.*, 3(2), 143–5, 1978.

72. Woyke, M., Cwajda, H., Wojcicki, J. and Kosmider, K. "Platelet aggregation in workers chronically exposed to carbon disulfide and subjected to prophylactic treatment with cynarex." *Med. Pr.*, 32(4), 261–264, 1981. (In Polish.)

73. Heckers, H., Dittmar, K., Schmahl, F.W. and Huth, K. "Ineffeciency of cynarin as therapeutic regimen in familial type II hyperlipoproteinaemia." *Atherosclerosis*, 26, 249–253, 1977.

74. Mancini, M., Oriente, P. and D'Andrea, L. "Hypocholesterolemic effects of quinic acid 1,4-dicaffeate in atherosclerotic patients." In: S. Garattini and R. Paoletti (eds.), *Drugs Affecting Lipid Metabolism (Proceedings of the Symposium on Drugs Affecting Lipid Metabolism)* Milan, 1960. Elsevier Publishing Company, Amsterdam, 1961, pp. 535–537.

DANDELION
(Taraxacum officinale)

Dandelion is a strong cholagogue and choleretic (for definitions, see the preceding section on artichoke). It is used specifically for the health of the liver and related organs and glands. Research has shown that it aids the body in recovering from many kinds of liver disease, including hepatitis and liver insufficiency. Related disorders of digestion, such as dyspepsia, have also been shown to benefit from the ingestion of dandelion. Several European proprietary liver remedies contain dandelion root. Another proven quality of dandelion is its diuretic action, attributable at least in part to the presence of potash in the herb. Besides its content of bitters, dandelion is high in inulin, a form of carbohydrate easily assimilated by diabetics and hence is a potential source of nutritional support for diabetics.

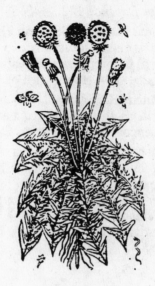

DANDELION

Dandelion is both a cholagogue and a choleretic

Dandelion is one of the three strongest-acting cholagogues known, the others being wormwood and *helichrysum arenarium*. It raises the secretion of bile by over 50 percent. In experiments with rats, dandelion affects the secretion of bile much like an injection of the animal's own bile would. Since rats do not have gall bladders, the herb must work directly on the liver.[1-4]

It is postulated that the active choleretic principles may be heterocyclic nitrogen-containing constituents. But experts in the area of dandelion research agree that the many properties of this herb are the result of interactions among its constituents rather than being a case of one chemical—one effect.[1,5]

Clinically, dandelion has been observed to benefit people with colitis, liver congestion, gallstones and several forms of liver insufficiency. In particular, chronic hepatitis and dyspepsia with insufficient bile secretion are susceptible to the effects of this herb.[6,7]

German medicines containing dandelion along with other herbs such as milk thistle and nettle have been used in clinical studies. In one trial, 19 cases of gallstones, acute and chronic bile duct and gallbladder inflammation, jaundice, dyskinesia of the bile duct and jaundice caused by complete obstruction by gallstones, showed more or less complete recovery within a period ranging from a few days to several days, depending upon the severity of the symptoms. Further tests on both healthy and sick subjects, using careful controls and sophisticated probes, found that the medicine significantly enhanced both the concentration and the secretion of bilirubin in the duodenum just minutes after adminstration.[5]

SAFETY DATA

Dandelion is generally regarded as safe by the FDA. Some people are allergic to dandelion and may experience hay fever or asthma.

REFERENCES

1. Maiwald, L. "Pflanzliche cholagoga." *Zhurnal Allgemein Medizin*, 59, 1304–1308, 1983.
2. Chabrol, E., Charonnat, R., et al., "Recherches experimentales sur l'action choleretique du neptal." *Comptes Rendus, Societe de Biologie*, 102(12), 991–992, 1930.
3. Chabrol, E., Charonnat, R., Maximin, M., Waitz, R. and Porin, J. "L'action choleretique des composees." *Comptes Rendus, Societe de Biologie (Paris)*, 108(12), 1100–1102, 1931.
4. Buessemaker, J. "Ueber die choleretische wirkung des loewenzahns." *Archiv der Exp. Pathol. und Pharmakologie*, 181, 512–513, 1936.

5. Faber, K., "Der Loewenzahn=Taraxacum Officinale Weber." *Pharmazie*, 13(7), 423–435, 1958.
6. Leclerc. *Phytotherapie*, Paris, 1927 (Cited in Buessemaker, op.cit., ref. 4).
7. Racz-Kobila, E., Racz, G. and Solomon, A. *Planta Medica*, 26, 212, 1974.

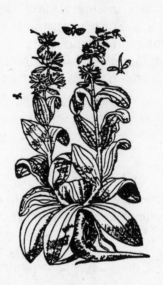

GENTIAN

GENTIAN ROOT
(Gentiana lutea)

Gentian root is one of the strongest bitters known. It is the standard to which all other bitters are compared. At dilutions of 1:12,000 it still has a bitter taste. Pure amarogentine, one of the constituents, is bitter at dilutions as high as 1:50,000.[1] Gentian embodies the best of all properties that bitters are known to possess: stomachic, cholagogue, choleretic, sialagogue (promoting the flow of saliva), secretagogue (stimulating secretions), appetite stimulant and digestive tonic. In dyspepsia and indigestion and several other forms of digestive disease, gentian has shown excellent results. It appears to be quite good at stimulating the secretion of pancreatic enzymes. As a cholagogue its action is reliable, but not particularly strong. It has antibacterial properties, and several of its components are anti-inflammatory. It stimulates the digestive system in general. Clinical or in vivo tests routinely demonstrate the plant's ability to promote secretion of all digestive juices. It has all of these good effects on digestion, yet is totally nonaggravating to the empty stomach.

Gentian root is a good cholagogue

Gentian has been shown to be a true cholagogue, but not one of the strongest—it raises bile secretion by about 20 percent. This action is due to its heterocyclic, nitrogen-containing constituents.[2]

Gentian root has strong action on all aspects of digestion

The ability of gentian extract to stimulate the appetite, promote the secretion of saliva and gastric, liver, pancreatic and intestinal juices and accelerate the emptying of the stomach, has been investigated and substantiated.[3]

In one important clinical trial, gentian, in a preparation that also included lesser amounts of cayenne, ginger root and wormwood, was very effective in relieving the symptoms of indigestion and heartburn in human subjects.[4]

Gentian root reflexively stimulates the gall bladder and pancreas, as well as the mucous membranes of the stomach, thus contributing to an increased secretion of digestive juices and enzymes.[5,6]

Administration of gentian preparations has been found to be most effective if it precedes mealtimes by about half an hour. But its activity begins about five minutes after reaching the stomach, as digestive juices begin to flow and the secretion of bile increases. Whatever level of digestive liquid is achieved in 30 minutes will be maintained for two to three hours without increasing further. This provides for better digestion of fats and proteins.[5,7]

Gentian has an effect on the vascular system: the abdominal organs are better fed by blood and there is a slight rise in blood pressure. This leads to a more rapid distribution of absorbed nutrients throughout the body.[8]

SAFETY DATA

Gentian root is generally recognized as safe and effective. Large doses have been known to cause a gastroenteritis-like irritation.[8] Some experts recommend that people with high blood pressure, and expectant mothers, should avoid the herb.[9]

REFERENCES

1. Weiss, R.F. *Lehrbuch der Phytotherapie*, Stuttgart, Hippokrates Verlag, 1960.

2. Maiwald, L. "Pflanzliche cholagoga." *Zhurnal Allgemein Medizin*, 59, 1304–1308, 1983.

3. Glatzel, H. and Hackerberg, K. "Roentgenological studies of the effect of bitters on digestive organs." *Planta Medica*, (1593), 223–232, 1967.

4. Glatzel, H. "Treatment of dyspetic disorders with spice extracts." *Hippokrates*, 40(23), 916–919, 1969.

5. Deininger, R. "Amarumbitter herbs: common bitter principle remedies and their action." *Krankenpflege*, 29(3), 99–100, 1975.

6. Yamamoto, A. In: *Enzymes In Food Processing*, 2nd edition, G. Reed, Ed. Academic Press, New York, 1975, p. 123.

7. Ivancevic, J. and Kadrnka, S. *Archiv fuer Pharmakologie und Experimentelle Pathologie*, 189, 557–567, 1938.

8. List, P.H. and Hoerhammer, L.H. *Hagers Handbuch Der Phar-*

mazeutischen Praxis, six volumes, Springer-Verlag, Berlin, 1968–1979, citation for Gentian.

9. Pahlow, M. *Das Grosse Buch der Heilpflanzen*. Graefe und Unzer GmgH. Munich, 1979, pp. 124–126.

GINGER
(Zingiber officinale)

Ginger root is one of those herbs put on the earth, it seems, for the primary purpose of maintaining the wellness of the gastrointestinal tract. It ameliorates dozens of ailments, including any form of nausea, gas, heartburn, flatulence, diarrhea, dizziness, vertigo—it doesn't matter much what the cause. Nausea from motion sickness, morning sickness, stomach flu and from almost any other source can be suppressed with ginger root. Indigestion, gas, heartburn, flatulence and virtually any other acute gastrointestinal condition can be successfully treated with ginger root. Dizziness, vertigo, and certain headaches can often be eliminated by the use of ginger root.

Ginger root is held by folk medicine to activate digestive processes, much as an enzyme would. Whether this is due to an intrinsic enzymatic property of ginger or to the herb's ability to activate gastric, pancreatic and intestinal enzymes has not been decided. The property itself, however, is not questioned by food scientists. Centuries of use of this spice have repeatedly demonstrated its digestion-stimulating action, in countries all over the world.

Ginger root eliminates and prevents nausea

Ginger root, in the powdered, encapsulated form, has been found more effective than dimenhydrinate (Dramamine) in preventing the nauseating symptoms of motion sickness. Human subjects, spun in a chair, were given either ginger root, dimenhydrinate or placebo 20 minutes before the trial. The psychophysical method of magnitude estimation was used to record subjective impressions of stomach feelings during the session. Statistical analysis of power functions obtained from subjective estimations showed significant differences between all groups, with ginger root being clearly superior. Other field trials and pilot studies revealed that for most people who are susceptible to motion sickness, two or three capsules one-half hour before a trip, two to three capsules at regular (one- to two-hour) intervals during the trip is usually sufficient to prevent the nausea that often accompanies travel. It is recommended that enough ginger root be ingested to cause a ginger aftertaste in the throat.[1,2]

Powdered, encapsulated ginger root is effective in preventing and relieving nausea and diarrhea associated with several other conditions, including morning sickness (up to 75 percent success rate), stomach flu, dizziness and vertigo (40 to 50 percent success rate).[2]

Ginger root helps prevent rises in blood cholesterol

Ginger root has a good hypocholesterolemic property. An oleoresin of ginger root, included in a hypercholesterolemic diet for rats at 0.5 to 1.0 percent, was significantly capable of preventing the rise in serum and hepatic cholesterol levels seen in control animals. It is thought that the herb interferes in cholesterol absorption from the intestine through a bile acid sequestering ability.[3]

THE BEST FORM OF GINGER ROOT

The best form in which to ingest ginger for effective application in the GI tract is the encapsulated powder. In this form you can take enough to do the job without having to experience any form of discomfort. Unencapsulated powder can burn the palate, although there are certainly people who use it this way and claim to actually enjoy the sensation! Most of us would just as soon avoid the pain, especially during a bout with stomach flu. Ginger teas and beverages are sometimes quite pleasant, but it is very difficult to ingest therapeutic amounts in this fashion. You simply cannot get enough into solution: Ginger tinctures can pack a wallop, but they, like the teas, leave the important fiber behind. Although I haven't conclusively demonstrated this principle yet, I am certain that much of the herb's effectiveness arises from the physical properties of the powder itself. Extracting the supposed active principles from the powder ignores the importance of the whole herb. Along these lines, we should be aware of the fact that nobody has so far definitely determined what principles of ginger root are totally responsible for its antinausea properties. Excellent standardized powdered whole ginger root is available.

The encapsulated powder is better than tinctures, teas, un-encapsulated powder, tea bags, and candied ginger root. But all of these forms will have some effect on nausea, and may be completely effective in mild conditions. Only the capsule will work for severe forms. I say this because I often hear people recommend a ginger tea for motion sickness. While the tea may work for mild cases, only capsules, in sufficient number, will handle moderate to severe motion sickness.

What about acute cases of nausea?

Ginger is the perfect remedy for acute nausea if you take enough to do the job. The biggest mistake people make in trying to use ginger root is not taking enough. Because herbs are mild-acting, it often takes considerable amounts to achieve quick therapeutic results. While ginger root in small amounts, and in combinations with other digestive herbs, has an excellent tonic effect, it can be used in much larger amounts during acute attacks of nausea, dizziness or vertigo. More than ten years of experience and research, involving observations in hundreds of cases, has produced the principles for ginger root application outlined in the next few paragraphs.

First, the ginger root rule of thumb: *Use it till you taste it.* This means that you have ingested enough when you can taste it, or feel a ginger root sensation somewhere in the esophagus, a few minutes after swallowing the capsules. If you don't feel the sensation, you should swallow a few more capsules. Ginger root has a kind of built-in dosage regulator. By the way, the ginger sensation does not get any worse if more capsules than necessary are swallowed. Thus, you do not have to fear overdosage. Follow the ginger root rule of thumb for optimum success.

Motion sickness. Used properly, ginger root will be effective for almost all cases of motion sickness. Severe cases: 4 400 mg capsules 20 minutes before the journey. Mild to moderate cases: 2 capsules 15 minutes before the journey. Everyone: use 2–4 capsules minimum whenever the slightest nauseating symptoms are felt. Do not wait too long. Do not give the nausea a chance to develop. Many people just take two capsules every ½ hour to 1 hour for the entire trip. Remember, these are just suggestions—use the ginger root rule of thumb to determine your individual requirements.

Morning sickness. The success rate with morning sickness has been substantially lower than with other forms of nausea, probably because pregnancy-associated morning sickness is a much more complicated condition. However, enough women do experience success to warrant a try by any expectant mother. Generally, the women who have the most success use about the same regimen. They take anywhere from 3 to 8 capsules before getting out of bed in the morning (have the water and capsules at hand), then remain in bed and keep taking the capsules as necessary until any nausea experienced upon waking is completely gone. Then, throughout the remainder of the day, they take 3–5 capsules at the slightest hint of nausea, relaxing quietly until it totally subsides.

Dizziness and vertigo. One of the side benefits of using ginger root to treat nausea is that it also eliminates dizziness, vertigo and headaches. The author is aware of about a dozen cases of people, unable to leave their homes, ride in a car or train for years due to dizziness, vertigo and nausea, who regained the ability to travel symptom-free after swallowing capsules of ginger root. Dizziness and vertigo can be eliminated with as few as 2–4 capsules taken periodically throughout the day.

Stomach flu. The greatest quantities of ginger root are ingested by people trying to eliminate nausea and prevent vomiting during a bout of 24-hour or 3-day gastroenteritis or flu. Most success is achieved by beginning to swallow capsules at the very first sign of nausea, or sooner, if you believe you have been exposed to flu organisms. People experience all the other symptoms of the flu, including severe lower back pain and fever, but do not get nauseated while using ginger root. Meanwhile, other people around them are nauseated and throwing up. For best success, make the ginger root rule of thumb the first fundamental law of the universe. Catch the disease early and don't skimp on the dosage. Remember, 12 capsules of powdered whole ginger root only equals a tablespoon of material.

SAFETY DATA

Large doses of zingerone, a constituent of ginger root, have produced experimental toxicity in lab animals, but the ingestion of zingerone as found in ginger root poses no threat to health, and it is generally regarded as safe by the FDA. Even very large doses have not been found to create a health hazard. The stimulatory nature of ginger root can produce increased cardiovascular activity of an innocuous nature.

REFERENCES

1. Mowrey, D.B. and Clayson, D.E. "Motion sickness, ginger and psychophysics." *The Lancet*, March 20, 655–657, 1983.

2. Mowrey, D.B. Unpublished field and clinical trials, presented in a paper at the Rocky Mountain Pyschological Association Convention, Denver, 1977; and in Phoenix, 1976.

3. Gujral, S., Bhumra, H. and Swaroop, M. "Effect of ginger (zingibear officinale roscoe) oleoresin on serum and hepatic cholesterol levels in cholesterol fed rats." *Nutrition Reports International*, 17(2), 183–189, 1978.

SCHIZANDRA
(Schizandra sinensis)

The oriental equivalent of milk thistle is schizandra. Though this herb has not been subjected to nearly the amount of research that milk thistle has, what work there is clearly suggests that schizandra affects many aspects of digestion, from stimulation of gastric juices to a tonic effect on the liver and gallbladder.

Like milk thistle, schizandra has been shown to render the liver immune to the toxic effects of various experimental poisons, including carbon tetrachloride. As in the case of milk thistle, this action is probably the result of short-circuiting the enterohepatic circuit that typically passes the toxin through the liver over and over again, resulting in massive damage.

For a fuller treatment of schizandra the reader is referred to the chapter on the immune system.

TURMERIC
(Curcuma longa)

Turmeric is an herb or spice with origins in ancient southern Asia. Turmeric adds not only flavor but color to many foods and prepared seasonings. In the West its culinary uses far outnumber its traditional medicinal uses. Turmeric is the primary ingredient in many varieties of curry powders and sauces. Curry is not a single spice, but a mixture of herbs and spices, the exact composition of which varies from one geographical location to the next (however, several varieties of curry may be found in the same geographical location). Other herbs used in curry include coriander, cumin, garlic, cayenne, fennel, fenugreek, anise, nutmeg, mace, cinnamon, cloves, black pepper, cardamon, ginger and onion.

The selection of herbs and spices for curry powders and sauces has a profound impact on the digestibility, absorbability and assimilability of all food eaten in conjunction with the curry. Liver, gallbladder, kidney and other organs respond dramatically to the presence of curry herbs.

A survey of the folklore literature of the world reveals that turmeric herb has been employed not only in the culinary arts of many nations but has also contributed a great deal to the medical systems of these nations. In China alone, turmeric is used "to remove blood stasis, promote and normalize energy flow in the body, and relieve pain . . . to act on the spleen and liver . . . in treating chest and rib pain, amenorrhea, abdominal mass, traumatic injuries, swelling, and carbuncles . . . treatment of hematuria [bloody urine], pain and itching of sores and ringworms, toothache, colic, flatulence, and hemorrhage."[1]

Throughout Asia one finds the herb being used as stomachic, stimulant, carminative, hematic or styptic, to treat jaundice and other liver troubles, for irregular menstruation of all kinds, for promoting circulation, dissolving blood clots, for relieving pain, diarrhea, rheumatism, coughs, tuberculosis, and so on. Turmeric is hardly ever used alone, but is found in hundreds of different medicinal formulas. One might say it is not viewed as a primary medicinal aid but as an important, perhaps indispensable, adjunct.

Turmeric possesses considerable cholagogue action

Sesquiterpenes in the essential oil of turmeric were isolated in 1926, and to them has been ascribed much of the therapeutic activity. However, a great deal of research has suggested that whole turmeric probably contains a wide variety of active principles.[2-6]

In 1936, the constituent curcumin was compared to whole extract and several other isolated constituents.[7] Curcumin, the isolated essential oil, and a component known as p-tolymethylcarbinol increased the secretion of bile, but in differing ways and under differing conditions. Thus, curcumin produced a rhythmic emptying of the gallbladder, the bile being dark and viscous, and the amount after any given contraction being small compared to the actual size of the gallbladder. The gallbladder would then immediately refill with bile and the cycle would repeat.

Tolymethylcarbinol produced a pure continuous increase in the secretion of bile with no distinguishable contractions. The emptying of the gallbladder had no effect or retrograde effect on the action of the chemical, and the bile was much clearer than that produced by curcumin.

The action of the whole alcoholic extract was very similar to that of tolymethylcarbinol. However, it is to be remembered that the content of tolymethylcarbinol in the total extract is too small to have produced the observed activity. The whole extract must have contained other substances with similar action to tolymethylcarbinol. The whole extract did not contain enough curcumin to produce the effects observed with the concentrate.

This study demonstrated that turmeric contains a variety of substances that exert an effect on the production and secretion of bile—i.e., cholagogic action. Quantitative and qualitative differences in action among the constituents would be observed in clinical settings. Use of whole herb could account for many of the traditionally observed medicinal and physiological effects. Asian researchers independently validated the same properties of turmeric.[7-9]

Summarizing the data from these studies, it can be shown that turmeric acts in the following ways to promote good gastrointestinal health:

1. Turmeric stimulates the flow of bile; several constituents have this property.

2. The increased flow of bile depends in part on the contraction of the gallbladder and in part on the increase in bile secretion, both of which are enhanced by turmeric.

3. The stimulation of bile depends mostly on the presence of the essential oil.

4. The flavonoids in turmeric cause the contraction of the gallbladder and thereby increase the effective emptying of this organ.

Turmeric has a synergistic action with other cholagogues

An interesting study compared the effects of a suspension of milk thistle (*Carduus marianus*), celandine (*Chelidonium majus*) and turmeric on choleretic activity in 28 healthy patients.

The cholagogic activity of celandine and milk thistle are known to be very limited. Even a very good cholagogue will only raise the production of bile in healthy humans by about 25–49 percent (though the effect can be much greater in experimental animals). In this case, however, the volume of bile rose by an incredible 369 percent compared to baseline levels. A similar extraordinary rise in the secretion of bilirubin was observed, 285 percent. These results indicate that the interactions among the principles of cholagogues are not simply additive, nor even multiplicative, but involve mechanisms that will require much more research before they are clearly understood.[13–15]

Turmeric has hepatoprotective action

Asian scientists also explored the ability of an alcohol extract of turmeric to prevent lesions to the liver induced by some potent toxin, such as carbon tetrachloride or galactosamine. The preparation provided highly significant hepatoprotective activity. However, much more work is needed before we will completely understand how turmeric's liver-protecting action works. What has been clearly demonstrated so far is that turmeric possesses antihepatotoxic activity on the order possessed by other liver-protective herbs such as milk thistle and licorice.[10–12]

Turmeric may prove useful in the treatment of gallbladder disease

Turmeric has been successfully employed in protecting the gallbladder against disease and in treating that organ when it ails. Gallstones (cholelithiasis), acute and chronic inflammation of the gallbladder (cholecystitis), and inflammation of the bile duct (cholangitis) are among the conditions effectively treated.[16] The anti-inflammatory and antibacterial properties of turmeric probably play a major role.

Turmeric has effects on the cardiovascular system

The several effects of turmeric on the cardiovascular system are reviewed in the chapter devoted to that subject.

SAFETY DATA

No toxicity has been observed at recommended dosages. In exceedingly high amounts, it has been observed to inflame the mucous linings of the stomach. Since this reaction is similar to that of cayenne on "innocent" tissue, it is possible that the stomach lining would adapt to the presence of turmeric over time, eventually exhibiting no inflammation at all to even very high doses.

REFERENCES

1. Leung, A.Y. *Chinese Herbal Remedies*, Universe Books, New York, 1984, p. 164.

2. Guttenberg, A. *Klin. Wschr*, 1926, p. 1998 (cited in Robbers, H. below).

3. Dieterle, H. and Kaiser, P. In: Arch. Pharmazie Ber., dtsch es., 270, 413, 1932.

4. Kalk, H. and Nissen, K. "Untersuchungen ueber die wirkung der cucuma (Temoe Lawak) auf die funktion der leber und der gallenwege." *Dtsch. Med. Wschr.*, 36, 1613, 1931. And Kalk, H. and Nissen, K. *Dtsch. Med. Wschr.*, 44, 1932 (cited in Robbers, H., below).

5. Franquelo, E. *Muench. Med. Wschr.*, 1933. p. 524 (cited in Robbers, H., below).

6. Grabe, F. *Naunyn Schmiederbergs Arc.*, 176, 673, 1934.

7. Robbers, H. "Ueber den wirkungsmechanismus der einzelnen

curcumabestandteile auf die gallensekretion." *Archiv fuer Experimental. Path. und Pharmacol.*, 181, 328–334, 1936.

8. Ramprasad, C. and Sirsi. M. *Journal of Scientific Indian Medical Research*, Sect. C, 15, 262, 1956.

9. Ramprasad, C. and Sirsi, M. *Journal of Scientific Indian Medical Research*, Sect. C, 16, 108, 1957.

10. Kiso, Y., Suzuki, Y., Konno, C., Hikino, H., Hashimoto, I. and Yagi, Y. "Application of carbon tetrachloride-induced liver lesion in mice for screening of liver protective crude drugs." *Shoyakugaku Zasshi*, 36, 238–244, 1982.

11. Kiso, Y., Tohkin, M. and Hikino, H. "Assay method for antihepatotoxic activity using carbon tetrachloride-induced cytotoxicity in primary cultured hepatocytes." *Planta Medica*, 49, 222–225, 1983.

12. Kiso, Y., Suzuki, Y., Watanabe, N., Oshima, Y. and Hikino, H. "Antihepatotoxic principles of curcuma longa rhizomes." *Planta Medica*, 49, 185–187, 1983.

13. Bauman, J. Ch., Heintze, H. and Muth, H.W. "Klinisch-experimentelle untersuchungen der gallen-, magen-, und Pankreassekretion unter den phytocholagogen wirkstoffen einer carduus marianus-chelidonium-curcuma-suspension." *Arzneimittel-Forschung*, 26, 98, 1971.

14. Zaterka, S. and Grossman, M.I. "The effect of gastrin and histamine on secretion of bile." *Gastroenterology*, 50, 500, 1966.

15. Maiwald, L. "Pflanzliche cholagoga." *Zhurnal der Allgemein Medizin*, 59, 304–308, 1983.

16. Luckner, et al. *Pharmazie*, 22, 376, 1967.

CHAPTER FIVE

The Musculoskeletal System

The musculoskeletal system consists of the bony skeleton of the body and the muscles attached to it. For the purposes of this book, we will define it as also including the tendons and ligaments, various other connective tissues and the skin. These additional structures do not fit easily into any of the traditional body systems, yet their health is just as important to maintaining a high quality of life as any of the other critical tissues of the body.

Those of us fortunate enough to possess an intact musculoskeletal system often take it for granted, yet it is one of the most marvelously designed inventions in the universe. It gives our bodies strength, support and flexibility and allows us to move from one place to another, a kind of miracle in itself. You just think "I want to go over there," and the next thing you know, you're moving in that direction; the feet come off the floor just so much, move just so much forward, avoiding a brick in your path, and come to rest on the ground with just so much force—you don't fall over, you don't pitch forward, you can depend on your other leg following smoothly, and so forth. We talk a lot about the human will; this is one place your will has almost complete freedom. We not only move about our environment, we talk, bend, look around, listen, write, sing and engage in thousands of other kinds of behaviors thanks to our ability to influence the action of muscles and bones.

And then there are the myriad involuntary behaviors that go on inside us continually, each of which depends on the protection of skeletal structures and the movement of muscles: e.g., breathing, digesting, heart beating, blood circulation.

It behooves us to keep this fantastic machine running well.

THE BONES

The skeletal system consists of over 200 bones, long, short, flat or irregular in shape, each with its own specific function. Here are some of the major functions:

1. Support for the soft tissues of the body.
2. Protection for internal organs like the heart, brain, lungs, and spinal cord.
3. Provision of a place for muscles to attach to allow movement, places which are, in essence, a series of internal, fully independent levers on which the muscles can pull.
4. Storage for minerals.
5. Manufacture (in the marrow) of red and white blood cells and platelets.

Structure of bone

Many people are surprised the first time they see a long bone of the body in cross-section. It isn't solid, but hollow, filled with soft kinds of stuff that don't look like bone at all. The shell of a bone consists basically of (1) a tough protective membrane on the outside called the periosteum, (2) a layer of compact bony material made of calcium, phosphorous, silicon, salts and other minerals, and (3) collagen, an organic protein. Channels called haversian canals, containing blood vessels, run through the bony layer. The interior of the bone contains a spongelike network of bone cells that provides some more strength without adding much in the way of weight. Some bones also contain marrow. The marrow contains mostly fat cells that do nothing but store fat unless the body loses a lot of blood; at that point these fat cells transform into cells with the ability to produce blood. Toward the ends of long bones occurs marrow with many red blood cells. In this marrow, red and white blood cells and platelets are formed on a regular basis.

JOINTS

Joints are just places where two bones meet, but they are minor wonders, because they determine the kind of movement through different planes and ranges that bones can do at those junctions. Joints contain the synovial fluid, which lubricates the bones and prevents friction and wear on them during movement. As a person gets older, the amount of this fluid gradually decreases and movement becomes harder and more painful as the joints stiffen.

There are several types of joints: (1) fixed joints, as in the skull, that lock the bones tightly together and do not allow movement at all; (2) hinged joints, as in the knee and elbow, that allow movement in just one direction; (3) ball and socket joints, as in the shoulder and hip, that permit circular movement; (4) pivot joints, as at the joint between the skull and vertebrae at the neck, that allow forward/backward and side-to-side movement; and (5) gliding joints, as in the ankle and wrist, that allow the kind of multiple movements possible in those joints.

Cartilage

The bones of infants and children are composed mainly of a firm, elastic, fibrous substance known as cartilage that is produced by cells called chondrocytes. As a child matures, this cartilage gradually gives way to bone cells. It is often said that children are much less susceptible to broken bones than adults. Cartilage doesn't break easily. The process whereby bone cells deposit crystals of calcium carbonate and calcium phosphate into the matrix, or ground substance of the bone, is called ossification. After ossification, the bone is now stronger than it was as cartilage but it is also more brittle.

During adolescence bones still contain cartilage at their ends, but by the mid-twenties the cartilage is fully ossified and bone growth ends. However, there is still a lot of cartilage in the body; a good deal of cartilage remains around the bones throughout life, and some of it remains extremely flexible; witness, for example, the nose and outer ear, the larynx and the trachea. At the ends of bones, cartilage forms tough, smooth, fibrous pads that help reduce the friction between the bones and act as shock absorbers for the bones. As this cartilage becomes worn, as in osteoarthritis, joint movement deteriorates. A special type of shock-absorbing cartilage is also found between the bones of the spinal column.

Connective tissue

Have you ever wondered how bones are held together? The answer is by strands of tough, yet flexible, fibers of connective tissue called ligaments. Ligaments surround joints, covering both the bones and the cartilage and holding the bones tightly together. Ligaments can stretch a little, and that allows the bones of the joint to move. Ligaments can be found outside the musculoskeletal system, providing support for various organs, including the bladder, liver, diaphragm and uterus, and helping to maintain the shape of the breasts.

Muscle fibers do not attach directly to bones. They attach to another kind of connective tissue called tendons, which attach to bones. When you contract a muscle it shortens, pulling the tendon, which moves the bone. Tendons are extremely strong and flexible, yet almost completely inelastic. They can be cylindrical, or can occur in wide sheets of fibers known as aponeuroses.

Tendons consist mainly of a tough, white, fibrous protein called collagen, and some blood vessels. Larger tendons also have a nerve supply. Even a slight attempt to stretch a tendon triggers a reflex contraction of the adjoining muscle and bone (e.g., the knee-jerk response). Collagen is the primary substance of the bone matrix upon which new bone growth and repair takes place. It is the most common protein in the body and its major structural protein. It is the stuff that holds the cells and tissues of the body together. Anything that keeps us from falling apart should be considered a major target for good health practices.

MUSCLES

Muscles provide the force needed to move the body or part of the body. Muscles make up from one-third to one-half of the body's total weight. Hundreds of muscles are found in every part of the body, from the large muscles in the thigh to the tiny muscles in the middle ear.

There are three types of muscle: (1) skeletal muscle, so called because it is attached to bone, but also called striated muscle in reference to its banded appearance, or voluntary muscle because we can move it at will; (2) smooth muscle, so called because it is attached to internal organs such as the stomach, but also known as involuntary muscle because it cannot normally be brought under conscious control. Smooth muscles control such things as blood pressure, movement of food through the digestive tract, contractions of the bile duct and so forth; and (3) the cardiac muscle. The cardiac muscle combines aspects of the other two types. It looks like some kind of striated muscle, but is involuntary, responding to the body's activity rather than to the will. It is attached to nothing but itself.

Skeletal muscles are classified according to the type of action they perform: (1) extensors open out a joint, flexors close it; (2) adductors draw a part of the body inward, abductors move it outward; (3) levators raise it, depressors lower it; (4) constrictors close an orifice when contracting—the orifice opens as they relax.

Skeletal muscles are made up of bundles of muscle fibers. A muscle fiber is made up of even smaller units called myofibrils which are in turn composed of the real heart of the system: microscopic filaments called actin and myosin, the proteins that control contraction. Bundles inside of bundles. Imagine that a muscle such as the biceps is a truck full of paper drinking straws. Inside the truck are large boxes of straws (which would correspond to separate bundles of muscle fibers); inside the large boxes are the smaller boxes that fit in the kitchen drawer (these correspond to a single muscle fiber); inside the box are the individual straws (which correspond to the myofibril); under a microscope you can see the individual paper fibers that make up the straw, some black, some white; these are the actin and myosin.

Each muscle fiber is supplied with one or more nerves that receive impulses from the brain or spinal cord. The impulse causes the nerve to secrete a neurotransmitter, a chemical called acetylcholine, which in turn initiates a series of chemical and electrical events, involving the passage of sodium, potassium and calcium ions in and out of muscle cells. These events result in the sliding of myosin filaments over the top of the actin filaments. (Imagine closing up the sections of an extendable ladder, or pushing the two halves of a deck of cards together after a shuffle.) This action causes the muscle to shorten in length. It's hard to believe how fast this series of events takes place. As I sit here typing this manuscript, with my fingers frantically flying over the keys in an effort to meet deadlines, I don't even really think about each and every movement, but they occur with deadly inaccuracy—they're even more inaccurate when I do think about it.

The complexities of muscle movement involve outgoing impulses of a thousand different kinds interacting with information transmitted back to the brain by sensory nerve fibers imbedded in muscles and tendons that relay information on relative stretch, position in space, plus other forces that may be acting on the body at the time.

Healthy muscle function depends on the tone of the muscle,

the chemical environment around the muscle and nerve cells, and the stress being exerted on muscles, ligaments, nerves and tendons.

Smooth muscle contractions rely on the same actin/myosin action as in the skeletal muscle. But the nerve supply to smooth muscle comes from the autonomic division of the nervous system. "Autonomic" implies automatic, which it is. Smooth muscle contractions and tone also depend upon the relative concentration of many different hormones, upon oxygen levels and on changes in pH.

The cardiac muscle is able to contract about 100,000 times every day. It looks like skeletal muscle but it is under the control of the autonomic nervous system and hormones.

THE SKIN

Not usually considered part of the musculoskeletal system, the skin, the largest organ of the body, nevertheless bears many structural and functional resemblances to bones and muscles. First of all, it helps give shape to the body and hold it together. Second, it is composed of many of the same connective tissues that occur around bones and muscles. Third, it offers protection to the internal organs.

The skin consists of a thin outer layer and a thicker inner layer (the epidermis and dermis, respectively). Below the dermis lies the subcutaneous tissue, composed mainly of fat cells.

The hair and nails are essential extensions of the skin, composed mainly of keratin, a hard protein substance. Keratin is the primary component of the epidermis. Pores are holes in the skin that contain extensions of the sweat glands located deep in the dermis. The dermis is also the home for sebaceous glands that produce sebum, an oily substance necessary to keep the skin soft and moist and also waterproof. Hairs arise in follicles located in the subcutaneous layer. The dermis is packed with blood vessels and lymph vessels, bringing nutrients and oxygen to all of the cells in the skin and removing wastes. Several different kinds of nerve cells innervate the skin—pain receptors, temperature receptors, touch receptors, pressure receptors, and others.

The relative thickness of the epidermis varies from one body part to another, being hard and thick on the soles and palms, yet extremely thin and soft on the eyelids.

The skin is the main protective organ of the body, shielding it from bacteria, injury, sun rays, and so on. It helps maintain body temperature within a narrow critical range. When the body is hot, the sweat glands produce the cooling perspiration, and the blood vessels dissipate more heat. When it's cold, the blood vessels of the skin contract, thereby conserving heat. The skin is also one of the primary ways the body has for getting rid of wastes—sweating.

DISORDERS OF THE MUSCULOSKELETAL SYSTEM

Bones

Nutritional The primary nutritional problems associated with bones are a lack of vitamin D and the mineral calcium. In children, rickets can develop. The counterpart in adults is called osteomalacia, and should not be confused with osteoporosis. It results in bones that are too soft to maintain their shape. They bend, leading to bad posture.

Degenerative With advancing age, the bones may begin to degenerate. In the case of osteoarthritis there occurs a very damaging wearing down where the bones of the joint rub on one another.

Hormonal During menopause, the secretion of estrogen stops. Since estrogen is so important in maintaining bone mass, the density of bone material without estrogen may decrease dramatically within a short time. Osteoporosis is also a natural part of aging. Without supplementation, the density in bones of people over 70 may only be about one-half to two-thirds normal. Low-density bones tend to become brittle and fracture and break very easily.

Injury Injuries to bones, especially fractures, are more serious than similar injuries to other tissues. They take longer to heal and they must be held rigidly in place to avoid faulty healing. The kind of nutritional support required for bones during healing is about the same as skin and connective tissue, but should be present in higher amounts.

Infection Infections in bones, such as osteomyelitis, or a bone abscess, can be very severe, since any inflammation can easily shut off blood flow to parts of the bone, leading to their death.

Fractures Broken bones are just what they sound like—actual breaks in the bony layer of the bone. Serious tearing of parts of the bone usually occurs also. Treatment usually involves putting the bones together as closely as possible to the original position, sometimes with pins and plates, immobilizing the bone, and waiting for it to heal itself.

Muscles

Injury This is the most common disorder of the musculoskeletal system. It leads to a lack of blood supply to the muscle with subsequent difficulties in functioning and even retaining the viability of individual muscle cells. Healing of injured muscle almost always creates scarring which shortens its natural length. Tears and sprains are very common. Blows to the muscle from blunt weapons can create internal bleeding, or hematoma formation. On rare occasions, bone can form in the hematoma (called myositis ossificans).

Genetic disorders So-called muscular dystrophies cause progressive disability and weakness through slow but systematic degeneration of muscle fibers. These may begin at birth or be triggered at some point later in life. They are often sex-linked, appearing only in males. Another genetic disorder is cardiomyopathy, a general term for inherited heart disease.

Infection   Gangrene is the primary infection affecting muscle tissue. It is usually a complication of injury, such as a deep wound that cannot receive the proper medical attention. Tetanus used to be a common muscle infection, but it is being slowly eradicated through inoculation. Myalgia, caused by the influenza B virus, is a rather common painful infection of muscle tissue. Trichinosis, acquired from eating raw pork, also attacks muscle fibers.

Tumors   Myomas are noncancerous tumors occurring in muscle tissue. The uterus is a favorite target of myomas (called fibroids). Cancerous tumors are called myosarcomas; they are rare.

Metabolic and hormonal disorders   Imbalances in the levels of hormones and electrolytes in and around the neuromuscular junction can lead to a variety of ailments. Low levels of potassium in the heart can lead to cardiac weakness and total failure. Low levels of calcium lead to nervous excitability and spasms. Either an excess or a depletion of thyroid hormone causes disorders in the muscles around the eyes, and adrenal exhaustion produces profound muscular weakness.

Impaired blood and oxygen supply   The major symptom of low blood supply is cramping. Serious muscular exertion that results in prolonged contraction of muscle fibers can restrict blood flow to certain muscles, lead to the buildup of lactic acid and other chemicals in the muscles and thereby create an environment conducive to cramping. Peripheral vascular disease also leads to a reduction of blood supply and can result in nocturnal cramps, or severe muscle pain during walking or exercising (claudication). Another example of this problem is angina pectoris in the heart muscle caused by coronary heart disease.

Autoimmune disorders   Myasthenia gravis is thought to be an autoimmune disorder. It is characterized by interrupted transmission of nerve impulses to muscles. Lupus erythematosus, rheumatoid arthritis, scleroderma and sarcoidosis are other autoimmune diseases that affect muscles.

Tendinitis Injuries can sometimes produce inflammation of a tendon. It can be painful, can restrict movement of the attached muscle, and may be marked by extreme tenderness. Examples are painful arc syndrome, characterized by pain in the shoulder when the arm is raised to a certain point, and tennis elbow, caused by inflammation around the bony prominence on the outer side of the elbow. Any activity that results in overexertion of the muscles that straighten the wrist and fingers produces an uncompromising strain on the tendons (e.g., gardening, tennis, home decorating).

Ruptured tendon The Achilles tendon is injured more often than any other tendon, usually because it is subjected to stretching due to sudden contractions of the calf muscles during such vigorous sports as track and field, baseball, basketball, football, and soccer. Baseball finger, tears of the tendons of biceps, wounds in the tendons of the hand, and arthritic ruptures of tendons in the hands are other common tendon injuries.

Torn ligaments Ligaments of the ankle joint and knee are often injured. Minor problems, such as sprains, do not actually tear the ligament, but still require medical attention. To tear a ligament clean from the bone, one has to subject it to a strong twisting stress, as might happen if the knee is suddenly turned while the weight of the body is on that leg. Football and soccer players are most susceptible to this injury. It often requires immobilization with a plaster cast in order to heal, and repeated injuries of this nature have ended the career of more than one professional athlete.

Sprain is defined as the tearing or stretching of a ligament that holds together the bone ends in a joint. It is usually caused by a sudden pull. Ankle sprains are the most common; they are caused by "going over" the outside of the foot in such a way that almost all of the weight of the body (plus gravity in case you are leaping into air) is placed on the ankle.

The Skin

Injuries Wounds, burns, scratches, insect bites, and animal bites lead the long list of possible injuries to the skin. Some are minor in nature, requiring only the barest of first aid measures, but others, such as serious burns, can be life-threatening. In between are numerous conditions that can produce scarring and serious infection.

Infections and inflammations As good a barrier as the skin is, it is nevertheless breached by viruses, bacteria, fungi, allergens, and parasites. The list of surface skin infections is almost endless, including chicken pox, warts, cold sores, herpes zoster, boils, cellulitis, erysipelas, impetigo, athlete's foot, ringworm, dermatitis, eczema, psoriasis and rashes. (These are more susceptible to prevention and treatment with immune system tonics than with the herbs discussed in this chapter.)

Tumors The skin is often attacked by benign tumors. However, more serious malignant cancers do also occur with regularity.

Autoimmune disorders Perhaps the most common autoimmune disorder of the skin is lupus erythematosus, mentioned in connection with the muscles. Another is vitiligo, characterized by white patches due to destruction of the skin's pigment layer of cells. Various rashes have autoimmune origins, as does scleroderma, a progressive hardening of the skin and other tissues.

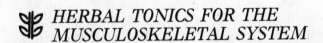

HERBAL TONICS FOR THE MUSCULOSKELETAL SYSTEM

The use of tonic herbs calls for choosing plant materials which contain a wide range of nutrients and other substances that this system can take advantage of in its efforts to mature and to heal itself in the event of injury or illness. It may come as some surprise to learn that there are plant materials that can speed up the healing of bone, connective tissue and skin. Many of these plants are only now beginning to be studied experimentally. We have just begun to scratch the surface of possible applications. The future looks very bright in this area.

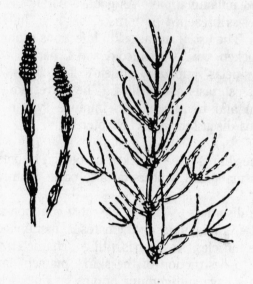

HORSETAIL

HORSETAIL
(Equisetum arvense)

One of the most important trace elements in human nutrition is silicon. It is used in the growth and repair of bone and tissue, and in other biological processes. Although silicon, in the form of quartz, is the most abundant mineral in the earth's crust, amazingly little is found in forms that the body will accept and utilize. Since the best sources of bioactive silicon are found in the plant kingdom, a goal of herbal research is to find and develop these into viable and effective health aids.

To be effective, silicon-containing substances must dissolve in water and must be digestible. These factors are of concern because silicon is seldom found as a pure element but in compounds, most of which do not dissolve and are not digestible.

Of all the silicon-containing foods presently known and being studied, horsetail is by far the best. Silicon occurs in this plant in probably the most soluble and bioactive form found in nature.

Horsetail (or shave grass or scouring rush), a component of herbal medicine for centuries, has recently been standardized to contain a large quantity of silicon, in the form of silica and silicic acid. Standardization is necessary because the content of silica compounds in horsetail varies considerably, depending upon where the plant grows, when it is gathered, how it is prepared (e.g., dried versus fresh), and even on who does the extracting. The best products now available consist of standardized horsetail in a base of whole horsetail herb to take advantage of the herb's other constituents, which include the saponin equisetonin, several flavoglycosides (including isoquercitrin, equisetrine and galuteolin), calcium, phosphorus, iron, carotene, thiamine, riboflavin, niacin, ascorbic acid, resin, starch, tannin, various acids and some sterols.

TRADITIONAL USES OF HORSETAIL

Externally, both the American Indians and the Chinese use horsetail to stop bleeding and accelerate the healing of wounds and broken bones. The effectiveness of horsetail in external applications is related to the solubility of silica in the fluids of wounds or in the poultice materials, and its absorption directly into blood and cells at the site of the wound.

Internally, horsetail is often used as a source of minerals, especially silica and calcium, in a form that can be easily used by the body in the production and repair of bone, skin and connective tissue. As a diuretic and astringent, it is widely used in the treatment of genitourinary problems such as gravel and inflammations. Europeans, Asians, and Americans use horsetail in the treatment of pulmonary tuberculosis, cystitis, cramps of the bladder, kidney stones, enuresis, lithiasis, dropsy, internal bleeding, fevers, eye diseases, nephritis, cystic ulceration, gonorrhea, gout, rheumatism, and miscellaneous hemorrhaging conditions of the bladder, kidneys and prostate. Horsetail has even found its way into folk medicine treatments for cancer.[3–5]

Horsetail helps mend injured connective tissue, skin and bones

Research in Europe has shown that horsetail stops bleeding and helps build up the blood. It also possesses good antibiotic action. Silicic acid, or horsetail tea, causes a slight rise in white blood cell count, and thereby enhances nonspecific resistance to diseases of many types. The use of horsetail to treat atherosclerosis is also currently being validated in European research.

Modern research has validated long-standing folk medicine practices of using horsetail to mend connective tissue and bone. Horsetail stimulates many cellular metabolic processes that are the basis for the repair of connective tissues and bone.[2]

Possible synergy among the many nutrients found in horsetail cannot and should not be ruled out. In fact, positive interactions are highly probable.

STANDARDIZATION OF HORSETAIL

The only plant that has been systematically subjected to rigid standardization for silicon content is horsetail. Standardization is important because it is very easy to destroy the organic nature of the silicon by accidentally separating the silicon from the organic material to which it was originally bound or by changing the nature of those bonds.

ROLE OF SILICON

Silicon is found throughout the human body, both inside and outside of cells. We get most of our silicon through the diet. Silicic acid in foods and beverages is readily absorbed into the bloodstream across the intestinal wall. Most is rapidly excreted in the urine. Only a small amount is ever utilized by the body. In the blood, silicon levels are very carefully regulated by homeostatic mechanisms.

Silicon is involved in the processes by which bone, cartilage, connective tissue and skin are formed. Connective tissues such as aorta, trachea, tendon, bone and skin and its appendages are unusually rich in silicon.[6]

The growth and repair of tissue requires a starting point, something to grow on—what is called a matrix. One of the ways silicon works is by helping to form and be a part of this matrix.

It is subsequently involved in the buildup of minerals on the matrix during the formation of the new bone or connective tissue. Silicon is also heavily involved in the metabolic processes of the matrix itself.[7]

Silicon is present in several important cells:

1. Osteoblasts. Bone-forming cells that are responsible for the deposition of calcium phosphate on the protein matrix of the bone during repair processes and during the transformation of cartilage into mature bone.

2. Chondroblasts. Cartilage-forming cells. Here, silicon stimulates the deposition of proteins and GAGs (GlycosAmino-Glycans—materials that form a major part of the structural framework of bone, skin and connective tissues) on the matrix. Some major GAGs are hyaluronic acid, chondroitin sulphate and keratin sulphate.

3. Fibroblasts. Fiber-forming cells. Here, silicon plays much the same role as in chondroblasts. These cells are also important in the biosynthesis of collagen.

There is evidence suggesting that when tissues are injured, the various types of tissue have a "pecking order" for obtaining silicon for repair. If bone, cartilage, collagen and GAG are all involved in the same injury, bone repair has precedence over the others. This means that the repair of the other tissues may be significantly retarded during bone repair unless more silicon is supplied in the form of supplements. Therefore, the historical use of horsetail to speed recovery from fractures, torn ligaments and related injuries makes good sense.

Silicon is also important in the formation of the fibrous tissues in joints that allow them to bend and flex with ease.

Bioactivity

It has been found that the chemical form of silicon may be an important determinant of bioactivity. Inorganic metasilicate (the kind of silicon used in most experimental research) is one of the most soluble forms of silicon, but several organic complexes possess a higher bioactivity. Moderate increases in blood silicon levels are obtained after feeding sodium metasilicate, but much higher levels are reached after feeding organic silicates.[8]

Scientists feel that silicon materials probably undergo differing rates of solubility, digestion, absorption and assimilation depending upon the chemical nature of the materials and their susceptibility to various digestive processes. The more bioactive forms of silicon are able to attach to a great variety of substances in the spaces around cells during bone growth, wound healing and similar processes, while the less active silicon species are excreted without contributing to health. It is important to note that no enhancers of silicon bioavailability are known.[1]

THE ROLE OF SILICON IN AGING

It has often been observed that the silicon content of the aorta, other arterial vessels, and the skin dermis decreases with age, as the incidence of atherosclerosis increases. The use of horsetail to treat arthritis and related inflammatory conditions may be related to an ability to replace lost silicon. In this light, a relationship has been discovered between silicon, age and endocrine balance. A decline in hormonal activity may be responsible for the change in silicon levels. Silicon, or horsetail, therapy could help to counteract this mechanism.[9-12]

Silicon may also be involved in the prevention of some forms of senility. According to one theory, some kinds of senility do not occur unless there is more aluminum in the bloodstream than silicon. As long as the silicon/aluminum ratio favors silicon, the detrimental effects of the aluminum, the ultimate "bad guy," are not seen.[13]

It has also been shown that aluminum adversely affects bone formation. Silicic acid counteracts this effect. If you eliminate silicon, you observe the toxicity of aluminum.

CONCLUSION

Silicon plays a vital role in the developmental growth and repair of bone, cartilage, skin, arteries, tendons, ligaments and other connective tissues throughout the body. The body appears to have homeostatic systems that regulate the amount and kind of silicon used. The chemical form of supplemental silicon is critical to its metabolic fate; the single most important factor governing assimilation and effective utilization is, of course, bioactivity. Inorganic silicon (e.g., sand) will be least assimilable, while forms that are ingested as plant material (e.g., horsetail) will be most assimilable. The single most bioactive and effective form of silicon available is found only in the plant horsetail and its standardized concentrates. Horsetail also contains a full complement of other valuable nutrients that can affect all phases of tissue repair processes.

SAFETY DATA

Horsetail is not toxic to humans, but has been known to have detrimental effects on livestock that have grazed on it for extended periods of time.

REFERENCES

1. Sanger, A.G. and Hodson, M.J. "Silica in higher plants." *Silicon Biochemistry*, Wiley Chichester (Ciba Foundation Symposium 121), 1986, pp. 90–111.

2. Weiss, R.F. *Herbal Medicine*. Beaconsfield Publishers, Ltd., Beaconsfield, England, 1988, pp. 223, 238, 315, 349.

3. List, P.H. and Hooerhammer, L.H. *Hagers Handbuch der Pharmazeutischen Praxis*, six volumes, Springer Verlag, Berlin, 1968–1979, citation for Equisetum.

4. Duke, J.A. *CRC Handbook of Medicinal Herbs*, CRC Press, Inc., Boca Raton, Florida, 1985.

5. Schindler, H. "Die inhaltsstoffe von heilpflanzen und pruefungs-methoden fuer pflanzliche tinkturen. 59. equisetum arvense." *Arzneim.-Forsch.*, 3(10), 541–542, 1953.

6. Carlisle, E.M. "Silicon as an essential trace element in animal nutrition." *Silicon Biochemistry*, Wiley, Chichester (Ciba Foundation Symposium 121), 1986, pp. 123–139.

7. Carlisle, E.M. "The nutritional essentiality of silicon." *Nutrition Reviews*, 40(7), 193–198, 1982.

8. Benke, G.M. and Osbon, T.W. "Urinary silicon excretion by rats following oral administration of silicon compounds." *Fd. Cosmt. Toxicol.*, 17, 123–127, 1979.

9. Birchall, J.D. and Espie, A.W. "Biological implications of the interaction (via silanol groups) of silicon with metal ions." *Silicon Biochemistry*, Wiley, Chichester (Ciba Foundation Symposium 121) 1986, pp. 140–159.

10. Dobbie, J.W. and Smith, M.J.B. "Urinary and serum silicon in normal and uraemic individuals." *Silicon Biochemistry*, Wiley, Chichester (Ciba Foundation Symposium 121), 1986, pp. 194–213; and "The silicon content of body fluids." *Scott. Med. J.*, 27, 17–19, 1982.

11. Loeper, J.E., et al. "Fatty acids and lipid peroxidation during experimental atheroma. Silicon's action." *Pathol. Biol.*, 32, 693–697, 1984.

12. Okuda, A. and Takahasi, E. *Nippon Dojo Hiryogaku*, 33, 1–8, 1962.

13. Solomons, N.W. "The other trace minerals." In: Solomons, N.W. and Rosenberg, I.H. (eds.), *Absorption and Malabsorption of Mineral Nutrients*, A.R. Liss, Inc., NY, pp 283–285.

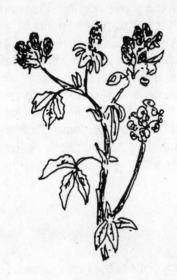

ALFALFA

ALFALFA
(Medicago sativa)

One of the things the body needs to repair and heal its many connective tissues, muscles and bones is a source of concentrated nutrition, a host of minerals, vitamins and other substances. Alfalfa contains an enormous quantity of nutrients, in a form that is easily digested and assimilated by man. It is up to 50 percent protein, contains a good quantity of beta-carotene, chlorophyll and octacosanol. Also present are saponins, sterols (beta-sitosterol, stigmasterol and alpha-spinasterol), flavonoids, coumarins, alkaloids, acids, vitamins (A, B1, B6, B12, C, D, E, K, niacin, pantothenic acid, biotin, folic acid), amino acids, sugars, minerals (calcium, phosphorus, potassium, magnesium, iron, zinc and copper), trace elements and other nutrients.[1,2]

Overall, alfalfa has a long-standing reputation as a most nutritious food, an appetite stimulant and vitality augmenter. Much of that reputation was gained during observations of its effect in livestock feed. Subsequently, alfalfa added to the diets of humans produced the same results. The ancient Arabs were the first to recognize the nutritional benefits of alfalfa; they called it the "father of all foods" (Al-fal-fa), but the American Indians were perhaps the first culture to discover its medicinal value.[3]

Herbalists have used alfalfa for many different purposes. Most of those applications bear a one-to-one correspondence to the various nutrients in the plant. The one word that keeps appearing is "tonic." The plant is a kidney tonic, liver tonic, "superlative restorative tonic," digestive tonic, prostatic tonic, reproductive tonic, musculoskeletal tonic, glandular tonic, and so forth.

CHLOROPHYLL

Alfalfa is, of course, one of the best sources of chlorophyll available. Chlorophyll extracts from plants have been shown to stimulate the growth of new skin tissue in wounds. In one study, 1,372 cases of experimentally induced wounds and burns were treated topically by 17 different ointments. Only the chlorophyll preparation showed consistently significant results.[14] Infected wounds did not show improvement in this study, but other studies using more concentrated chlorophyll preparations have reported anti-infectious activity in addition to healing action.[15] Chlorophyll has also been shown to increase the effectiveness of penicillin by as much as 35 percent.[16] Chlorophyll is especially active in recalcitrant wounds that refuse to heal under normal treatment. French scientists have shown that alfalfa can reduce tissue damage caused by another modern hazard: radiotherapy.[17] Radiation burns have been repaired by other plants that contain significant amounts of chlorophyll, suggesting that this substance may be the common active constituent.[18]

Tonics are said to affect the very life blood of the body, to rejuvenate, make new, refresh. It is intriguing to speculate about the relationship between photosynthesis, which intimately involves chlorophyll, and respiration, or breathing, which depends upon the presence of hemoglobin. A chlorophyll molecule is amazingly similar to a molecule of hemoglobin, differing mainly in a substitution of an atom of iron in hemoglobin for an atom of magnesium in chlorophyll. Both molecules are biosynthesized from the same protoporphyrin. And protoporphyrin synthesis is identical in both mammalian reticulocytes and plant chloroplasts. Hemoglobin is responsible for transporting oxygen, acquired through respiration, to the tissues of the body; photosynthesis is the only chemical source of oxygen on the planet. Equally important for the life blood of humans and other nonplant organisms is the carbohydrate manufacturing function of photosynthesis. Photosynthesis is the major exogenous source of carbohydrates, and hence of carbon and energy. Photosynthesis is the process whereby solar energy is converted into a form utilizable by life forms. Chlorophyll is the light absorber. Loosely speaking, it takes energy from the sun. Hemoglobin gives it back, also loosely speaking. But the analogy is real. For it is the exhaled CO_2, the end product of respiration, that is photochemically reduced to carbohydrate during the process of photosynthesis.

It is interesting to note that the primary act of photosynthesis is typically described as the excitation of the chlorophyll molecule to a higher energy state through the absorption of radiant light. Everything that follows is essentially a domino effect. The same idea can be applied to the transfer of the oxygen molecule from hemoglobin to the cells of the body—an excitation that results in a higher energy state. It is also interesting that the series of events that follows the transformation of chlorophyll to an activated molecule in plants is almost exactly the same series of events that characterizes the respiratory chain in animals, i.e., a series of electron transfer steps through oxidation and reduction, involving the cleavage of water (through oxidation), the formation of NADPH and ATP, and so forth.

We might also note a couple of anomalies in these schemes. Hemoglobin is not the only substance responsible for transporting oxygen to the tissues of living organisms. Others exist, all of which are very similar to hemoglobin in structure. As a class, they are called "respiratory pigments." We normally think of hemoglobin as red, but in some invertebrates, the respiratory pigment is green! We also tend to think of hemoglobin as being restricted to the animal kingdom, but hemoglobin has been found in some plants (such as in the root nodules of legumes).

The point of this discussion is a simple one: though we don't know enough about the intimate mechanisms of photosynthesis as compared to animal respiration to suggest functional equality between chlorophyll and hemoglobin, the parallel functions currently uncovered, as well as the lack of concrete distinguishing features (other than iron versus magnesium) strongly suggest the likelihood of some kind of dietary importance in chlorophyll that springs from its similarity to hemoglobin.

Alfalfa diminishes the symptoms of arthritis and rheumatism

Alfalfa has traditionally been one of the best herbal treatments for arthritis, gout and rheumatism. Clinical research suggests that at least one or two persons in ten will respond very well to the use of alfalfa, experiencing an almost total reduction in painful symptoms. Another, less definable, fraction of the population will experience partial relief. So the herb is definitely worth a try. Alfalfa's antirheumatic effect is probably due in part to its extremely high nutritive value.[4-7] But it might also be a function of the plant's ability to affect lipid metabolism. Alfalfa has a proven cholesterol-lowering effect. Steroidal anti-inflammatory action is suggested by its content of plant steroids, and by some research that found an estrogenic effect on ruminants (grazing animals). Although the treatment of arthritis is difficult at best, the use of alfalfa over the long term could significantly help many people deal with this ailment.[5-10]

Other properties

Alfalfa has also been shown to possess antibacterial action against gram negative bacteria (such as *Salmonella typhi*), and it contains at least one protein with known antitumor activity. It is important to realize that alfalfa is also fiber. As such it has been shown, along with bran and pectin, to bind and neutralize various types of agents carcinogenic to the colon. Finally, some work suggests that alfalfa induces activity in a complex cellular system that inactivates dietary chemical carcinogens in the liver and small intestine before they have a chance to do the body any harm. This system, called the microsomal mixed-function oxidase system, actually increases the metabolism of potential carcinogens, e.g., polycyclic hydrocarbons, resulting in their degradation before they have a chance to do any damage. In other words, by increasing the activity of carcinogens, this system ironically reduces the probability that their activity will result in cancer.[11-13]

SAFETY DATA

Given the fact that alfalfa has been used for centuries without any significant toxicity being reported, it is highly unlikely that therapeutic amounts pose a threat. Routine screening tests have been uniformly negative.

REFERENCES

1. Duke, J.A. *CRC Handbook of Medicinal Herbs*, CRC Press, Inc., Boca Raton, Florida, 1985, pp. 220–221.

2. Pedersen, M. *Nutritional Herbology*, Pedersen Publishing, Bountiful, Utah, 1987, pp. 70–73.

3 Kohler, G.O. "The unidentified vitamins of grass and alfalfa." *Feedstuffs*, August 8, 1953.

4. Lucas, C. and Power, L. "Dietary fat aggravates active rheumatoid arthritis." *Clin. Res.*, 29(4), 754a, 1981.

5. "Calcium pantothenate in arthritic conditions." *Practitioner*, 224, 208–211, 1980.

6. McDuffe, F.C. Arthritis Foundation. As reported in *Med. World News*, July 22, 1985.

7. Skoldstam, L. "Fasting and vegan diet in rheumatoid arthritis." *Scand. J. Rheumatol.*, 15(2), 219–221, 1987.

8. Cookson, F.B., Altschul, R. and Fedoroff, S. "The effects of alfalfa on serum cholesterol and in modifying or preventing cholesterol-induced atherosclerosis in rabbits." *J. Athero. Res.*, 7, 69–81, 1967.

9. Cookson, F. B. and Fedoroff, S. "Quantitative relationships between administered cholesterol and alfalfa required to prevent hypercholesterolemia in rabbits." *Br. J. Exper. Path.*, 49, 348–355, 1968.

10. Malinow, M.R., et al. "Comparative effects of alfalfa saponins and alfalfa fiber on cholesterol absorption in rats." *Amer. J. Clin. Nutr.*, 32, 1810–1812, 1979.

11. Bickoff, E.M., et al. "Tricin from alfalfa-isolation and physiological acitivity." *J. Pharm. Sci.*, 53(11), 1411–1412, 1964.

12. Tyihak, E. and Szende, B. "Basic plant proteins with antitumor activity." *Hung. Teljes* 798, 28 Aug. 1970.

13. Wattenberg, L.W. "Effects of dietary constituents on the metabolism of chemical carcinogens." *Cancer Research*, 35, 3326–3331, 1975.

14. Smith, L.W. and Livingston, A.E. "Chlorophyll. An experimental study of its water soluble derivatives in wound healing." *Amer. J. Surg. New Series*, vol. LXIII(3), 358–369, Dec., 1943.

15. Smith, L.W. "Chlorophyll: An experimental study of its water-soluble derivatives. IV. The effect of water soluble chlorophyll derivatives and other agents upon the growth of fibroblasts in tissue culture." *J. Lab. Clin. Med.*, 1, 541, 1953.

16. Smith, L.W. and Livingston, A.E. "Wound healing." *Am. J. Surg.*, 67, 30–39, 1945.

17. De Froment, P. "Unsaponifiable substance from alfalfa for pharmaceutical and cosmetic use." *Fr. Demande* 2,187,328., 22 Feb., 1974.

18. Holmes, G.W. and Mueller, H.P. "Treatment of post-irradiation erythema with chlorophyll ointment." *Am. J. Roentgenol. Rad. Ther.*, 50, 210–213, 1943.

DEVIL'S CLAW
(Harpagophytum procumbens)

Devil's claw has become a primary treatment for arthritis and rheumatism. Secondarily, it is often used to treat gastrointestinal problems, much in same manner that our Western bitters are used. The plant originated in South Africa, but its use has made its way to America via the British Isles. It is generally regarded as both safe and effective, and works mainly as an anti-inflammatory agent. In Africa, in the Kalahari Desert and Namibian steppes, the root is used as a treatment for indigestion, blood diseases, fever, pain and pregnancy-related problems.

For external use, devil's claw root is made into ointments for skin rashes, wounds and the like. Diabetes, hepatitis, kidney and bladder deficiency, nervous malaise and respiratory ailments are all treated with devil's claw preparations.

Devil's claw in arthritis and rheumatism: anti-inflammatory effects

Since the end of World War II, devil's claw has been used in medical institutions throughout southern Africa, and in some hospitals and clinics in Germany, as a treatment for inflammatory diseases. Most of these trials have been partially to totally effective. The first published report of this early research appeared in 1958. In that paper, devil's claw was reported to be effective in reducing inflammation and swelling in experimentally-induced arthritis. Using simple water extracts, the researcher was able to reduce swelling from 300-800 percent in a matter of days.[1]

By 1962, the active component, harpagoside, had been identified,[2] and in 1970 this compound was subjected to a rigorous pharmacological screening trial in which the anti-inflammatory property was validated.[3] Whole devil's claw preparation was found to be superior to pure harpagoside, both were found to be safe; furthermore, the antiarthritic effect was found to not be due to any painkilling property of the plant, since it had none.[4] Meanwhile, other reports were appearing reporting good clinical results. In one case, over 100 patients were treated with either pure devil's claw or with a combination of herb and standard treatment.[5] Evidence for lack of toxicity continued to accumulate. Other important chemicals have been identified: harpagide, procumbide, beta-sitosterol, stigmasterol, fatty acids, triterpenes and flavonoids.

An early review paper on devil's claw suggested that the plant was a good stimulant of the lymphatic system, with detoxifying effects that extended to the whole organism, and provided evidence from clinical studies involving close to 400 persons that the plant was indeed effective for most of the conditions treated by folk medicine, especially as pertaining to the liver, gallbladder, bladder and kidneys.[6]

More recent studies have found that devil's claw preparations are generally well suited for the treatment of chronic rheumatism, arthritis, gout, spondylosis-induced lower back pain, neuralgia, headaches, and lumbago.[8,9] One study found that its anti-inflammatory effects equaled those of pyrazolone derivatives and the commonly prescribed antiarthritic phenylbutazone.[3] Analgesic effects of a subjective nature are reported, but objective tests are ambiguous on this point. Relief of pain is probably a side benefit of reduced inflammation. Improved motility in the joints is often reported, as well as improved feeling of well-being. Currently, physicians in Europe are injecting devil's claw extract directly into arthritic joints, where it acts much like cortisone in terms of reducing inflammation.[10] As is the case with most arthritis treatments, not everybody benefits, but there are enough who do to warrant further investigation of this plant, and to recommend it as a possible treatment option.

Not all studies have reported success. For example, in one case, 13 patients exhibiting various kinds of arthritis, for whom conventional therapy had failed, were given devil's claw tablets (410 mg/3x daily for six weeks) without positive results.[7] Simultaneous rat studies likewise produced negative results, even though indomethacin was effective. The lack of toxicity of harpagophytum was again established in these trials. But the lack of positive effect is hard to explain when compared to the many other reports. The use of a highly selective group of subjects may have contributed to the failure. At any rate, it is obvious that much more experimental and clinical work needs to be done on this plant.

The British Pharmacopoeia recognizes devil's claw as having anti-inflammatory, antirheumatic, analgesic, sedative and diuretic properties, and as being good for rheumatism, arthritis, gout, myalgia, fibrositis, lumbago, and pleurodynia, and suggests combining it with menyanthes, apium, gaultheria and dioscorea in the treatment of rheumatism.[13]

Devil's claw has good gastrointestinal properties

Not much research has been done in this area, but it has been established that devil's claw root possesses a bitter value equal to that of the main Western bitter, gentian root.[10] It would therefore be expected to possess similar gastrointestinal properties. Indeed, in the few reported studies on GI problems, harpagophytum proved effective in treating such complaints as dyspepsia and conditions relating to the proper functioning of bile salts, the gallbladder, and the enterohepatic circuit. [11] In a related manner, the herb helps to regulate cholesterol and fatty acid levels in the blood. As one author points out, devil's claw may be the perfect treatment for elderly people with arthritis, obesity and hyperlipemia.[12]

SAFETY DATA

The data supporting the safety of devil's claw are quite extensive, including concomitant toxicity tests with the experimental and clinical work, as well as studies designed specifically to test for toxicity, all of which validate its safety and reveal a complete lack of toxicity.[8] Nevertheless, reports of adverse side effects have been circulated by the British government.

REFERENCES

1. Zorn, B. "Uber die antiarthritische wirkung der harpagophytumwurzel." *Zeitschrift fur Rheumaforschung*, 17, 134-138, 1958.

2. Tunman, P. and Lux, R. "Zur kenntnis der inhaltsoffe aus der wurzel von h.p." *Deutscher Apotheker-Zeitung*, 1274-1275, 1962; and 395-396, 1963.

3. Eichler, O. and Koch, C. "Uber die antiphlogistiche, analgetische und spasmolytische wirksamkeit von harpagosid." *Arzneimittel-Forschung*, 20(1), 107-109, 1970.

4. Schmidt, S. "Phytotherapie beim rheumatischen formankreis." *Erfahrungsheilkunde*, 5, 152-154, 1973/5.

5. Schmidt S. "Rheumatherapie mit harpagophytum." *Therapiewoche*, 72, 1072-1074, 1972.

6. Seeger, P.G. "Harpagophytum, ein wirksames phytotherapeutikum." *Erfahrungsheilkunde*, 8, 1973.

7. Grahme, R. and Robinson, B.V. "Devil's claw (harpagophytum procumbens): pharmacological and clinical studies." *Annals of the Rheumatic Diseases*, 40(6), 632, 1981.

8. Caprasse, M. "Description, identification et usages therapeutiques de la 'griffe du diable': harpagophytum procumbens DC." *Pharm. Belg.*, 35(2), 143-149, 1980.

9. Erdoes, A., Fontaine, R., Friehe, H., Durand, R. and Poeppinghaus, T. "Beitrag zur pharmakologie und toxikologie verschiedener extrakte, sowie des harpagosids aus harpagophytum procumbens DC." *Planta Medica*, 34, 97-108, 1978.

10. Weiss, R. F. *Herbal Medicine.* Beaconsfield Publishers, Ltd, Beaconsfield, England, 1988, pp. 265-267.

11. Zimmerman, W. "Erfahrungen mit harpagophytum." *Physikalische Medizin und Rehabilitation*, 18, 317-319, 1977.

12. Hoppe, H. "Einfluss der droge harpagophytum procumbens DC auf diabetes mellitus mit fettstoffwechselstorungen." *Erfahrungsheilkunde*, 7, 230-233, 1974.

13. *British Herbal Pharmacopoeia*, British Herbal Medical Association, West Yorks., 1983, p. 111.

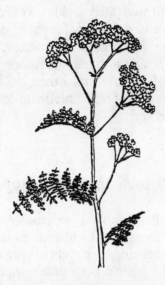

YARROW

YARROW
(Achillea millifolium)

Yarrow is a common bitter, and is used as such in the folklore of Europe and North America. It contains an essential oil which in turn consists mainly of cineol, azulene and proazulene. The bitter substance is known as achilleine. Yarrow is used to treat inflammatory conditions of the joints, but has also found wide application in the treatment of dyspepsia, and is broadly classified as a cholagogue, as are most bitters. There is research to support this claim. Due to the presence of the volatile oil, yarrow is also a good antibiotic and spasmolytic agent. Cineol itself has been shown to be antiseptic, expectorant and carminative, again conforming to the pattern for essential oils.

Yarrow is a cholagogue

The cholagogue activity of yarrow may be due to the presence of unsaturated fatty acids. At least it has been observed that unsaturated fatty acids have good cholagogue effects, and that they are present in yarrow. It is often difficult to discover exactly why a given substance has cholagogue action; in the case of yarrow and other unsaturated fatty acid-containing plants, such as milk thistle, at least this one connection has been observed.[1-3]

Yarrow has some antibiotic properties

Yarrow is often applied externally to help heal skin wounds. Its effectiveness may be attributed to good antimicrobial action. In routine screenings, extracts of yarrow have shown some antibacterial activity against both gram negative and gram positive bacteria.[4,5]

Yarrow is anti-inflammatory and antiarthritic

There is published evidence indicating that yarrow has antipyretic, anti-inflammatory and hemostatic properties. These effects would also tend to support the use of this plant in the treatment of painful inflammation of tissues and joints. The American Indians were the first to recognize the ability of yarrow to reduce the pain and swelling of joint disease. They passed this knowledge on to the early settlers. Ever since, yarrow has been one of the most popular treatments of arthritis and related conditions. It is doubtful that everyone, or even a majority of people, will respond significantly to yarrow. It is asking too much of just one plant that it contain the nutrients needed and utilizable by everyone with arthritis. But for that 10–20 percent or so who will respond to it, it is a gift from heaven.[6-9]

SAFETY DATA

Contact dermatitis, photosensitization and other allergic reactions may occur in sensitive individuals.[10]

REFERENCES

1 Maiwald, L. "Pflanzliche cholagoga." *Zhurnal Allgemein Medizin*, 59, 1304-1308, 1983.

2. Goetz, H.G. "Cholagoga. Pharmazeutische praxis." Supplement to: *Die Pharmazie*, 9, 193, 1971.

3. Chabrol, E., Charonnat, R., Maximin, M., Waitz, R. and Porin, J. "L'action choleretique des composees." *C.R. Societe de Biologie* (Paris), 108(12), 1100-1102, 1931.

4. D'amico, M.L. "Richere sulla presenza di sostanze ad azioneantiviotica nelle piante superiori." *Fitoterapia*, 26(1), 77-79, 1950.

5. Goranov, K., et al. "Clinical results from the treatment of hemorrhagic form of periodontosis with a complex herb extract and 15% DMSO." *Stomatologia*, 65(6), 25-30, 1983.

6. Goldberg, A. S., et al. U.S. Patent 3,552,350, 1970; *Chem. Abstract* 73, 102048w, 1970.

7. Goldberg, A.S. and Mueller, E.C. *Journal of Pharmaceutical Science*, 58, 938, 1969.

8. Chandler, R.F., et al. "Herbal remedies of the Maritime Indians: sterols and triterpenes of achillea millefolium L. (yarrow). J. *Pharm. Sci.*, 71(6), 1982.

9. Kudrzycka-Bieloszabska, F.W. and Glowniak, K. *Diss. Pharm. Pharmacol*, 14, 449, 1966.

10. Mitchell, J.C. *Recent Advances In Phytochemistry*, Vol. 9. V.C. Runeckles (ed.), Plenum Press, New York, 1975, p. 119.

SAW PALMETTO BERRIES
(Serenoa repens)

Saw palmetto berry is an old American tonic that has gained recent attention among individuals wishing to build muscle tone and bulk. John Lloyd, a famous early American medical botanist, observed that animals fed on these berries grew sleek and fat. This same observation was made by many early settlers searching for fodder and nutritional supplements for their livestock. Much early research demonstrated saw palmetto's effect on body weight, general health and disposition, tranquilization, appetite stimulation and reproductive health. Saw palmetto berries' main effect appears to be on the digestive system, to stimulate appetite and provide excellent nutrition. The plant's own array of constituents seem ideally suited for strengthening the musculoskeletal system.

Saw palmetto berries contain plant steroids

Dried saw palmetto berries contain high concentrations of free and bound sitosterols, including the very active beta-sitosterol. When a solution was injected under the skin of animals, it exhibited hormonal activity of some kind, though not enough research has been directed at this action to explain its nature. One might speculate that the presence of such high concentrations of sitosterols, together with other principles in the berry, forms the basis for biological activity in man. Needless to say, a great deal more research would be required to verify such a mechanism.[1] (For more on saw palmetto, see the section on the male reproductive system.)

SAFETY DATA

Saw palmetto berries have no known toxicity.

REFERENCES

1. Elghamry, M.I. and Haensel, R. *Experientia*, 25, 828–829, 1969.

WILD YAM
(Dioscorea spp.)

Wild yam root has been used for hundreds of years to treat rheumatism and arthritis-like ailments. The discovery of steroidal glycosides (diosgenin) in the root validated this ancient practice.

Yams are the best source of steroidal precursors

Most species of yams contain large amounts of plant steroids, primarily diosgenin, a saponin precursor in the synthesis of progesterone. Without the yams, the industrial complex would not be able to meet the worldwide demand for synthetic corticosteroids. But with them, scientists can derive animal or human steroids in a fairly straightforward multistep process. Wild yams are the only really good source of plant steroids for such purposes. Agave and yucca are two other sources, neither of which equals wild yam.

Diosgenin provides about 50 percent of the raw material for steroid synthesis.[12] Stigmasterol, from soybeans and other herbs, comes about as close as any other plant sterol to being useful in steroid synthesis, but yields what is better called a semi-synthesis. It must be emphasized that there is not an equivalency between diosgenin and human steroids. It takes many synthetic steps to get from one to the other. If yam has steroidal effects on the body, it is not because it contains steroidal hormones, but because the steroidal precursors have similar effects. The body does not recognize them or mistake them for its own hormones, but uses them in a similar manner.

Yams have anti-inflammatory and antiarthritic action

Research has shown that yam, yam extract and/or diosgenin possess good to excellent anti-inflammatory action. In one series of studies, yam was found to induce a short-lived decrease in blood pressure and an increase in coronary flow when injected intravenously into rabbits. Also in rabbits, the saponins of yam, fed orally, prevented large increases in blood cholesterol levels. The good therapeutic effect of dioscorea saponins on patients with atherosclerosis combined with hypertension was confirmed in clinical practice.[9–11, 13]

Yams and DHEA

Another important use for wild yam root has surfaced in recent years, involving the presence of dehydroepiandosterone, or DHEA, a substance apparently that, unlike the sex hormone precursors, is identical to a hormone produced in the adrenal glands of mammals. DHEA is the most abundant steroid circulating in the plasma of normal human adults. The purpose of this substance has remained a mystery throughout most of the history of mankind. Now researchers have discovered an inverse relationship between blood levels of DHEA and the risk of developing obesity, atherosclerosis and cardiovascular disease.[1, 2, 4] Furthermore, plasma levels of DHEA appear to be linked to all disease-related causes of premature death, not just cardiovascular disease.[5, 6] The relationship appears to be one of cause and effect. Lower DHEA levels actually cause premature death. Plasma levels of DHEA drop approximately 6.5 micrograms per deciliter of blood for each year of life. Men in their 70s have DHEA levels 10–20 percent lower than men in their 20s. And men with higher levels live longer.[3]

DHEA works by inhibiting the synthesis of fatty acids and cholesterol. Animal studies have shown that DHEA administration delayed aging, inhibited obesity and lowered cholesterol levels in the blood. The implication is clear: though DHEA levels might naturally decrease with age, supplementation can keep them high enough to delay the effects of aging.

The British Herbal Pharmacopoeia recognizes wild yam root as a spasmolytic, mild diaphoretic, anti-inflammatory, anti-rheumatic and cholagogue, for use in the treatment of intestinal colic, diverticulitis, rheumatoid arthritis, muscular rheumatism, cramps, intermittent claudication, cholecystitis, dysmenorrhea, and ovarian and uterine pain. Bilious colic and rheumatoid arthritis are specific indications for the use of yam.[14]

SAFETY DATA

The use of wild yam as a food supplement in normally recommended amounts is safe. Users of larger amounts may run the risk of metabolic changes due to the presence of dietary DHEA. Pregnant women should avoid it. DHEA may interfere with the metabolism of alcohol and barbiturates in the liver. ·

REFERENCES

1. Gordon, G. and Bush, D. *New England Journal of Medicine*, 315, 1519-1524, 1986.

2. Drucker, W.D., Blumberg, J.M., et al. "Biologic activity of dehydroepiandrosterone sulfate in man." *Journal of Clinical Endocrinology*, 35, 48-54, 1972.

3. Simonova, J., Gregorova, I. and Sonka, J. "Metabolicke komplekace otylosti-pokus o jejich ovlivneni dehydroepiandrosteron sulfatem." *Sbornik Lek.*, 75, 27-30, 1973.

4. Fassati, P., Fassati, M., et al. "Treatment of stabilized liver cirrhosis by dehydroepiandrosterone sulphate." *Agressologie*, 14(4), 259-268, 1973.

5. Sonka, J., et al. "Defekt des dehydroepiandrosteron—ein neues syndrom?" *Endokrinologie*, 47, 152-161, 1965.

6. Sonka, J., et al. "Serum lipids and dehydroepiandrosterone excretion in normal subjects." *Journal of Lipid Research*, 9, 769-772, 1968.

7. Coleman, D.L., Leiter, E.H. and Applezweig, N. "Therapeutic effects of dehydroepiandrosterone metabolites in diabetes mutant mice." *Endocrinology*, 115, 239-243, 1984.

8. Gansler T.S., Muller, S. and Cleary, M.P. "Chronic administration of dehydroepiandrosterone sulphate reduces pancreatic beta-cell hyperplasia and hyperinsulinemia in genetically obese zucker rats." *Proc. Soc. Exp. Biol. Med.*, 180, 155-162, 1985.

9. Sokolova, L.H. "Effect of saponins on the development of experimental atherosclerosis." *Farmakologia i Toxikologia*, 21(6), 85-90, 1958.

10. Shulutko, I.B., Tugbaeva, L.Y. and Nesterov, V.A. "Therapeutic efficiency of dioscorea saponins in the treatment of patients with atherosclerosis." *Drugs of Plant Origin*, A.D. Turlova (ed.), Moscow: Medgiz, 1962, pp. 143-145. (In Russian.)

11. Sokolova, L.N., Kichenko, V.I., et al. "Diosponine—a new drug for treatment of patients with atherosclerosis." *Med. Prom.*, 7, 43-48, 1961. (In Russian.)

12. Weiss, R.F. *Herbal Medicine*. Beaconsfield Publishers, Beaconsfield, England, 1988, pp. 330-331.

13. Lewis, D.A. *Anti-inflammatory Drugs from Plant and Marine Sources*, Birkhouse Verlag, Berlin, 1989, pp. 201-202.

14. British Herbal Pharmacopoeia, British Herbal Medicine Association, West Yorks, England, 1983, pp. 78-79.

ECHINACEA
(Echinacea sp.)

Often overlooked amid all the attention echinacea draws as an immunotonic is this herb's profound effect on maintaining and healing the connective tissues of the body. By inhibiting the enzyme hyaluronidase, echinacea prevents the pathogenic destruction of connective tissue. It also stimulates the repair of connective tissue by marshaling all the forces that typically regulate that process. These actions and others are reviewed in greater detail in the section on echinacea in the chapter on the immune system. While reading that information, keep in mind how important all those actions are in regard to musculoskeletal health.

LICORICE ROOT
(Glycyrrhiza glabra)

Licorice can be recommended for just about everybody, for male and female alike, young and old, well or sick. It is the grand tonic of the world, in this author's opinion.

For that reason, I recommend it as an important tonic in the maintenance of the musculoskeletal system. The amazing anti-inflammatory actions of licorice root extend to the entire surface area of the body, both outside and inside. Not only the skin, but the mucous membranes of the gastrointestinal tract yield to the soothing and healing action of licorice root. The plant reinforces the body's ability to withstand attack from virtually any kind of pathogen, and should therefore be considered a tonic for the musculoskeletal system.

If one is looking for a broad-spectrum tonic to protect, maintain health, and heal injuries, there is no herb better than licorice root. For a full discussion of this plant, the reader is referred to the chapter on the immune system.

SARSAPARILLA
(Smilax sp.)

Smilax has enjoyed a long reputation as a blood purifier and tonic. One of the characteristics of herbal medicine is the belief that while the body is experiencing the healing process, waste materials accumulate rapidly in the blood. If the accumulation occurs more rapidly than the body can get rid of the debris, toxins and metabolic wastes, congestion occurs. The congestion interferes with the delivery of nutrient substances to the site of healing and thereby retards recovery; the congestion may also lead to other problems involving autointoxication, constipation, acne, etc.

The blood purifier is an herb that facilitates the removal of wastes from the blood, either by promoting better circulation, or improving liver and kidney action, or by insuring regular bowel movements, or by opening the pores of the skin. One of the most dramatic indications of a blood purifier at work is the rapidity with which many kinds of skin problems clear up. Smilax, for example, has been shown to have a dramatic impact on the rate of healing of psoriasis.[1]

The tonic action of smilax contributes to the overall health of the entire body in ways not yet discovered, but often observed. For a further review of smilax, the reader is referred to the chapter on the male reproductive system.

SAFETY DATA

Smilax has never been known to display toxicity, even with long-term use.

REFERENCES

1. Thurman, F.M. "The treatment of psoriasis with sarsaparilla compound." *New England Journal of Medicine*, 227, 128-133, 1942.

CHAPTER SIX

The Female Reproductive System

✿ The female reproductive system comprises the organs that allow women to produce ova (eggs), to have sexual intercourse, to take care of and nourish a fertilized ovum until it develops into a full grown fetus, and to give birth.

Most of the female reproductive organs lie within the pelvic cavity. Every month ova are released from the ovaries of sexually mature women. The ovaries are two small egg-shaped glands. They also secrete sex hormones such as estrogen and progesterone which control the reproductive or menstrual cycle. Another important reproductive structure is the uterus, a hollow, pear-shaped organ lying between the bladder and the rectum. The ova are carried to the uterus via the fallopian tubes. If they unite with a spermatozoon on this journey, fertilization takes place.

Sperm reach the fallopian tubes from the vagina, a muscular chamber at the bottom of the birth canal, by way of the cervix, which projects into the top of the vagina.

PUBERTY

Fertility begins at puberty. It is signaled by the onset of menstruation. (It ends with the cessation of menstruation, i.e., at menopause.) Puberty is that time when secondary sexual characteristics appear and sexual organs mature, allowing reproduction to take place. Physical and emotional changes characterize puberty and adolescence, which occur somewhere between 10 and 15 years of age. It is initiated by pituitary hormones known as gonadotropins; these stimulate the ovaries to begin or increase secretion of estrogen hormones.

Secondary sexual characteristics in girls include development of breasts, pubic and underarm hair, widening of the pelvis, increases in fat, and the onset of menstruation. Puberty is said to be complete when menstrual periods become regular and predictable.

MORE ON ESTROGENS AND PROGESTERONE

One of the two main groups of hormones essential for female sexual development and healthy functioning of the reproductive system, estrogens play an important role in the total health of a woman during her life from puberty on. Estrogens are produced mainly in the ovaries, but to some degree in the adrenals. During pregnancy, they may be produced in the placenta. Progesterone increases the deposition of fats and increases the production of sebum in the glands of the skin.

Progesterone, produced in the ovaries, is also an important hormone for the health of the female reproductive system. It is produced during the second half of the menstrual cycle, and by the placenta during pregnancy. Following ovulation, progesterone levels increase and cause the endometrium (the lining of the uterus) to thicken in preparation for receiving an ovum that has been fertilized. Should fertilization not occur, the production of progesterone and estrogen decreases and the endometrium is shed along with the unfertilized egg during menstruation.

Progesterone assures that a fetus develops in a healthy manner by maintaining the health of the placenta. A fall in progesterone at the end of pregnancy helps initiate labor.

MENSTRUATION

Menstruation refers to the cyclical shedding of the endometrium or uterus lining. It is indicated by bleeding. Menstruation occurs only during the fertile years of a woman's life (puberty to menopause). When the body stops producing eggs or ova, menstruation ceases.

Menstruation is under the control of hormones, estrogen during the first part of the cycle, progesterone during the second half. Other hormones regulate specific parts of the menstrual cycle.

The story begins in the ovaries, almond-shaped glands that lie on either side of the uterus. The ovaries contain cavities known as follicles in which egg cells develop. The ovaries produce most of the body's supply of female sex hormones.

The ovaries lie just below openings in the fallopian tubes. Mature eggs from the ovaries enter the fallopian tubes following ovulation. Ovulation refers to the development and release of an ovum from a follicle. It is regulated by hormones, and occurs midway through the menstrual cycle. Follicle stimulating hormone (FSH) is responsible for stimulating the growth of the ova during the first half of the cycle. Then luteinizing hormone (LH) kicks in and stimulates the release of just one ovum (normally). Then the follicle forms a mass of tissue called the corpus luteum that in turn secretes progesterone during the second half of the cycle (see above).

Once the ovum enters the fallopian tube it travels along until met by a sperm traveling up the tube from the uterus. If none happens to be there during transit of the tube, the ovum is shed during menstruation. The fallopian tube is about three inches long and is lined with fingerlike projections called fimbriae, and hairlike projections called cilia, that sweep the ovum along. Muscular contractions of the fallopian tubes themselves also help the egg along in its journey toward the uterus, a trip that lasts about two weeks.

MENOPAUSE

Technically, this term refers to the cessation of menstruation as a result of decreased estrogen production, but it actually covers a sometimes quite lengthy period of time when menstruation becomes relatively irregular and the production of female sex hormones goes through periodic fluctuations in intensity and quality. The result might be a decade of unsettling physiological and psychological symptoms.

Somewhere in a woman's life, usually between the ages of 45 and 55, the follicles cease to produce ova; this leads to a decrease in estrogen production. Without the influence of estrogen, an increase in the level of gonadotropin hormones and androgens may occur. More than half of menopausal women experience hot flashes and night sweats to one degree or another. These symptoms may last for up to five or more years. Over 20 percent will experience significant vaginal dryness. In all women, the vagina itself will shrink and lose elasticity and become more susceptible to infection.

During and after menopause, the skin thins and dries as the sebaceous glands lose much of their capacity to secrete oils. This leads to a drying out and increase in brittleness of body and scalp hair.

One of the most troublesome aspects of menopause is the loss of calcium from the bones. Over a period of several years this can lead to severe osteoporosis (brittle bones). Menopause may also produce hypertension and hypercholesterolemia (increase in blood cholesterol levels) which may, in turn, produce atherosclerosis and increase the risk of stroke or coronary heart disease.

One of the more serious constellations of health problems women face during their lives occurs following menopause. Without the continued production of estrogens, the vagina may dry up, the skin lose its natural softness, the breasts sag, hot flashes increase, and the bones lose their strength (osteoporosis). Many women elect to ingest synthetic estrogens to help counteract these changes. Unfortunately, the side effects from these drugs can also be damaging. Breast tenderness and enlargement, bloating, weight gain, nausea, reduced sex drive, depression, headaches, and vaginal bleeding are common. They also increase the risk of blood clots (which could precipitate strokes), and increase the tendency toward hypertension.

In menopause, progesterone drugs are usually combined with the estrogen drugs to reduce the risks of cancer of the uterus from the estrogens, but progesterone drugs themselves have unpleasant side effects, including headache, swelling, weight gain, loss of appetite, dizziness, blackouts, rash, irregular periods, breast tenderness, and ovarian cysts.

The use of herbs helps many women avoid the necessity of using estrogenic and progesteronic drugs.

DISORDERS OF THE FEMALE REPRODUCTIVE SYSTEM

Amenorrhea

Amenorrhea is the lack of menstruation. It can be primary (menses having never occurred) or secondary (menses not occurring in someone who has had regular periods before). Primary amenorrhea may be the result of the large inherent variability in the normal age of onset of puberty, from 11 to 14 (there are factors that can increase that range to 10-17 or older, such as activity in sports or dance, weight loss, illness, stress, anxiety and depression). Primary amenorrhea may also result from endocrine system problems, such as a pituitary or adrenal tumor, or hypothyroidism, or Turner's syndrome, in which one female sex chromosome is missing, and there are other rare causes.

Secondary amenorrhea can be caused by pregnancy, the period following pregnancy, menopause, stress, strenuous physical activity, illness, sudden change in lifestyle, and use of birth control pills. There are other causes that indicate serious underlying illness; if you suspect this is the case, see a doctor immediately.

Menorrhagia

This condition is defined as heavy periods in which more than average amounts (2 fluid ounces) of blood are lost. Menorrhagia may be the rule in some women, but for most women bleeding should cease in about five days, with the heaviest loss occurring during the first three days. The first question you need to answer is "Have my periods always been heavy?" If the answer is yes, then the cause may be something as simple as a thicker-than-usual lining of the uterus. If your answer is no, then the next question is "Might the use of an IUD be responsible?" If the answer is no, and if you have had only one heavy period, and if that period was also somewhat late in arriving, the probability is good, though not extremely high, that you just experienced an early miscarriage (but sometimes a normal period can be late and heavy).

If your periods have become not only heavier but also more painful, this may be an indication of fibroids (benign growths) of the uterus, or endometriosis. If your periods have become not only heavier, but are lasting longer than they used to, fibroids may again be the problem.

Dysmenorrhea

Dysmenorrhea refers to painful periods. Many women experience it, usually as cramps in the lower abdomen. Such pain is seldom a sign of ill health, but if the pain is much greater than normal, it can be a signal of something going wrong. If the pain has recently become much more severe than normal, you first need to rule out the possibility of IUD-induced pain. If your periods have become heavier than normal, as well as more painful, endometriosis may be indicated.

If the pain is accompanied by lower back pain usually occurring between periods and/or by abnormal vaginal discharge, this may indicate an infection of the fallopian tubes.

If none of these syndromes seems to apply, then your pain may be normal for you, but that doesn't mean you have to live with it. The use of tonic herbs and herbal analgesics may bring significant relief.

Metrorrhagia

This is a somewhat archaic term for irregular vaginal bleeding, i.e., at times other than during the normal menstrual period. The periods may themselves be irregular, or the bleeding may occur between regular periods. Irregular periods can be expected during the time following the onset of puberty and just before menopause. They can also occur occasionally for unknown reasons, perhaps related to diet and stress. Bleeding between periods can be a sign of serious problems and must not be taken lightly. Also, vaginal bleeding during pregnancy should be brought to the attention of your physician.

If the bleeding is like that of your normal period and you are over 40, it probably signals the approach of menopause.

If the bleeding is not like normal, and it only occurs following intercourse, it may signal some minor abnormality of the cervix or it could signal more serious cervical disease. Obtain a diagnosis. If you are over 40, and it has been several months since your last regular period, it may mean you have entered menopause, or it may signal the presence of anything from a minor vaginal disorder to cervical cancer. Obtain a diagnosis immediately. An IUD will often cause spotting between periods. In and of itself, such bleeding is no cause for alarm.

Ovarian Cysts, Cancer and Other Disorders

These are abnormal, fluid-filled swellings occurring in the ovary. They are usually benign, and many disappear without treatment. They may cause abdominal discomfort, painful intercourse and menstrual problems (amenorrhea, menorrhagia and dysmenorrhea). More serious cysts may require surgical removal.

The symptoms of ovarian cancer may resemble those of cysts, but it is much more dangerous. Ovarian cancer is the fourth leading cause of death by cancer in women. If you suspect the presence of cancer, obtain a competent diagnosis.

Turner's syndrome is a rare chromosomal abnormality that results in the absence or failure of normal development of the ovaries. Oophoritis is a simple inflammation of the ovaries and may be caused by the mumps virus or other infections. About one out of 20 women will experience ovarian failure in which the ovaries simply cease to work; this often results in premature menopause.

Disorders of the fallopian tubes

Salpingitis is the term used to refer to inflammatory disorders of the fallopian tubes that usually occur following bacterial infections. Salpingitis is a common cause of infertility.

Ectopic pregnancy is the development of an embryo outside of the uterus. It usually occurs in the fallopian tube. The tube may rupture and hemorrhage as a result.

Endometriosis

Endometriosis is a condition in which fragments of the lining of the uterus, endometrium, attach to and begin to grow on parts of the body outside of the uterus. They are usually found on organs within the pelvic cavity. Endometriosis is most common in women between the ages of 25 and 40, and may often cause infertility. The fragments probably find their way into the pelvic cavity by traveling up the fallopian tubes and out into the cavity. The problem is that these pieces of endometrium continue to respond to the menstrual cycle as if they were still in the uterus, and during menstruation begin to bleed. The blood has nowhere to go and its accumulation usually leads to the formation of painful cysts.

Premenstrual syndrome (PMS)

PMS is the constellation of physical and emotional symptoms that occur in many women during the week or two before menstruation. It usually begins in conjunction with ovulation and continues until the onset of menstruation. It is estimated that more than 90 percent of all women will experience PMS at some time during their reproductive years. The syndrome can be serious enough to interfere with social and work relationships. Symptoms include but are not limited to severe tension, irritability, fatigue, depression, headaches, backaches and stomachaches.

A Nobel prize will probably go to the person who discovers a certain cure for PMS. Until then we must muddle along as best we can. Dozens of theories of PMS abound and hundreds of different treatments have been suggested. But the ultimate cause is not understood, and a treatment that works for every woman has not been invented. Here are some of more effective steps: avoidance of salt, caffeine and chocolate; supplements of vitamins B6 and E, evening primrose oil, oral contraceptives (they work by eliminating the normal menstrual cycle), and progesterone. Megavitamin therapy is popular. The use of tonic herbs works for many women.

Vaginal yeast infections

PMS is a serious concern, but equally distressing to many women are periodic, sometimes continuous bouts of vaginal infection, usually due to a fungus known as *Candida albicans*. This infection is also known as candidiasis, and occurs in the mucous membranes. When it occurs in the mouth, it is known as thrush. Candida is a normally occurring microorganism of the vagina and mouth, but its growth is usually controlled by the presence of bacteria. During antibiotic therapy these bacteria can be destroyed, thereby allowing the fungus to grow uncontrolled. A weakened immune system, especially in patients with AIDS, in patients being treated with immunosuppressant drugs, and in persons with chronic immune problems such as chronic fatigue syndrome, etc., may also create conditions that encourage the growth of Candida. Other conditions that foster growth of the fungus are diabetes, pregnancy, and birth control pills. Antifungal drugs are a popular, although often unsatisfactory, treatment. Alternative measures emphasize dietary factors and the use of antifungal herbs.

❧ HERBAL TONICS FOR THE FEMALE REPRODUCTIVE SYSTEM

Tonic herbs can be very useful to women in the prevention and treatment of menstrual disorders to help stimulate the onset of menstruation, control its flow, regulate the cycle, and make it less painful. These herbs should serve as adjuncts to good diagnostic procedures, clinical treatment, and food supplements.

Herbal tonics are well suited for aiding treatment of menstrual problems because they are mild-acting, do not drastically affect the hormonal balance of the body, and may help restore normal function.

One should try to use both single herbs and herbal combinations. Combining herbs assures the gradual accumulation of active principles from each herb without a concomitant rise in concentration of any unwanted constituents that may reside in any one plant. For example, licorice root may be used for almost all female complaints; yet the use of copious amounts of this herb may lead to hypertension in some people. You can avoid this problem and still get excellent physiological activity by combining moderate amounts of licorice root with other herbs. Likewise, there are herbs that may relax the uterus in small amounts and cause cramps in large amounts. By combining small amounts of each of these herbs you get an increasing relaxant effect without the risk of cramps.

Combining also draws upon the possibilities of synergy and other beneficial interactions among the various herbs.

DONG QUAI

(Angelica chinensis, A. polymorpha, A. acutiloba and other members of the Chinese angelica family)

Next to *Panax ginseng*, the root of dong quai is undoubtedly the most honored and respected herb in China, and is quickly gaining an equal reputation among users in the rest of the world. Experts estimate that dong quai has been used by the Chinese for at least 2,000 years. It is described in a pharmacopoeia written in 544 A.D. It is said to have Yin qualities, while ginseng has Yang qualities. Dong quai is used medicinally as a tonic, cardiotonic, respiratory tonic and liver tonic. It is used to promote circulation, to regulate the menstrual cycle and stop discomforts of menstruation. That means it's good for PMS. In Western herbal terms, it is used for dysmenorrhea (painful menstruation), metrorrhagia (too much menstruation) and amenorrhea (too little, or no, menstruation). Dong quai is also often recommended during pregnancy to ease delivery, reduce pain and discomfort and eliminate complications as much as possible. Many Chinese herbal formulas, of ancient origin and generations of use, contain dong quai. Most of the actions of dong quai depend on the presence of coumarins, phytosterols, polysaccharides, and flavonoids.

Dong quai contains phytoestrogens with potential estrogenic action

Dong quai contains estrogenic substances that may exert some regulating effect on estrogen levels and on estrogenic biological mechanisms. They seem to enhance estrogenic effects when estrogen levels are too low, and compete when levels are too high. This would be in keeping with the idea of a menstrual tonic. It is doubtful if dong quai has any direct estrogenic effects.[1,2,9]

Dong quai has smooth muscle relaxing, antibiotic and analgesic properties

Substantial pharmacological research has validated these properties in dong quai. Anticramping, hypotensive, tonic, anti-asthmatic, analgesic, anti-inflammatory and antiarthritic properties in the root have all been demonstrated by basic research. It has also been shown to be effective against several strains of microorganisms, especially fungi such as *Candida albicans*, the primary causative agent in vaginal yeast infections. This constellation of properties would help explain the plant's sometimes dramatic effect on the PMS symptoms.[1,5,7,9]

Dong quai has opposing (tonic) actions on the uterus and other medicinal effects

Two fractions of dong quai have opposite actions on the uterus. The volatile oil inhibits contractions, while the non-volatile component stimulates them. In a lengthy series of studies, Chinese physicians have determined that several formulas based on dong quai were effective in a variety of clinical situations, including amenorrhea, dysmenorrhea, sterility, susceptibility to miscarriage, uterine bleeding, uterine convulsions, anemia, ovarian functional disorders, climacteric disorders, blood stasis and toxemia of pregnancy.[13,4,8,9]

Dong quai enhances metabolic and humoral actions

In animal studies dong quai enhanced metabolism, increased oxygen utilization in the liver, and increased the metabolism of glutamic acid and cysteine. It was suggested that these effects depended on the presence of vitamin B12 and folic acid in the preparation. Dong quai also reduced or prevented vitamin E deficiency-induced disease in rats. These results again suggest reasons why dong quai is effective in treating PMS.[14,7,9]

Dong quai has cardiovascular properties

Studies have shown that dong quai is hypotensive through a dilation of blood vessels. This action is attributed to coumarins, which have been shown in other studies to dilate coronary arteries, possibly by blocking calcium channels. Coumarins also act as vasodilators and antispasmodics; however, some may act as central nervous system stimulants. One part of dong quai's tonic effect is thus explainable. Dong quai also inhibits platelet aggregation, probably through the presence of ferulic acid.[1,9,12–14]

Dong quai has immune-system enhancing properties

An antiallergy property of dong quai has been investigated fairly thoroughly. The plant operates in one way by stimulating B lymphocytes and T lymphocytes. Related coumarins have also demonstrated considerable immune-enhancing effects; it is reasonable on that basis to assume that dong quai also possesses such properties. Among those effects is the ability to enhance and activate white blood cells. The polysaccharides in dong quai have also been implicated in immune stimulation. They stimulate interferon production, leukocyte production and have anti-cancer properties.[3,5,6,10,11,13]

SAFETY DATA

Cases of dong quai toxicity are quite rare, and very mild when they are reported. Some people appear to be allergic. Due to presence of coumarins, some persons may become photosensitized and develop dermatitis.[14]

In a decision that borders on the incredible, the Canadian government has banned the sale of dong quai for food use in that country.

REFERENCES

1. Zhu, D.P.Q. "Dong Quai." *American Journal of Chinese Medicine*. 15(3-4), 117-125, 1987.
2. Lou, Z.H. "Abnormal menstruation and pre-menstrual syndrome." *Journal of New Traditional Chinese Medicine*, Kwang Chow TCM College, 5, 47-48, 1984.
3. Kumazawa, Y., Mizunoe, D. and Otsuka, Y. "Immunostimulating polysaccharides separated from hot water extract of angelica acutiloba Kitagawa (Yamato Tohki)." *Immunology*, 47, 75-83, 1982.
4. Yamada, H., Kiyohara, H., et al. "Studies on polysacharides from angelica auctiloba." *Planta Medica*, 48, 163-167, 1984.
5. Yamada, H., Kiyohara, H., et al. "Studies on polysaccharides from angelica acutiloba, IV. Characterization of anticomplementary arabinogalactan from the roots of angelica acutiloba Kitagawa." *Molecular Immunology*, 22, 295-304, 1985.
6. Berkarda, B., Bouffard-Eyuboglu, H. and Derman, U. "The effect of coumarin derivatives on the immunological system of man." *Agents and Actions*, 13, 50-52, 1983.
7. Ohno, N., Matsumoto, SI., Suzuki, I., et al. "Biochemical characterization of a mitogen obtained from an oriental crude drug, tohki (angelica acutiloba Kitagawa)." *J. Pharm. Dyn.*, 6, 903-912, 1983.
8. Harada, M., Suzuki, M. and Ozaki, Y. "Effect of Japanese an-

gelica root and peony root on uterine contraction in the rabbit in situ." *J. Pharm. Dyn.*, 7, 304-311, 1984.

9. Yoshira, K. "The physiological actions of tang kuei and cnidium." *Bulletin of the Oriental Healing Arts Institute*, 10, 269-278, 1985.

10. Sung, C.P., Baker, A.P., et al. "Effects of angelica polymorpha on reaginic antibody production." *Journal of Natural Products*, 45, 398-406, 1982.

11. Haranaka, K., Satomi, N., et al. "Antitumor activities and tumor necrosis factor producibility of traditional Chinese medicines and crude drugs." *Cancer Immunol. Immunother.*, 20(1), 1-5, 1985.

12. Xu, L.N., Yin, Z.Z. and Lin, M. "The antithrombotic effect of Dang Gui (angelica senensis) injection and its clinical trial." In *Abstracts of International Symposium on Traditional Medicine and Modern Pharmacology*, Beijing, 1986, p. 104.

13. Hsu, H.Y. "Application of Chinese herbal formulas and scientific research. I." *Oriental Healing Arts International Bulletin.*, 11(2), 87-96, 1986.

14. Tu, J.J. "Effects of radix angelicae sinensis on hemorrheology in patients with acute ischemic stroke." *Journal of Traditional Chinese Medicine*, 4(3), 225-228, 1984.

GINGER
(Zingiber officinale)

Ginger root has often been employed in the alleviation of PMS symptoms, nausea during pregnancy, and irregular, painful menstruation. It is perhaps the best medicinal agent for many symptoms experienced by women due to the minor hormonal fluctuations of everyday life, including headaches, dizziness, upset stomach, cramps, and it will help to activate the medicinal properties of other herbs with which it is combined. Ginger tones up most parts of the female reproductive system without causing cramps or other discomforts. Women with PMS routinely express their appreciation for this plant.[1-4]

Other effects of ginger root are noteworthy, though not directly applicable to the female reproductive system. For a review of some of these see the chapter on the digestive system.

Ginger root eliminates and prevents nausea

See the section on ginger in the chapter on the digestive system for a discussion of ginger root's use in the treatment of nausea, including morning sickness.

SAFETY DATA

Large doses of zingerone, a constituent of ginger root, have produced experimental toxicity in lab animals, but the ingestion of zingerone as found in ginger root poses no threat to health. It is generally regard as safe by the FDA.

REFERENCES

1. Mowrey, D.B. *The Scientific Validation of Herbal Medicine*, Keats Publishing, New Canaan, Conn. 1986.
2. Backon, J. "Ginger: inhibition of thromboxane synthetase and stimulation of prostacyclin: relevance for medicine and psychiatry." *Med. Hypoth.*, 20, 271-278, 1986.
3. Mustafa, T. and Srivastava, K.C. "Ginger (zingiber officinale) in migraine headache." *J. Ethnopharmacol.*, 29, 267-273, 1990.
4. Suekaswa, M., et al. "Pharmacological studies on ginger. I. Pharmacological actions of pungent constituents, (6)-gingerol and (6)-shogaol." *J. Pharm. Dyn.*, 7, 836-848, 1984.

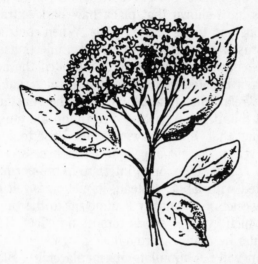

BLACK HAW

BLACK HAW and CRAMP BARK
(Viburnum prunifolium, V. opulis)

Black haw first came to the attention of the medical establishment when early American physicians observed its use by the North American Indians, who used it primarily as a uterine tonic and as an effective treatment for menstrual disorders. Early American physicians became extraordinarily proficient in the application of the herb and recommended it to women of all ages to tone the entire reproductive system. Black haw was official in most pharmacopoeias during the 19th century for the treatment of dysmenorrhea, threatened abortion and asthma.

Black haw bark has spasmolytic and uterine relaxant properties

A series of *in vitro* and *in vivo* tests on guinea pig, rat and human uterus have shown that black haw bark extracts reduce the contractions and tonus of the uterus. When contractile activity in the uterus was induced with estrogen injections, crude extracts of black haw bark significantly inhibited the action. The researchers then isolated at least four principles that were very active uterine relaxants. It appeared that the substances selectively relaxed the uterus by acting directly on the muscle. These results indicate that black haw inhibits hypertonicity of the uterus. However, it doesn't appear to cause excessive relaxation in a uterus of normal tone, or to interfere in the normal contractions associated with labor. Instead, its action is felt during the months and weeks of pregnancy leading up to the time of delivery, during which event it exerts almost no effect. Thus it will help relieve uterine cramps throughout pregnancy (and at other times also) but will not stimulate uterine flaccidity. Black haw is now commonly used in Europe, where herbalists maintain that it stabilizes the tonus of the uterus and reduces the severity of contractions.[1-6]

Black haw would be expected to help women recover and maintain normal function in the uterus. It should be particularly effective where there is a history of menstruation disorders, PMS, anemia of pregnancy, disrupted menstrual cycles, and disorders of sexual performance.

Black haw bark may prevent threatened abortions

In 19th-century Canada and the United States black haw was used to halt the course of threatened abortions. It is still used for that purpose in Europe, where prominent naturopaths enthusiastically endorse its use, even to the point of using it to counteract the effects of abortifacient drugs.

Crampbark has many of the same properties as black haw

The Indians also used the bark of another species of viburnum to remedy the complaints associated with what we now call PMS and the severe cramps of labor. This plant was so effective that they called it crampbark. It is generally used in much the same manner as black haw bark: as a uterine sedative, antispasmodic and emmenagogue, and to relieve spasmodic muscular cramps, uterine and ovarian pain and dysfunction, metrorrhagia of menopause, and threatened miscarriage.

Crampbark contains most of the same chemicals as black haw bark and would therefore be expected to have much the same characteristic action. Since the Indians used the two together, and since early American physicians and current European physicians have respected that tradition, the two are recommended by this author also.

SAFETY DATA

Black haw and crampbark possess no known toxicity. The berries are poisonous. Use of bark only is recommended.

REFERENCES

1. Hale, E.M. *The Special Symptomatology of the New Remedies.* Philadelphia, 1877, citation for Viburnum.

2. Youngken, H.W. *Textbook of Pharmacognosy.* 5th ed. Blakiston, Philadelphia, 1943, citation for Viburnum.

3. List, P.H. and Hoerhammer, L. *Hagers Handbuch der Pharmazeutischen Praxis.* Volumes 2-5, Springer-Verlag. Berlin, 1968-1979, citation for Viburnum.

4. Hoehammer, L., Wagner, H. and Reinhardt, H. "Chemistry, pharmacology and pharmaceutics of the components from vibur-

num prunifolium and V. opulus." *Botanical Magazine* (Tokyo), 79, 510-525, 1966.

5. Hoerhammer, L., Wagner, H. and Reinhardt, H. "New methods in pharmacognosy, XI. Chromatographic evaluation of commercial viburnum drugs." *Deutsche Apotheker Zeitung*, 105(4), 1371-1372, 1965.

6. Jarboe, C.H., Schmidt, C.M., Nicholson, J.A. and Zirvi, K.A. "Uterine relaxant properties of viburnum." *Nature*, 212(5064), 837, 1966.

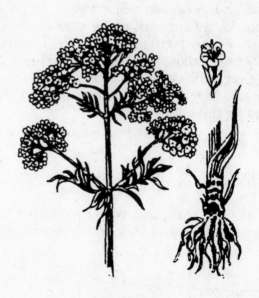

VALERIAN

VALERIAN ROOT
(Valeriana officinalis)

Valerian root has been used for centuries to calm upset nerves, treat mood problems, pain, headache and various other symptoms that remind one of PMS. It achieved great notoriety in 18th-century Europe as a cure for female hysteria, or "vapors," in young girls and in the elderly. In medieval times, valerian was so popular it became known as "all-heal." It is currently one of the most popular orthodox antispasmodic medications in Russia, Germany and other parts of the world, including North America.

The root is used to treat insomnia, nervous tension, anxiety, muscle cramps and spasm, muscle pain, headache, stress, menstrual pain and discomfort, hysteria, epilepsy (as an anticonvulsant), autonomic nervous disorders of all kinds (including hypochondria), hypertension, a wide variety of gastrointestinal disorders, and so forth. In herbal terms, it is antispasmodic (muscle relaxant), calmative (sedative, depressant), a nervine (tranquilizer), carminative (good for upset stomach and digestion) and anodyne (pain reliever).

Valerian root relieves cramps, menstrual discomfort and PMS

Menstrual pain and discomfort will yield to valerian root best if caused or aggravated by nervousness. High-strung people experiencing PMS will benefit more from valerian root than women whose PMS is more organic in nature.[1] The same applies to gastrointestinal problems such as dyspepsia and ulcers. Valerian targets the nervous system components of these and other conditions. Stress, muscle spasms, nervous exhaustion, headaches with nervous components, heart problems involving nervous tension, insomnia, and even whooping cough are the kind of disorders for which valerian is best suited.[2,6,7]

Valerian root counteracts the effects of stress

Clinical observations of the last couple of decades have almost uniformly shown that valerian root preparations appear to stabilize the autonomic nervous system in psychosomatic patients and those with disorders of the autonomic nervous system. These kinds of disorders are rarely diagnosed in the United States. In Germany, however, clinicians are more sensitive to subtle dysfunctions of the autonomic nervous system, and recognize these as the basis for a great many cases of functional insufficiency including anxiety, insomnia, hysteria, ulcers, exaggerated nervousness, PMS, post-menopausal depression, etc. Valerian root products produce a clear increase in performance coupled with moderate sedation; therefore, motor coordination, concentration ability and reasoning skills increase, but without any hypnotic or depressive symptoms.[1,2,3,8] These effects may be summarized as stress reduction.[4] In one German study with 70 hospitalized patients diagnosed as having dysregulation of the autonomic nervous system arising from various causes, valerian extract suppressed and regulated all symptoms, and produced a mildly relaxing sedative effect; it was especially effective in relieving symptoms of restlessness and tension.[5]

SAFETY DATA

Whole standardized, guaranteed potency valerian root is without toxicity. Purified extracts of the root may contain high concentrations of specific constituents for which safety data is not known.

REFERENCES

1. Broeren, W. *Pharmakopsychiatr. Neuropharmakol.*, 2, 1, 1969.
2. Straube, C. "The meaning of valerian root in therapy." *Therapie der Gegenwart*, 107, 555-562, 1968. (In German.)
3. Buchtala, M. *Hippokrates*, 12, 466-468, 1969.
4. Moser, L. "Medicine for stress behind the wheel?" *Deutsche Apotheker Zeitung*, 121, 2651-2654, 1981.
5. Boeters, U. "Behandlung vegetativer regulationsstoerungen mit valepotriaten." *Muenchener Medizinishce Wochenschrift*, 37, 1873-1876, 1969.
6. Tresser, V.E. "Psychopharmaka in der HNO-Praxis - Erfah-

rungen mit einem neuartigen phyto-ataraktikum." *Hippokrates: Zeitschrift fuer Praktische Heilkunde*, 40, 314-316, 1969.

7. Dumnova, A.G. "Treatment of primary arterial hypertension in children and adolescents." *Pediatriya*, 50(11), 79-81, 1971. (In Russian.)

8. Kempinskas, V. "On the action of valerian." *Farmakologiia i Toksikologiia*, 2, 305-309, 1964. (In Russian.)

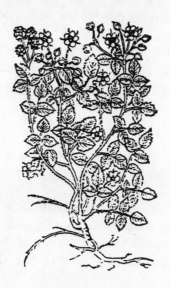

RED RASPBERRY

RED RASPBERRY
(Rubus idaeus)

A hot tea preparation of raspberry leaf is said to temper the effects of runaway hormonal production in women, as might occur during menstruation, pregnancy and delivery. Raspberry leaf prevents the typical hypergrowth effects of chronic gonadotrophin on ovaries and uterus, and relaxes uterine muscles. In several species of animals, raspberry tea concentrates relaxed the smooth muscle of the uterus if it was "in tone," and caused contractions in the muscle if it was relaxed. This implies the existence of a normalizing effect in raspberry leaf. The relaxing response would probably ease delivery, a use for which raspberry leaf has been famous for years.

Cold raspberry leaf tea has an antidiarrheal property that is probably due to the astringent tannic acid principles it contains. The ability of the herb to remedy extreme laxity of the bowels may be due to a combination of the astringent property and the effects of the herb on smooth muscle. The astringent principles are also responsible for the herb's external effectiveness in treating sores, itches and so forth, and for the effectiveness of a strong tea as a refreshing gargle and mouthwash. The astringency of this herb is also exploited in the treatment of dysentery, internal bleeding, ulcers and chronic skin disease.[1,2]

Raspberry leaf has normalizing effects on the uterus

Experiments in which gonadotrophin was administered chronically to young female rats, causing increased weight of ovaries and uterus, showed that simple water extracts of raspberry leaf significantly inhibited that effect, even though they did not abolish it.[3,4]

The extracts also diminished contractions of rat uterus and inhibited the effect of TSH on the thyroid gland. Concentrates of an infusion of the dried raspberry leaf were tested on the *in situ* uterus of cat and rabbit and on isolated uterus of the dog, cat, rabbit and guinea pig. *In situ* and isolated intestine was also used. The leaf was shown to contain a principle readily extracted with water which relaxes the smooth muscle of the uterus and intestine when it is in tone, but the same principle (or possibly another) causes contraction of the uterus of the rabbit in situ and of the isolated uteri of the cat, rabbit and guinea pig when these are not in tone. The investigators hypothesize that the relaxation response probably accounts for traditional therapeutic use in menstrual disturbances and during the birth process.[5]

The actions of red raspberry are tonic in the best meaning of that word. The plant can be used to help maintain the tone of the uterus in a position of homeostasis. This can be especially advantageous during bouts of PMS.

SAFETY DATA

Red raspberry leaf has no known toxicity.

REFERENCES

1. List, P.H. and Hoerhammer, L.H. *Hagers Handbuch Der Pharmazeutischen Praxis*, Springer-Verlag, Berlin, 1968-1979, citation for Rubus.
2. Martindale. *The Extra Pharmacopoeia*, The Pharmaceutical Press, London, 1977.
3. Burn, J.H. and Withell, E.R. "A principle in raspberry leaves which relaxes uterine muscles." *The Lancet*, 2 (6149), 13, 1941.
4. Kurzepa, S. and Samojlik, E. "Badanie wplywu wyciagow niektorych roslinrodziny rosaceae na aktywnosc gonadotropowa i tyreotropowa uszczurow." (The effect of extracts from some rosaceae plants upon the gonadotrophic and thyrotrophic activities in rat.) *Endokrynologia Polska*, 15(2), 143-150, 1963.
5. Noble, R.L. The report of the proceedings, Sixth International Conference On Planned Parenthood, 14-21 February, 1959, 243-250, Vigyon Bharan, New Delhi, India.

LICORICE ROOT
(Glycyrrhiza glabra)

Licorice root is one of the most biologically active herbs in the world, wherein it has found extensive therapeutic use. It has also been the subject of an enormous amount of research. Although we are only interested in properties that affect female reproductive physiology, a quick review of the other properties of licorice will be presented to give the reader some idea of the immense potential underlying the frequent ingestion of this plant.

Licorice root is an effective treatment for stomach ailments

Licorice exerts a soothing action on the mucosal surfaces of the GI tract, and is frequently used to help these tissues heal.

Licorice root derivatives, glycyrrhetinic acid (GLA), deglycrrhizinated licorice (DGL), and carbenoxolone sodium (CS) have all been experimentally proven as among the best anti-ulcer medications available. Whole licorice and its derivatives appear to have the ability to inhibit gastric acid secretion with the advantage of being devoid of other adverse anticholinergic properties.[1-3]

CS is the only drug treatment for ulcers that has unequivocally been shown to be effective in man.[4-7] However, CS potentiates the side effects of pure licorice root extract and GLA; therefore many physicians choose to use DGL, which is nearly as effective but exhibits no side effects.[8-13] This author feels that use of *whole* licorice root is probably the wisest course.

Licorice root helps prevent and heal skin problems

The conditions that increase the occurrence of acne-like symptoms during certain stages of the menstrual cycle may be affected by the consumption of licorice root. The anti-inflammatory properties of the root have been considered responsible for its effectiveness in the treatment of numerous skin disorders, including eczemas, dermatitis, impetigo, and traumatized skin. GLA has often been compared to hydrocortisone for its anti-inflammatory action in various skin problems. Other conditions could be listed for which licorice root has been an effective topical treatment, including atopic, subacute and chronic eczematous conditions, itching dermatoses, pruritus, acute impetigo; infantile eczema and eczema; seborrheic, infective, sensitization, contact, neuro-, and exfoliative dermatitis; pustular psoriasis; impetigo; and lichen simplex.[14-23]

It should be mentioned that the antipyretic (fever-reducing) effects of GLA have been shown equal to those of the widely used sodium salicylate.[24-25]

Licorice root has anticholesterol activity

Licorice root and/or its derivatives have been shown to reduce cholesterol levels, but overdose can lead to hypertension and sodium retention. (See the heading "Toxicity" for a discussion.)[26, 27]

Licorice root is used to increase the health of the liver

Assuming that certain symptoms of PMS are caused by the buildup of toxic metabolic substances in the body, licorice root may be useful in increasing the liver's ability to filter out some of these toxins. In the treatment of liver diseases (e.g., hepatitis and cirrhosis), GLA has proven extremely promising. In Chinese medicine, licorice is often used as a remedy for jaundice and is considered a great liver detoxifier. Experimental work has validated the usefulness of licorice in the treatment of hepatitis, cirrhosis, and related liver disorders.[28-32]

Licorice root as an antiasthma agent

The anti-inflammatory effect has been employed in the treatment of asthma, and the herb has proven antitussive and expectorant actions. The demulcent and expectorant properties of licorice are well accepted. For this reason, licorice is often found in cough drops, lozenges and syrups.[33-38]

Licorice is a good tonic for the adrenal glands and Addison's disease

Licorice appears to both mimic and potentiate the action of the adrenal-corticosteroids, though it also differs in action from these chemicals in several important ways.

Licorice components have been found to exert a positive effect on the course of serious adrenal insufficiency, even in Addison's disease, which is characterized by near-total adrenal exhaustion. There is evidence that that effect depends on the presence of a small amount of glucocorticoid. In other words, if the disease has advanced to the stage of complete adrenal exhaustion, licorice will be most beneficial if combined with a small amount of cortisone. Since the traditional treatment is the use of increasingly large amounts of cortisone, the ability to greatly reduce the dosage through the addition of licorice root represents a very attractive alternative.[39-41]

Licorice possesses antiarthritic properties

The antiarthritic property of GLA and of aqueous extracts of licorice have also been shown. Other inflammatory diseases also respond well to licorice root. Comparisons of licorice root to hydrocortisone are frequently made in the medical literature of England, China and other countries.[42-45]

Licorice has antimicrobial action

In relation to the immune system, licorice root and its derivatives have recently shown extremely promising results as interferon inducers, especially in the treatment of hepatitis; the herb finds hepatitis also through other immune-stimulating effects. [46-48]

Glycyrrhizic acid, at concentrations well tolerated by uninfected cells, inhibits both growth and cytopathic effect of vaccinia, herpes simplex, Newcastle disease, and vesicular stomatitis viruses while being ineffective on poliovirus. It is suggested that glycyrrhizic acid interacts with virus structures (conceivably proteins) producing different effects according to the viral stage affected: inactivation of free virus particles extracellularly; prevention of intracellular uncoating of infecting particles; impairment of the assembling ability of virus structural components. [49]

Ethanolic extracts of the powdered roots of commercial licorice showed reproducible antimicrobial activity in vitro against *Staphylococcus aureus*, *Mycobacterium smegmatis* and *Candida albicans*. The use of licorice root continues to be one of the most common treatments for chronic vaginal yeast infection. [50]

Licorice has estrogenic action

Licorice root is often used for its supposed estrogenic properties. As it turns out, 90 percent of the available research shows estrogenic properties, while 10 percent has not found such effects. The first report of licorice root's estrogenic property was made in 1950, when a steroid estrogen with an absorption spectrum identical to estriol was extracted. [51]

Since then, several investigators have found estrogenic activity in licorice root. Stigmasterol and beta-sitosterol have been identified as the probable active components. [52-54]

Licorice root proved to be highly estrogenic as shown by the mouse uterine weight method. With 3 doses of 25 mg each of the alcohol extract, the estrogenic activity was significantly higher than that produced by estradiol monobenzoate. A higher dose of 50 mg daily for 3 days had a lower estrogenic value, which suggests an antihormone factor in the extract. Extracts showed an inhibitory action on the spontaneous movement of the uterus at diestrus, estrus, and pregnancy. [55]

An extract of licorice was found to have a strong estrogenic effect as it increased uterine development in immature rats and acted synergistically with estradiol by intensifying its action on uterine development, when 2 mg of GLA was combined with 0.1 microgram of estradiol.[56,57]

There has been one dissenting voice in the research on the estrogenic properties of licorice root. In this study, GLA was found to be devoid of estrogenic activity in the absence of endogenous estrogen, and, in fact, was antiestrogenic in that it antagonized exogenous estrogen in doses which did not interfere with somatic growth or the estrogenic effect on pituitary trophic hormone.[58] These findings could be evidence for the tonic effect of licorice.

SAFETY DATA

From time to time one reads about purported licorice toxicity. These cases almost invariably involve potent extracts of the plant found in some licorice candies. The tonic property of the plant is absent, and so one action or another is allowed to come through without the balancing action of the other constituents. In passing it should be noted that any potential for toxicity in this herb can be completely counteracted by a simple potassium supplement in the diet.

About 20 percent of the population is sensitive to the effects of ingesting high amounts of licorice extract. In these people, excess potassium is removed from the body, and sodium is retained. The symptoms, mainly hypertension and edema, mimic those that occur when too much of the hormone aldosterone is secreted by the adrenal glands. For this reason the licorice syndrome is called pseudoaldosteronism. Most victims of this condition either ingested large quantities of licorice extract-containing candy, were under treatment with carbenoxolone (an extremely concentrated extract), or had preexisting edematous tendencies which were exacerbated by the licorice candy. (Note that we are talking about European candies here; American licorice contains very little or no licorice extract.)

An illustrative case: A 53-year-old man was admitted to

the hospital exhibiting several of the lesser symptoms of pseudo-aldosteronism. He was a heavy salt and water user so that he was predisposed to having problems, even though he was in otherwise excellent health for his age. He ate 700 grams of licorice candy during the nine days prior to admission, which purportedly pushed him over the edge into pseudoaldosteronism. Minimal treatment was required to restore him to good health.[59]

The sodium and water retention properties of licorice extracts were first noticed in 1946, when a doctor found that about 20 percent of patients treated with these extracts acquired edema. Since then, it has been shown that licorice intoxication is able to induce hypertension with features of primary hypermineralocorticism. The principle of licorice responsible for the syndrome is called glycyrrhetinic acid (GLA).[60-62]

The toxicity of licorice has been greatly exaggerated by well-meaning quasi-herbalists and media types. Candy flavored with licorice extract has led to poisoning in individuals who habitually consumed half a pound to a pound or more daily, and in individuals who, for one reason or another, are extremely sensitive to the licorice extract (as found in ulcer cures and laxatives). But ingestion of the whole herb, as would be found in capsule, tea or stick form, has not resulted in any significant toxicity. Pseudoaldosteronism can be easily prevented by the use of a high-potassium, low-sodium diet. Although no formal trial exists demonstrating an absolute protective effect, patients on carbenoxolone who normally consume high-potassium foods and restrict sodium intake, even those with preexisting hypertension and angina, have been reported to be free from sodium-retaining side effects.[63]

As a general cautionary measure, persons with a history of hypertension, renal failure, or the current use of cardiac glycosides, may wish to avoid the use of licorice root altogether.

REFERENCES

1. Takagi, K., Watanabe K. and Ishii, Y. "Peptic ulcer inhibiting activity of licorice root." *Proc. Int. Pharmacol. Meeting,* 7(2), 1-15, 1965.

2. Anderson, S. "Protective action of deglycyrrhizinised liquorice on occurrence of stomach ulcers." *Scandinavian Journal of Gastroenterology,* 6(8), 683-686.

3. Brogden, R.N., Speight, T.M. and Avery, G.S. "Deglycyrrhizinised liquorice: a report of its pharmacological properties and therapeutic efficacy in peptic ulcer." *Drugs,* 8(5), 330-339, 1974.

4. Lewis, J.R. "Carbenoxolone sodium in the treatment of peptic ulcer." *Journal of the American Medical Association,* 229(4), 460-462, 1974.

5. Sircus, W. "Progress report on carbenoxolone sodium." *Gut,* 13, 816-824, 1972.

6. Nagy, G.S. "Evaluation of carbenoxolone sodium in the treatment of duodenal ucler." *Gastroenterology,* 74, 7-10, 1978.

7. Cliff, J.M. and Milton-Thompson, G.J. "A double blind trial of carbenoxolone capsules in the treatment of duodenal ulcer." *Gut,* 11, 167-170, 1970.

8. Turpie, A.G.G., Runcie, J. and Thompson, T.J. "Clinical trial of deglycyrrhizinated liquorice in gastric ulcer." *Gut,* 10, 299-302, 1969.

9. Anderson, S., Brany, F., Caboda, J.L.F. and Mizuno, T. "Protective action of deglycyrrhizinated licorice on the occurrence of stomach ulcers in pylorous-ligated rats." *Scandinavian Journal of Gastroenterology,* 6, 683-686, 1971.

10. Cooke, W.M. and Baron, J.H. "Metabolic studies on deglycyrrhizinated licorice in two patients with gastric ulcer." *Digestion,* 4, 264-268, 1971.

11. Tewari, S.N. and Wilson, A.K. "Deglycyrrhizinated licorice in duodenal ulcer." *Practitioner,* 210, 820-823, 1973.

12. Millar, J.H.D., et al. *British Medical Journal,* 1, 765, 1973.

13. Wison, J.A.C. "A comparison of carbenoxolone sodium and deglycyrrhizinated liquorice in treatment of gastric ulcer in the ambulant patient." *The British Journal of Clinical Practice,* 26, 563-566, 1972.

14. Adamson, A.C. and Tillman, W.G. "Hydrocortisone." *British Medical Journal,* 1501, Dec 17, 1955.

15 Colin-Jones, E. "Glycyrrhetinic acid." *British Medical Journal,* 161, Jan 19, 1957.

16. Mccallum, D.I. "Glycyrrhetinic acid." *British Medical Journal*, 1239, Nov 24, 1956.

17. Sommerville, J. "Glycyrrhetinic acid." *British Medical Journal*, 282-283, Feb 2, 1957.

18. Kuroyanagi, T. "The effect of prednisolone, 6-mercaptopurine and glycyrrhizin on skin homotransplantation in rats." *Arerugi*, 16(10), 676-679, 1967.

19. Cunitz, G. "On the effect of succus liquiritae.: *Arzneimittel-Forschung*, 18, 434-435, 1968.

20. Tangri, K.K., Seth, P.K., Parmar, S.S. and Bhargava, K.P. "Biochemical study of the antiinflammatory and antiarthritic properties of glycyrrhetic acid." *Biochem. Pharmacol.*, 14(8), 1277-1281, 1965.

21. Nikitina, S.S. "Data on the mechanism of anti-inflammatory action by glycyrrhizic acid and glycyrrhetic acid from glycyrrhiza." *Farmikol. I Toksikol.*, 29(1), 67-70, 1966.

22. Amagaya, S., Sugishita, E., et al. "Comparative studies of the stereoisomers of glycyrrhetinic acid on anti-inflammatory activities. *Journal Pharm. Dyn.*, 7, 923-928, 1984.

23. Nasyrov, K.M. and Lazareva, D.N. "Study of the anti-inflammatory activity glycyrrhizin acid derivatives." *Farmakol. i Toksiko.*, 43(4), 399-404, 1980.

24. Saxen, R.C. and Ghalla, T.N. "Antipyretic effect of glycyrrhetic acid and imipramine." *Japanese Journal of Pharmacology*, 18(3), 353-355, 1968.

25. Aleshenshaya, E.E., Aleshkina, Y.A., et al. "Pharmacology of glycyrrhiza glabra (licorice) preparations." *Farmikol. i Toksikol.*, 27(2), 217-222, 1964.

26. Donomae, I. "Gycyrhizzin acid." *Nippon Rinsho*, 19, 1369-1372, 1960.

27. Nakamura, M.Y., Ishiara, T., et al. "Effects of dietary magnesium and glycyrhizzin on experimental atheromatosis of rats." *Japanese Heart Journal*, 7(5), 474-486, 1966.

28. Ichioka, H. "The pharmacological action of glycyrrhizin. III. The effect on the bile secretion in rabbits." *Gifu Daigaku Igakubu Kiyo,* Gigu University School of Medicine, 15(3), 810-812, 1968.

29. Ichioka, H. "The pharmacological action of glycyrrhizin. II. The effect on urinary excretion of bilirubin in rabbits' ligated common bile duct." *Gifu Daigaku Igakubu Kiyo*, Gifu University School of Medicine, 15(3), 580-589, 1968.

30. Ichioka, H. "The pharmacological action of glycyrrhizin. I. The effect on the blood bilirubin level in rabbits ligated common bile duct." *Gifu Daigaku Igakubu Kiyo*, Gifu University School of Medicine, 15(3), 792, 1968.

31. Zhao, M.Q., Han, D.W., Ma, X.H., Zhao, Y.C., Yin, L. and Li, C.M. "The preventive and therapeutic actions of glycyrrhizin, glycyrrhetic acid and crude saikosides on experimental cirrhosis in rats." *Yao Hsueh Hsueh Pao*, 18(5), 325-331, 1983.

32. Nakagawa, K. and Asami, M. "Effect of glycyrrhizin on hepatic lysosomal systems." *Japanese Journal of Pharmacology*, 31, 849-851, 1981.

33. Kuroyanagi, T. and Sato, M. "Effect of prednisolone and glycyrrhizin on transfer of experimental allergic encephalomyelitis." *Allergy*, 15, 67-75, 1966.

34. Leung, A. *Encyclopedia of Common Natural Ingredients Used in Food, Drugs and Cosmetics*. John Wiley & Sons, New York, pp. 220-223.

35. Anderson, D.M. and Smith, W.G. "The antitussive activity of glycyrrhetinic acid and its derivatives." *Journal of Pharmacy and Pharmacology*, 13, 396-404, 1961.

36. Takagi, K. and Fukao, T. "Effects of some drugs on capillary-permeability in the anaphylaxis of the mouse. *Japanese Journal of Pharmacology*, 21, 455-465, 1971.

37. Miyoshi, H. "Antidotal value of glycyrrhizin." *Nisshin Igaku*, 39, 358-365, 1952.

38. Chang, L. "Preliminary report on using glycyrrhiza in combination with antituberculosis drugs in pulmonary tuberculosis." *Jen. Min. Pao Chien*, 3, 235-238, 1959.

39. Molhuysen, J.A., Gerbranby, A.J., et al. "A licorice extract with deoxycortone-like action." *Lancet*, 259 (6630), 381-386, 1950.

40. Groen, J., Willebrands, P.H., et al. "Extract of licorice for the treatment of Addison's disease." *New England Journal of Medicine*, 244, 474-475, 1951.

41. Borst, J.G.G., Holt, S.P., De Vries, L.A. and Molhuysen, J.A. "Synergistic action of liquorice and cortisone in Addison's and Simmond's disease." *Lancet*, 1, 657-663, 1953.

42. Tangri, K.K., Seth, P.K., Parmar, S.S. and Bhargava, K.P. "Biochemical study of the anti-inflammatory and antiarthritic properties of glyccyrrhetic acid." *Biochim. Pharmacol.*, 14(8), 1277-1281, 1965.

43. Gujral, M.L., Sareen, K., Phukan, D.P. and Amma, M.K.P. "Antiarthritic activity of glycyrrhizin in adrenalectomized rats." *Indian Journal of Medical Science*, 15(8), 625-629, 1961.

44. Whitehouse, M.W., Dean, P.D.G. and Halshall, T.G. "Uncoupling of oxidative phosphorylation by glycyrrhetic acid, fusidic acid and some related triterpenoid acids." *Journal of Pharmacy and Pharmacology*, 19(8), 533-544, 1967.

45. Hench, P.S., Kendall, E.C., Slocum, C.H. and Polly, H.P. "Further studies concerning the participation of the adrenal cortex in pathogenesis of arthritis." *Proceedings Of The Mayo Clin.*, 24, 181, 1949.

46. Fujisawa, J., Watanabe, Y. and Kimura. "Therapeutic approach to chronic active hepatitis with glycyrrhizin." *Asian Medical Journal*, 23, 745-756, 1980.

47. Iwamura, K. "Ergebnisse der therapie mit dem medikament strong neo-minophagen c der chronisch aggressiven hepatitis in Japan." *Therapiewoche*, 30, 5431-5445, 1980.

48. Greenberg, H.B., Polland, R.B., et al. "Effect of human leukocyte interferon on hepatitis B virus infection in patients with chronic active hepatitis." *New England Journal of Medicine*, 295, 517-522, 1976.

49. Pompei, R., Pani, A., Flore, O., Marcialis, M.A. and Loddo, B. "Antiviral activity of glycyrrhizic acid." *Experientia*, 36, 304, 1980.

50. Mitscher, L.A., Park, Y.H., Clark, D. and Beal, J.L. "Antimicrobial agents from higher plants, antimicrobial isoflavanoids and related substances from glycyrrhiza glabra L. Var. Typica." *Journal of Natural Products*, 43(2), 259-269, 1980.

51. Costello, G.H. and Lynn, E.V. "Estrogenic substances from plants: I. Glycyrrhiza. *Journal of the American Pharm. Association*, 39, 177-180, 1950.

52. Shiata, I. and Elghamry, M. *Zbl. Veterinaermed*, 10, 155, 1963.

53. Vah Hulle, C. "Ueber die oestrogene wirkung der suessholz-wurzel." *Pharmazie*, 25, 260-261, 1970.

54. Murav'ev, I.A. and Kononikhina, N.F. "Estrogenic properties of glycyrrhiza glabra." *Rastitel'nye Resursy*, 8(4), 490-497, 1972.

55. Shihata, I.M. and Elghamry, M.I. "Estrogenic activity of glycyrrhiza glabra with its effects on uterine motility at various stages of the sex cycle." *Zentr. Vemterinaermed.*, Ser A, 10, 155-162, 1963.

56. Sharaf, A. and Gomaa, N. *Medicine and Medicament Courier*, 11, 29, 1965.

57. Sharaf, A. and Gomaa, N. "Gycyrrhetic acid as an active oestrogenic substance separated from glycyrrhiza glabra (liquorice)." *Egyptian Journal of Pharm. Science,* 16(2), 245-251, 1975.

58. Kraus, S.D. "Glycyrrhetinic acid—a triterpene with antioestrogenic and anti-inflammatory activity." *Journal of Pharmacy and Pharmacology,* 12, 300-306, 1960.

59. Chamberlain, T.J. "Licorice posioning, pseudoaldosteronism, and heart failure." *Journal of the American Medical Association*, 213(8), 1343, Aug 24, 1970.

60. Revers, F.E., *Nederl. T. Geneesk.*, 90, 135, 1946.

61. Conn, J.W., Rovner, D.R. and Chohen, E.L. *Journal of the American Medical Association*, 205, 80, 1968.

62. Ulmann, A., Menard, J. and Corvol, P. "Binding of glycyrrhetinic acid to kidney mineralcorticoid and glucocorticoid receptors." *Endrocinology,* 97(1), 46-51, 1975.

63. Baron, J., Nabarro, J., Slater, J. and Tuffley, R. "Metabolic studies, aldosterone secretion rate and plasma renin after carbenoxolone sodium as biogastrone." *British Medical Journal,* 2, 793-95, 1969.

BLACK COHOSH
(Cimicifuga racemosa)

Black cohosh was introduced to American medicine by the Indians, who called it squaw root in reference to one of its common uses, the treatment of uterine disorders. Among clinical findings are that it promotes and/or restores healthy menstrual activity, soothes irritation and congestion of the uterus, cervix and vagina, relieves the pain and distress of pregnancy, contributes to quick, easy and uncomplicated deliveries, and promotes uterine involution and recovery. In support of the clinical findings, research has found hypotensive principles, vasodilatory, estrogenic, anti-inflammatory and uterine contractile activity. Though the exact mode of action remains a mystery, black cohosh appears to act both directly on the tissues of the reproductive system and indirectly through the nervous system. The plant is a primary nerve and smooth muscle relaxant.

Black cohosh is hypotensive

This herb has a general hypotensive property that is due to the presence of active, water-insoluble resin. It has been hypothesized that the active principle of the resin influences circulation directly through the central nervous system and indirectly through an inhibition of vasomotor centers involving the handling of some forms of vertigo and auditory problems (one of the few remaining medically recognized uses for black cohosh is to relieve auditory tinnitus).[1]

The active principle has been identified tentatively as acteina. Research has shown that this chemical does not affect the periphery or the ganglionic synapses of the somatic nervous system, but has the effect in animal tests of decreasing the vasomotor reflexes caused by clamping and unclamping the carotid arteries. Further, the pure chemical has a hypotensive effect in rabbits, even in very low doses.[2]

In 1831, a report described four successive cases of chorea sancti viti (St. Vitus' dance) successfully treated with black cohosh. A couple of the cases were well advanced, with severe symptoms. The herbal cure took only a few days in each case. The doctors had no idea how the cure worked, but speculated that it acted directly on the nerves. It was emetic on occasion, seldom purgative, never diaphoretic or diuretic. An editor's note described yet another case of successful treatment.[3]

Black cohosh has estrogenic and hypoglycemic action

Substances with estrogenic action have been found in black cohosh, but there does not appear to be a large enough concentration to justify the extravagant estrogenic claims sometimes made for the plant. Since the state of the research on black cohosh is still rather primitive, it is probable that many, if not most, of the active principles have not yet been identified or tested.[4]

Some hypoglycemic activity is exhibited by black cohosh, but its clinical significance has not yet been evaluated experimentally.[5]

Black Cohosh has anti-inflammatory and antibiotic properties

Anti-inflammatory and antibiotic principles have been detected in black cohosh. These properties would be expected to interact in a synergistic manner with other plants that affect the female reproductive system. In fact, black cohosh is one of the most frequently found herbs in herbal combinations of all kinds.[6-7]

It should be mentioned that not all studies have been favorable. At least one study found very little sedative effect on the brain and neuromuscular apparatus. It had no action on isolated intestinal or uterine muscle beyond a depressant and poisonous property of the oily constituent. The positive results of other studies, however, throw this study into question, and an accusation of selective testing could be made.[8]

SAFETY DATA

Black cohosh is considered by the FDA as an herb of undefined safety. No known toxicity exists.

Large doses are certainly emetic. No evidence exists to indicate that the hypotensive property of the whole herb adversely affects living organisms.

REFERENCES

1. Salerna, G. "La cimicifuga racemosa nel campo otoiatrico: ricerche sperimentali." *Minerva Otorinolaringologica*, 5(12), 140-147, 1955.

2. Genazzani, E. and Sorrentino, L. "Vascular action of acteina: active constituent of actaea racemosa L." *Nature*, 194(5), 544-545, 1962.

3. Young, J. "Observations on the remedial powers of the cimicifuga racemosa in the treatment of chorea." *American Journal of Medical Science*, 9, 310-315, 1831.

4. Costello, et. al. *Journal of the American Pharmaceutical Association*, 39, 177, 1950.

5. Farnsworth, N.R. and Segelman, A.B. *Tile Till*, 57, 52, 1971.

6. Benoit, P.S., et al. *Lloydia*, 39, 160, 1976.

7. Nishikawa, H. "Screening tests for antibiotic action of plant extracts." *Japanese Journal of Experimental Medicine*, 20, 337-349, 1949.

8. Macht, D.I. and Cook, H.M. "A pharmacological note on cimicifuga." *Journal of the American Pharmaceutical Association*, 21(4), 324-330, 1932.

CHASTEBERRY
(Vitex agnus castus)

Vitex has a reputation as an anaphrodisiac that dates back to the Greeks and Romans, maybe earlier. At the same time, it is said to increase the efficiency of the female reproductive system. These data strongly suggest a tonic action in the plant. It has been used as a febrifuge, diaphoretic, emmenagogue, glactagogue, tonic, vulnerary and diuretic.

Vitex is currently enjoying great popularity, especially in Europe, where research has been making strides in discovering the mode of action of the plant. European manufacturers are constantly coming out with new and improved extracts of vitex and prescribing them for specific indications, most of which deal with hormonal imbalances in women.

Vitex contains agnuside, acubin and other iridoid glycosides, flavonoids, and a small amount of essential oil. None of these have been firmly identified as the principle active constituent, and some researchers feel that the properties of the herb must be the result of interactions and synergy among the various constituents.

Vitex helps to restore hormonal balance

Vitex works directly on the diencephalo-hypophyseal system, that is, through the pituitary gland, or master gland of the body. Any substance that affects the pituitary will have definite impact on hormonal functions throughout the system. In this case, one primary action of vitex is an increase in the production and secretion of luteinizing hormone, and an inhibition of the release of follicle-stimulating hormone. Thereby comes a change in the estrogen-gestagen ratio in favor of the gestagens, and hence a favorable hormonal influence on the corpus luteum. Vitex would therefore be an important factor in reestablishing hormonal balance in such conditions as corpus syndrome insufficiency (hyper- or polymenorrhea), and in premenstrual syndrome (PMS), involving hyperfolliculinism. Another important action of vitex, as yet not well studied, is an enhancement of prolactin biochemistry.

In clinical settings, vitex has been successfully used to treat acne and premenstrual herpes on the lip, and an effect has been noted on premenstrual effusions in the knee joint. Premenstrual water retention was successfully treated, as was secondary amenorrhea.[1-3]

Vitex has also been shown to be an effective lactagogue; women treated with vitex were able to breast-feed better than untreated mothers.[3,4]

Preparations of vitex in Europe are commonly prescribed for women suffering from breast inflammation, PMS, cyclic migraine, various imbalances of the menstrual cycle, unusual circumstances of puberty, and so forth.[5]

SAFETY DATA

No side effects have been reported with long-term use, i.e., for periods exceeding one year.

REFERENCES

1. Amann, W. *Therapie der Gegenwart,* 106(1), 124, 1967.
2. Amann, W. *ZFA,* 55, 48-51, 1979.
3. Amann, W. *ZFA,* 58, 228-231, 1982.
4. Weiss, R.F. *Herbal Medicine.* Beaconsfield Publishers, Ltd, Beaconsfield, England, 1988.
5. Braun, H. and Frohne, D. *Heilplanzen-Lexikon fuer Aerzte und Apotheker.* Gustav Fischer Verlag, Stuttgart, New York, 1987.

CHAPTER SEVEN

The Male Reproductive System

The male reproductive system comprises the organs that allow men to have sexual intercourse and to fertilize ova with sperm. Sperm and male sex hormones are produced in the testes, a pair of ovoid glands suspended in a pouch known as the scrotum. Sperm travels from each testis into the epididymis, along coiled tubes where they mature and are stored. Shortly before ejaculation, the sperm are propelled from the epididymis into another long duct called the vas deferens in which they travel to the seminal vesicles, a pair of sacs that lie behind the bladder. These sacs secrete seminal fluid which combines with the sperm to form semen.

Semen travels from the vesicles in two ducts to the urethra, a tube that provides passage for urine as well. These ducts pass through the prostate gland, a chestnut-shaped organ located beneath the bladder. The prostate actually surrounds the upper portion of the urethra. Prostatic secretions are added to the semen. At orgasm, semen is ejaculated from the urethra through the penis into the vagina.

PUBERTY

Male sexual capability, or virility, begins at puberty. Puberty is that time when secondary sexual characteristics appear and sexual organs mature, allowing reproduction to take place. Physical and emotional changes characterize puberty and adolescence, which occur somewhere between 10 and 15 years of age. It is initiated by pituitary hormones known as gonadotropins; these stimulate the testes to begin or increase secretion of androgens such as testosterone. Under the influence of the androgens, the boy experiences a sudden increase in the rate of growth of the testes and scrotum. This is followed by the appearance of other secondary sexual characteristics, such as the appearance of pubic, underarm and facial hair. Testosterone stimulates the production of sperm and causes the seminal vesicles and prostate gland to mature. Testosterone also produces the characteristic growth and distribution of hair on face, chest and abdomen. The larynx enlarges, the vocal cords elongate and thicken, and the pitch of the voice drops. Finally, a distinct widening of the shoulders takes place.

MORE ON ANDROGENS

It should be noted that androgens have an anabolic effect; that is, they raise the rate of protein synthesis and lower the rate at which it is degraded. This is what increases the bulk of muscles in the chest and shoulders, and accelerates growth. At the end of puberty, the androgens signal the long bones to stop growing. Androgens are also responsible for the typical male aggressive behavior. Acne due to an accumulation of excessive sebum results from androgen production, and these hormones may also be responsible for male-pattern baldness.

Since the adrenal glands also secrete androgens in both sexes, in amounts that normally have little consequence, manipulation of this process in women through drug therapy can result in the development of some of the secondary sexual characteristics of men, as well as amenorrhea (absence of menstruation). Abuses of this process are most commonly seen in athletes.

THE PROSTATE

Of special interest to men is the prostate gland, since the benign or malignant enlargement of this gland is one of the most common ailments in men as they grow older.

The prostate is a solid, chestnut-shaped organ that surrounds the upper, or first, part of the urethra. The prostate gland consists of an inner zone which produces secretions that help moisten the urethra, and an outer zone in which seminal secretions are produced. The seminal vesicles pass through the prostate to enter the urethra. Under the influence of androgens at puberty, the prostate begins to mature, reaching full size and weight by about the age of 20. But after the age of 50, it begins to enlarge further. Disorders of the prostate are rare before the age of 30.

DISORDERS OF THE MALE REPRODUCTIVE SYSTEM

Prostate Problems

As just mentioned, enlargement of the prostate may begin again at about age 50. This second stage may lead to serious problems, eventually resulting in surgical removal of the prostate gland. Between the ages of 30 and 50, many men experience *prostatitis*, or inflammation of the prostate due to bacterial infection, which should be distinguished from enlargement problems.

Prostatitis   Inflammation of the prostate resulting from bacterial infection, usually originating in the urethra. It may or may not be sexually transmitted. Causes pain when passing urine, and increases frequency of urination. May cause fever. May produce discharges from the penis. Pain in lower abdomen, rectum, lower back, and blood in urine are common. Genuine prostatitis may be rare; it is felt that most cases are functional, or neurotic, in nature.

Benign prostatic hypertrophy(BPH)   Often called enlarged prostate, or adenoma of the prostate. An increase in size of inner zone of the prostate gland in men over 50. The cause is unknown, though there is reason to suspect hormonal influences. Symptoms come on gradually, and result from a compression and distortion of the urethra (sometimes called infravesical obstruction), causing urinary problems, as described below.

Urine retention. The inability to empty the bladder; may be partial or complete. Produced by BPH and prostatitis (among other causes) that constrict the urinary tract due to pressure. Causes severe pain in lower abdomen. May lead to urinary tract infection and kidney damage.

Incontinence. Uncontrollable, involuntary urination that occurs in this case due to overflow of small quantities of urine. There is urge-incontinence—the desire to go; and overflow incontinence.

Polyuria, or frequent urination. Results when bladder muscle becomes overdeveloped in attempting to force urine through obstructed urethra. Produces an overactive bladder. Frequent urination is a sign that bladder muscle failure is imminent, and that surgery is required. May occur either in the daytime or at night.

Dysuria. Pain, discomfort, and difficulty in passing urine. A typical symptom of BPH. Sometimes described as a burning or scalding feeling. Preceded by difficulty in starting urination.

Strangury. Pain after the flow of urine has stopped, with a strong desire to continue.

Nycturia or nocturia. Incontinence or frequent urination during the night. An enlarged prostate obstructing the normal flow of urine will often cause the bladder to be full at night.

Cancer of the Prostate A malignant growth in the outer zone of the prostate. May produce an enlarged prostate with all of the typical symptoms. But must be distinguished from *benign* enlargement of the prostate.

Urethritis

Inflammation of the urethra due to infection, irritation or injury.

Impotence

Deficiency in sexual performance or in virility. Can have physiological or psychological roots. Stress, fatigue, anxiety, depression, or guilt can lead to impotence. Only about 10 percent of all cases of impotence are caused by physical problems. Among them are diabetes, spinal cord damage, alcoholism, drugs of various kinds and altered circulation due to age. Low levels of testosterone are implicated in a minority of cases.

❧ HERBAL TONICS FOR THE MALE REPRODUCTIVE SYSTEM

Since ancient times man has used brews and potions composed of herbs and roots, bark and berries to help maintain virility. In actuality, few plants have been shown to really affect the production of androgens. However, there are certain plants whose reputation for nurturing the various organs of the reproductive system have been validated by research and clinical application. These materials can provide significant benefits to the men wise enough to use them. The term "tonic" implies an ability to restore homeostasis no matter which way it departs from normal. In the case of male reproductive physiology, however, there is little call for "less." Ninety nine per cent of requests are to get "more." In fact, the concept of the "over-sexed" male probably involves more psychological variables than physiological. The herbs recommended for the male reproductive system may, therefore, not be tonics in the true sense of the term, because there is virtually no data to demonstrate their ability to reduce aspects of male reproductive physiology. It is doubtful many men would quibble on this point.

PYGEUM
(Pygeum africanum)

Scientists at a European firm recently completed almost two decades' worth of research on a plant they discovered in the ethnobotany of tropical Africa. The plant is called pygeum. Although pygeum appears to have been described for the first time in botanical texts of the second half of the 18th century,[1,2] its utilization as a medicinal plant presumably dates to some remote era, when it was the custom of certain isolated peoples of southern Africa to prepare teas by powdering the bark, dispersing it in water or milk, and administering it for both minor and serious complaints.

Pygeum is a large evergreen tree, which can reach a height of over 100 feet, and is marked by deeply fissured bark that constitutes the medicinal part of the plant. Research has established this remedy as an effective treatment for benign prostatic hypertrophy.

Clinical trials utilizing pygeum began in the 1970s. These early trials were generally pretty sloppy, as most early medical research tends to be, but the main finding was consistent: pygeum significantly and reliably affected the course of benign prostatic hypertrophy.[3-8]

Researchers began simultaneously to identify the different chemical fractions of the plant with suspected activity. Another series of animal and clinical trials was thereupon undertaken, the purpose of which was to clarify the action of each of the classes of constituents.[9-12]

Over the years, pygeum research techniques improved, as did the chemical analysis, extraction and standardization procedures, until the whole research effort reached a point in the last three or four years that is about as close to medical, technical and scientific perfection as one is likely to find in this field. Thus, pygeum lays legitimate claim to the status of a guaranteed potency herb (see the chapter on the cardiovascular system for more on guaranteed potency herbs). Recent animal and clinical trials are classic examples of randomized, placebo-controlled, double blind, elegantly instrumented, measured and statistically analyzed experimentation.

Active constituents of pygeum

Pygeum contains three groups[13] of lipid-soluble components with effects on prostate disease. These are summarized as follows:

Phytosterols: beta-sitosterol, beta-sitosterol-3-0-glucoside, beta-sitosterone.

Physiological action: Reduces prostaglandin-mediated inflammation (anti-inflammatory).

Pentacyclic triterpenoids: ursolic acid, 2-alpha-hydroxyursolic acid, oleanolic acid, crataegolic acid, friedelin.

Physiological action: reduces swelling due to water accumulation in prostate (anti-edema).

Linear alcohols: n-tetra-cosanol, n-docosanol, and their particular ester derivatives, such as n-docosyl trans-ferulate.

Physiological action: lowers cholesterol levels in prostate (hypocholesterolemic).

Pygeum reduces inflammation

Much attention has been focused on the phytosterols in pygeum, since past experience strongly suggests that these are responsible for much of the observed activity. Phytosterols are abundant in the plant kingdom; they occur in half of the common grains, in oil of corn, in the oil of soy beans, in saw palmetto and pumpkin seeds, and in the bark of pygeum.

While it was formerly thought that the phytosterols were able to reduce the size of prostate adenoma, the main action turns out to be anti-inflammatory—subjectively, a decrease in inflammation could be perceived as an actual reduction in size.

The precise mode of action involves the inhibition of the biosynthesis of prostaglandins, especially epithelial levels of prostaglandins E2 and F2-alpha, those crucial mediators of the inflammatory process.[14-16] Patients with BPH normally show extremely elevated levels of prostaglandins; in a period of several days to several weeks under the influence of pygeum phytosterols, these levels drop significantly. Clinical studies have routinely observed reduced prostatic prostaglandin levels and the alleviation of many cases of local hyperemia (excess blood) and vasal congestion.

It should be noted that some authors maintain that beta-sitosterol works by actively competing with some of the body's own substances that have similar chemical structures during the metabolism of androgens, with the result of sensitizing prostatic cells to the hormonal stimulation. The result is a reawakening of sleeping gonadal activity. This assumes, of course, that decreased gonadal activity is responsible for BPH, an important theory, but one not ascribed to by all investigators.

Pygeum reduces swelling

Recent research suggests that the presence of phytosterols cannot account for pygeum's total observed activity.[17] We must search further. Enter the pentacyclic triterpenoids (TPs) of pygeum. These substances, particularly ursolic acid and oleanolic acid, may be characterized by one special pharmacological action, evidenced by their response to traditional models of experimental inflammation: an effective antiedema, or diuretic, action.[18]

In addition, or in particular, the TPs have been found to inhibit the action of enzymes involved in the initial phases of the inflammation.[19] TPs strengthen the integrity of small veins and tiny capillaries, thereby putting the brakes on to some of the typical inflammatory processes that result in edema.[20]

In BPH, inflammation and edema are two of the major functional signs. They can range from hardly noticeable to very painful and obstructive. The gradual loss of the functional properties of the tissues that support the vascular bed can be reversed by the application of pygeum TPs. The antiexudative, and therefore antiedema, action of the pygeum TPs rests squarely on the capacity of ursolic acid and oleanolic acid to inactivate inflammatory enzymatic activity.

We see that the TPs have considerable power to complement the antiprostaglandin activity of the phytosterols, even though at this time it would be best to view their activity as ancillary and supportive.

Pygeum reduces cholesterol levels

Finally, we need to consider the action of the linear alcohols and ferulic esters, which is to profoundly alter the course of BPH by inhibiting the absorption and metabolism of cholesterol.[21,22] That particular concept—that cholesterol levels in enlarged prostates were not just coincidentally abnormally high, but that in fact the cholesterol contributed to the pathology—had been around for awhile, but largely overlooked.[23,24] Due to pygeum research, the theory is now enjoying a revival.[25]

And so a triad of pathological conditions emerges, each of which is ameliorated by one or more fractions of pygeum. The plant appears to be specially designed for fighting the symptoms and causes of BPH. Ultimately all the components of pygeum have been found to behave in a complementary and synergistic manner in terms of their effects on BPH. For the first time, there is real hope of some reversal in this condition, not just control of symptoms.

Pygeum has been successful in clinical trials

A standardized lipophilic extract of pygeum, as a raw substance and under a couple of different trade names, has been subjected to scores of clinical trials, a few of which are reviewed here. The typical daily dose is 200 mg, divided into two doses, over a period of four weeks to two months. Most of the later studies employ good protocol: double-blind, placebo-controlled, statistically evaluated, with attention being paid to both efficacy and safety: but even the earlier studies demonstrate strong pygeum effects. Efficacy was established by observing and measuring effects on several parameters: dysuria, nycturia, diurnal and nocturnal polyuria (frequent urination), perineal (abdominal) heaviness, residual urine, volume of the prostate, voiding volume, peak flow and time mean. Safety was established by routine blood chemistry tests, clinical signs and self-report by patient.

- Eighty percent of 25 patients with BPH or cervicoprostatic adenomatosis showed significant improvement in symptoms (micturition, and in 5 cases also the volume of the prostate) after 100 mg/day for 30 days.[26]
- Thirteen of 18 patients with BPH, and 3 of 7 patients with prostatitis, reported good results in amelioration of dysuria and polyuria.[27]
- In 27 patients with BPH and one with chronic prostatitis, all but three experienced significant symptomatic improvement after 6 weeks at 100 mg/day. In general, the worse the symptoms, the less chance for recovery.[28]
- After 60 days of receiving 75 mg/day in three divided doses, 60 percent of 20 patients reported significant improvement in dysuria and polyuria. Twenty percent reported no improvement.[29]

- Out of 52 patients, 22 had very good regression, and 14 acceptable regression, of symptoms ranging from urinary disturbances, such as dysuria and polyuria, to signs of bladder neck urethral obstruction. All patients were surgical candidates. Treatment was 75 mg divided into three administrations.[30]
- In a couple of the earliest trials on BPH patients, only 57-60 percent success was seen, but the treatment periods in most cases were fairly short, ranging from 10 to 50 days.[31,32] Since that time, controls and protocol have steadily improved.
- Against a placebo control, typical symptoms of BPH yielded significantly better to pygeum in 55 patients, aged 59-83. Only 10 percent of the patients reported no change, while a full 70 percent experienced very good results.[33]
- Out of 42 patients, aged 53-84, with obstructive urodynamic syndrome of prostatic origin, 19 experienced amelioration of diurnal polyuria, 31 experienced amelioration of nycturia and 21 showed improvement in residual urine after micturition. Treatment was 150 mg daily for 45 days.[34]
- In a double-blind, placebo-controlled study in 120 patients, significant changes were found in symptoms of nocturnal frequency, difficulty in starting micturition and incomplete emptying of the bladder. This study nicely portrayed confounding from placebo effects, since 50 percent of the placebo patients experienced improvement. It is very difficult under such circumstances to demonstrate statistical significance. That the researchers were able to do so highlights the strength of the pygeum treatment.[35]
- In an open trial on 104 outpatients, aged 18-45, affected by prostatitis of different origin secondary to infections, 89 percent experienced very good improvement in symptoms such as dysuria, polyuria, strangury and pains in the pelvis.[36]
- Thirty typical elderly BPH patients were treated for three

months with 100 mg daily. All 30 experienced statistically significant improvement in symptoms.[37]

- In 39 cases of BPH (mean age 70 years) 200 mg daily for 60 days produced significant improvement in 75 percent of the patients, compared to controls.[38]
- Twenty BPH patients, aged 51-89, were divided into two groups, pygeum and control. Pygeum patients experienced significantly greater reduction in dysuric symptoms after 60 days with 200 mg/day.[39]
- Another placebo-controlled trial, involving 40 men with prostatic hyperplasia (enlargement due to oversecretion of hormones), found significant improvement in more than 60-80 percent of the patients following 200 mg daily treatment for 2 months.[40]
- In a recent open trial, the effects of pygeum on various male genital infections was assessed. Significant relief of symptoms and improvement in indices of a sexual and reproductive nature were observed.[41]

Many other similar studies could be cited, but these should suffice to suggest the effectiveness of pygeum. BPH, prostatitis and related conditions, especially if functional in nature, are all amenable to safe and efficacious treatment with pygeum. Many patients even report improvement in such parameters as appetite, weight gain and mood. Four to six weeks of treatment are usually all that are necessary, but treatment may be repeated if desired.

SAFETY DATA

In all tests, animal and human, no significant toxic effects were observed and tolerance for the herb was excellent in every study. No meaningful side effects of any kind were observed. Some gastric disturbances have been noted, but these do not amount to more than 1 percent of the hundreds of patients treated. Even very elderly patients in generally poor condition could tolerate prolonged periods of treatment without side effects.

Pygeum has no contraindications; its action is not hormonelike, and it may therefore be used even in cases lacking a differential diagnosis between benign adenoma and cancer.

REFERENCES

1. Bentham, G. and Hooker, J.D. *Genera Plantarum*, Vol. I: 610, Reeve and Co., London, 1862.

2. Oliver, D. *Flora of Tropical Africa*, Vol. II: 375. Reeve and Co., London, 1871.

3. Lange, J. and Muret, P. "Experimentation clinique du V 1326 dans les troubles prostatiques." *Bordeaux Med.*, 11, 2807, 1970.

4. Grevy, A. and Favre, J.P. "Nouvelle therapeutique dans les troubles mictionnels d'origine prostatique ou cervicale chez l'homme." *Med. Int.*, 5, 3, 1970.

5. Viollet, G. "Experimentation clinique d'un nouveau traitement de l'adenome prostatique." *Vie Medicale*, 23, 3457, 1970.

6. Gallizia, F. and Gallizia, G. "Trattamento medico dell'ipertrofia prostatica con un nuovo principio fitoterapico." *Recentia Medica*, 9, 461, 1972.

7. Marcoli, M, D'Angelo, L., Frigo, G.M., Lecchini, S. and Crema, A. "Antiinflammatory and antiedemigenic activity of extract of pygeum africana in the rat." *New Trends Adrol. Sciences*, 1, 89, 1985.

8. Mondy, M. "Considerations sur les possibilites de traitement medical de l'adenome prostatique. Etude en particulier de l'action du V 1326." Thèse Clermont-Ferrand, 1971.

9. Lhez, A. and Leguevage, G. "Essai clinique d'un nouveau complexe lipido-sterolique d'origine vegetale dans le traitement de l'adenome prostatique." *Vie Medicale*, 26, 5399, 1970.

10. Legramandi, C., Ricci Barbini, V., Fonte, A. and Giudici, L. "Importanza del pygeum africanum nel trattamento delle prostatiti cronich abatteriche." *Gazz. Med. It.*, 143, 73, 1984.

11. Dufour, B., Chouquenet, Ch., Revol. M., Faure, G. and Jorest, R. "Etude controlee des effets de l'etrait de pygeum africanum

sur les symptomes fonctionnels de l'adenome prostatique." *Ann. Urol.*, 18, 193, 1984.

12. Wemeau, L., Delmay, J. and Blankaert, J. "Le Tadenan dans l'adenome prostatique." *Vie Medicale*, 14, 585, 1970.

13. Actually, a fourth class of potentially important chemicals exists, the C12-C24 fatty acids, but they appear to have no discernible effect on the prostate gland.

14. Zahradnik, H.P., Schillfahrt, R., Schoening, R., Ebbinghaus, K.D. and Dunzendorger, U. "Prostaglandin-gehalt in prostataadenomen nach behandlung mit einem sterol." *Fortschrifte der Medizin*, 98, 69, 1980.

15. Bauer, H.W. and Bach, D. "Prostaglandin esu E2 in prostatitis and hyperplasia of the prostata." *Urol. Int.*, 41, 139, 1986.

16. Bach, D., Walker, M. and Zahradnich, H.P. "Phytosterol lowers the prostaglandin concentration in prostate exprimate." *Therapiewoche*, 35/38, 4292, 1985.

17. Menchini-Fabris, G.F., Giorgi, P., Andreini, F., Canale, D., Paoli, R. and Sarteschi, M.L. "Nuove prospettive di impiego del pygeum africanum nella patologia prostato-vesicolare." *Archivo Italiano Urol.*, 60, 313, 1988.

18. Marcoli, M. et al., op. cit.

19. Kozay, K. et al. "Inhibition of glucosyl-transferase from streptococcus mutans by oleanolic acid and ursolic acid." *Caries Research*, 21, 104, 1987.

20. Specifically, the TPs halt the process of plasma exudation. Exudation is the discharge of fluid from blood vessels during the inflammatory process. Small blood vessels passing through inflamed tissue become wider and more permeable, allowing fluids and cells to escape, resulting in swelling, or edema. Tissue glucosamino-glycans in fact attach in the initial stages of the inflammatory process to enzymes, especially glucose-transferase and beta-glucouronidase, that biochemically break the bonds that unite disaccharides present in the polysaccharide structures of the vessel wall glucosamin-glycands, with the result that vessel walls become very leaky.

21. Nakayama, S. et al. "Effects of gamma-oryzanol and its related compounds on triton induced hyperlipidemia in rats." *J. Showa Med. Assoc.*, 46, 359, 1986.

22. Sakamoto, K., et al. "Effects of gamma-oryzanol and cycloartenol ferulic acid ester on cholesterol diet induced hyperlipidemia in rats." *Japanese Journal of Pharmacology*, 45, 559, 1987.

23. Swyer, G.I.M. "The cholesterol content of normal and enlarged prostates." *Cancer Research*, 2, 372-375, 1942.

24. Schaffner, C.P., Brill, D.R. and Singhal, A.K. "Presence of epoxycholesterols in the aging human prostate gland as a risk factor in cancer." *Cancer Detection and Prevention*, 3, 134, 1980.

25. Schaffner, C.P. "Effect of cholesterol-lowering agents." In: *Benign Prostatic Hypertrophy*, Springer-Verlag, New York, 1983, p. 295.

26. Guillemin, P. "Essai clinique du V 1326, ou Tadenan, vis-a-vis de l'adenoma prostatique." *Med. Pratic.*, N. 386, 75, 1970.

27. Lange and Muret, op. cit.

28. Wemeau, L. et al., op.cit.

29. Viollet, G., op.cit.

30. Lhez and Leguevage, op.cit.

31. Thomas, J. and Rouffilange, F. "Action du Tadenan sur l'adenoma prostatique." *Rev. Int. Serv. Sante des Armees de Terre, de Mer et de l'Air*, 43, 43, 1970.

32. Rometti, A. "Traitement medical de l'adenoma prostatique par le V 1326." *La Provence Med.*, 38, 49, 1970.

33. Huet, J.A. "Les affections de la prostate sujection du troisieme age." *Med. Interne*, 5, 405, 1970.

34. Colpi, G. and Farina, U. "Studio dell 'attivita dell' estratto cloroformio di coreteccia di pygeum africanum nella terapia della sindrome ostruttiva uretrale da prostatopatia non cancerosa." *Urologia*, 43, 441, 1976.

35. Dufour, B. et al., op.cit.

36. Legramandi, C. et al., op.cit.

37. Zurita, I.E., Pecorini, M. and Cuzzoni, G. "Tratamento da hipertrofia prostatica com extracto de prunus africana. Resultados obtidos em 30 pacientes." *Rev. Bras. Med.*, 41, 48, 1984.

38. Ranno, S., Minaldi, G. and Viscusi, G. "Efficasicia e tollerabilita del trattamento dell' adenoma prostatico con Tadenan 50." *Progresso Medico*, 62, 165, 1986.

39. Frasseto, G., Bertoglio, S. and Mancuso, S. "Studio sull' efficacia e sulla tollerabilita del Tadenan 50 in pazienti affette da ipertrofia prostatica." *Progresso Medico*, 42, 49, 1986.

40. Bassi, P., Arbitani, W. and De Luca, V. "Standardized extract of pygeum africanum in the treatment of benign prostatic hypertrophy." *Minerva Urologica*, 39, 45, 1987.

41. Menchini-Fabris, G.F., Giorgi, P., Andreini, F., Canale, D. and Paoli, R. "Nuove prospettive de impiego del pygeum africanum nella patologia prostato vesicolare." *Arch. It. Urol.*, 60, 313, 1988.

PUMPKIN SEED
(Cucurbita pepo)

The primary use of pumpkin seed is as an anthelmintic and vermifuge (to counter internal parasites), but the seed also has a reputation, extending into cultures as diverse as native American Indian and native African, for being a nonirritating diuretic, and a valued nonirritating treatment for benign enlargement of the prostate gland. A cytotoxic principle has also been identified that is used to fight cancer-induced enlarged prostate.

Pumpkin seed may counteract enlarged prostate

The seed embryo contains an anthelmintic compound which is also able to arrest cell division at metaphase, and may also be responsible for the observed effectiveness of pumpkin seed in cases where it is used to treat hypertrophy of the prostate gland. Anthelmintic properties against *Allolobophora fetida* have also been found in watery emulsions of the fresh seed, and anthelmintic properties have been found in the oil (which is high in both saturated and unsaturated fatty acids, including oleic, palmitic, stearic and linoleic), and in the whole seed.[1-5]

SAFETY DATA

Pumpkin seed has proved a mixed blessing for livestock owners. On the one hand, it is very nutritious, containing substantial amounts of vitamin C., niacin, riboflavin and thiamine, oils, and other nutritious substances. On the other hand, there are reports of animals (cattle, sheep, poultry, and ostrich) fed large amounts of pumpkin seed developing a kind of inebriation that involves loss of coordination in the extremities. The inebriation becomes habit forming and difficult to break.[1,2]

In humans, no reports of toxicity have been made, and the seed is ingested by people all over the world without incident.

REFERENCES

1. Steyn, D. G. Onderstepoort *J. Vet. Science,* 5, 79, 1935.
2. Burtt, D.J., *Transv. Agric. J.,* 2, 96, 278, 1903-1904.
3. Rath, E. *Archiv. Experimental Path. Pharmak.,* 142, 157, 1929.
4. Sanfillipo, G. *Bollitino Soc. Ital. Biol. Sper.,* 6, 490, 1931.
5. Duke, J. *Business of Herbs,* Sept/Oct, 1985.

SARSAPARILLA
(Smilax officinalis)

Smilax is another herb with a reputation as a remarkable tonic and male rejuvenator. This herb has been receiving considerable attention lately, but not of a research nature. Rather it has become a favorite of the body-building crowd. Is there any justification for this interest?

As a tonic, smilax has been used primarily to increase vitality and virility, and is used throughout Central and South America and some parts of southern North America to treat the symptoms of sexually transmitted diseases. This practice has even spread to Europe.

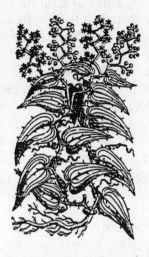

SARSAPARILLA

Herbal treatments for syphilis, especially those involving smilax, were historically very popular, mainly because the standard medical treatment was mercury. Mercury treatment was unpopular among the common people due to serious side effects. Sarsaparilla, on the other hand, was just as good a treatment without side effects. An interesting situation, reported in *Green Pharmacy: A History of Herbal Medicine*, occurred in military operations during 1812, when cases of syphilis treated with smilax by Portuguese doctors recovered more quickly than cases treated with mercury by British doctors.[5] Chinese physicians verified the antisyphilis property of sarsaparilla. In clinical observations, its effectiveness on primary syphilis was rated at 90 percent. Allowing for some halo effect, the results are still staggering.[1] This may help explain how the herb came to used that way in Europe. It was simply effective.

Other countries that use smilax for venereal disease include China, Thailand, the Philippines, Malaysia, Viet Nam and Cambodia. This kind of worldwide concurrence on the effects of a plant is good evidence in itself for the validity of the claim. Worldwide opinion also concurs on other uses for smilax, including an anti-inflammatory effect in arthritis and gout, and a detoxification effect in cancer and skin disorders.

The effectiveness of smilax in the treatment of skin disorders, such as the acne of adolescence caused by raging androgens, has received some experimental support.[6]

The tonic effect of smilax may be the result of its ability to stimulate the removal of accumulated waste products from the cells, blood and lymph. These actions would tend to increase the health of the entire body and increase vitality, which would be felt as increased energy and endurance. This is, of course, an overly simplified scheme, but until we learn more about the specific mode of action of sarsaparilla, we have to make do with generalizations.

One final note: Smilax contains a wide variety of saponins, mainly sarsasapogenin, smilagenin, sitosterol and stigmasterol. These substances commonly occur in plants with immune-enhancing action, in the adaptogens, in tonics, and in herbs used for their nutritive value. Smilax saponins have not been investigated thoroughly, but they may hold the key to the popularity of the plant for body-building purposes. Sarsaparilla saponins have, for example, been used in the synthesis of sex hormones.[2-4]

SAFETY DATA

Like all tonic herbs, smilax is perfectly safe to use on a daily basis in reasonable amounts. It has no known toxicity.

REFERENCES

1. *An Encyclopedia of Traditional Chinese Medicinal Substances (Ahong Yao Da Ci Dian)*, Jiansu College of New Medicine, 1977,

made available for English readers by Bensky, D.; Gamble, A. *Chinese Herbal Medicine Materia Medica*, Eastland Press, Seattle, 1986, pp. 144-145.

2. Leung, A.Y. *Encyclopedia of Common Natural Ingredients Used in Food, Drugs, and Cosmetics*, John Wiley & Sons, New York, 1980, pp. 293-294.

3. Morton, J.F. *Major Medicinal Plants: Botany, Culture, and Uses*, Charles C Thomas, Springfield, Illinois, 1977, p. 374.

4. Claus, E.P., Tyler, V.E. and Brady, L.R. *Pharmacognosy*, 6th edition, Lea & Febiger, Philadelphia, 1970, citation for Smilax.

5. Griggs, B. *Green Pharmacy: A History of Herbal Medicine*, Jill Norman & Hobhouse, London, 1981, pp. 41-42.

6. Thurman, F.M. "The treatment of psoriasis with sarsaparilla compound." *New Engl. J. Med.*, 227, 128-133, 1942.

SAW PALMETTO
(Serenoa repens)

Saw palmetto berries are an old American tonic. John Lloyd, a famous early American medical botanist, observed that animals fed on these berries grew sleek and fat. This same observation was made by many early settlers searching for fodder for their livestock. Once the fame of these berries reached medical researchers, the berries were investigated and their effects verified. Much research, especially in the 1870s, demonstrated the berry's effect on body weight, general health and disposition, tranquilization, venereal disease, appetite stimulation and reproductive health.

Eventually, pressure from within the medical establishment led to the inclusion of the herb in the National Formulary and the *U.S. Pharmacopoeia*. It was dropped from the USP in 1916 and the NF in 1950 as the enthusiasm of the medical profession for natural agents dwindled. Contributing to its demise was the fact that nobody had found any active principle in the herb (beyond what were thought to be some relatively inactive plant steroids) that could account for its observed actions. Had the plant been a native of Europe, there is a good chance that it would have been thoroughly investigated during the '50s and '60s. But like most native American species, once the era of modern medicine arrived, it failed to attract the kind of research attention that it seemed to deserve.

Saw palmetto helps prevent and treat benign prostatic hypertrophy

Eventually, the word on saw palmetto did reach Europe, and researchers there have carried out quite extensive research in recent years. Like pygeum, serenoa extract, concentrated and purified in the best tradition of guaranteed potency herbs, dramatically reduces the size of the enlarged prostate and restores function. The berry contains an oil composed of sterols and various saturated and unsaturated fatty acids. In Europe, and now in America, the purified fat-soluble extract is used medicinally. In whole berry, the sterolic fraction, contained in the fat-soluble extract, makes a major contribution to the action of the extract; it is composed of beta-sitosterol, stigmasterol, sycloartenol, and other substances.[1-7]

Saw palmetto affects the metabolism of testosterone

Just as proponents of pygeum rely on certain theories of what causes enlarged prostate that coincide with observed actions of pygeum, serenoa advocates bring forward theories that coincide with the suspected action of this plant. For example, it has been observed that serenoa prevents the conversion of testosterone to dihydrotestosterone (DHT); it also appears to interfere with the ability of DHT to bind to receptor sites on the membranes of prostate cells and their nuclei. In view of the fact that significant improvements in the symptoms of benign prostatic hypertrophy occur under the influence of serenoa, one is justified in theorizing that the original cause of the disease was the accumulation of DHT. Too much DHT could cause the prostate cells to divide and multiply at a rate in excess of normal, thereby leading to an enlargement of the gland.

In one double-blind, placebo-controlled study, serenoa extract was given to 110 patients suffering from BPH. The frequency of nocturnal urination decreased by over 45 percent, the rate of flow increased by over 50 percent, and the residual urine decreased by 42 percent. Those patients receiving the placebo experienced no significant change.[2]

In other studies, patients receiving the standardized serenoa extract demonstrated consistently better improvement in all aspects as compared to controls.[3-7]

Unlike pygeum, the data for serenoa do not provide good evidence that a cure has taken place, but only that symptoms have been relieved, sometimes more quickly than seen with pygeum. A combination of pygeum and saw palmetto, then, should provide quick symptomatic relief of pain and inflammation, followed by a gradual but certain reduction in swelling and elimination of the root cause of the problem.

SAFETY DATA

Saw palmetto berries have no known toxicity, and are generally regarded as safe by the FDA.

REFERENCES

1. Champault, G., Patel, J.C. and Bonnard, A.M. "A double-blind trial of an extract of the plant serenoa repens in benign prostatic hyperplasia." *Br. J. Clin. Pharmacol.*, 18, 461-462, 1984.

2. Carilla, E., Brailey, M., Fauran, F. et al. "Binding of permixon, a new treatment for prostatic benign hyperplasia." *J. Steroid Biochem.* 20, 521-523, 1984.

3. Boccafoschi, R. and Annoscia, S. "Comparison of serenoa repens

extract in patients with prostatic adenomatosis." *Urologia*, 50, 1257-1268, 1983.

4. Tasca, A., et al. "Treatment of obstructive symptomatology caused by prostatic adenoma with an extract of serenoa repens. Double-blind clinical study vs. placebo." *CR Ther. Pharmacol. Clin.*, 4(25), 15-21, 1985.

5. Crimi, A. and Russo, A. "Extract of serenoa repens for the treatment of the functional disturbances of prostate hypertrophy." *Med. Praxis*, 4, 47-51, 1983.

6. Champault, G., et al. "Medical treatment of prostatic adenoma. Controlled trial: PA 109 vs placebo in 110 patients." *Ann. Urol.*, 18, 407-410, 1984.

7. Cirillo-Marucco, E., et al. "Extract of serenoa repens (permixon R) in the early treatment of prostatic adenomatosis." *Urologia*, 5, 1269-1277, 1983.

MUIRA-PUAMA
(Liriosma ovata)

Few in number are the plants that seem to have a reliable reputation as true aphrodisiacs. Perhaps the most powerful of these, yohimbe, contains alkaloids that the government feels are unsafe for human consumption; its sale is therefore forbidden in several states. Without access to yohimbe, one must look elsewhere for this property. There is no lack of material to fill the void. Snake oil remedies abound, and confusion, dishonesty, and hyped-up placebo razzmatazz carry the day. Out of this mess, one plant, virtually unknown to most Americans, appears to have risen above the competition. The plant is called muira-puama. And though not much is known scientifically about the plant, all indications would lead one to believe that here is a material with the potential for making an important and significant contribution to the health of the male reproductive system. There is no evidence that the plant is a true tonic, in the sense of this book, but, as indicated earlier, we feel justified in a liberal approach to the subject of this chapter.

Muira-puama is a native folk medicine of Brazil. It is used as an astringent, and particularly as an aphrodisiac. European explorers observed this action and brought it back to Europe, where it has become part of the herbal medicine of England. In the United States, users are fewer in number than in England and South America, but the plant's reputation is beginning to grow among men interested in stimulating and maintaining virility.

The conservative *British Herbal Pharmacopoeia* contains a short chapter on muira-puama because of its long history of use in that country. The book recognizes muira-puama as an astringent, aromatic, and reluctantly acknowledges its possible aphrodisiac action. It is also recommended for use in the treatment of dysentery and impotence.[1]

The Italians, known for their romanticism, are more supportive of the aphrodisiac properties; they freely cite obscure references to the central nervous system tonic action of the plant, and are liberal in their comparisons of muira-puama to yohimbe. Early sources can be rallied in support of yohimbe-like action of muira-puama, but recent investigations are, sadly, lacking.[2-6]

SAFETY DATA

Muira-puama is nontoxic in therapeutic doses.

REFERENCES

1. *British Herbal Pharmacopoeia*, British Herbal Medicine Association, West York, England, 1983, pp. 132-133.

2. Duke, J.A. *CRC Handbook of Medicinal Herbs*, CRC Press, Inc., Boca Raton, Florida, 1985, p. 398.

3. Goell, cited by Frerichs, Arend and Zornig, in List, P.N. and Huerhammer, L.H., *Hagers Handbuch der Pharmazeutischen Praxis*, Springer-Verlag, Berlin, 1968-1979, citation for Liriosma.

SIBERIAN GINSENG, ELEUTHERO
(Eleutherococcus senticosus)

Siberian ginseng, along with most other species of ginseng, has an ancient reputation for stimulating male virility. The Chinese, in particular, have prized the root Asian ginseng for that purpose since the beginnings of recorded history, paying at times more for the root than its weight in gold. In fact, when supplies of native ginseng were running low in the early 19th century, American entrepreneurs made quite a bundle selling wild American ginseng to the Chinese to replenish their supply.

One can argue that there is no such thing as an aphrodisiac, but what benefits to sexual performance might be obtained from a substance that Russian athletes routinely ingested during international sporting events in order to benefit from its stimulating action? Placebo effect? Then what about the 1984 double-blind placebo controlled study that found that after one month of using Siberian ginseng sprinters and long distance runners experienced a significant increase in performance?[1]

Siberian ginseng helps combat the effects of stress

To the extent that virility is a function of a man's ability to cope with stress, Siberian ginseng should help. It has been found to provide a protective action against various stressors, including vigorous labor[2] and adrenal exposure to environmental stressors.[3] It also helps the body's cells manufacture life sustaining and energy-enhancing biochemicals[4] and even has an anti-cancer action.[5]

There are data that suggest that eleuthero has a significant impact on gonadotropic hormones and an anabolic effect on the production of sperm and testosterone. These data come from animal studies but man is, after all, an animal.

There is also data to suggest that eleuthero helps the body adapt to the changing conditions of everyday life, especially as they involve mental and physiological stress. Among the conditions that have been researched are stress from cold, exercise, noise, motion, heat, and even decompression. This kind of adaptation will certainly carry over in the one's sex life. Current thought suggests that the primary locus of action is on the adrenal glands.

A review of the research on the hormonal actions of eleuthero as well as its other properties can be found in the chapter on the nervous system.

REFERENCES

1. Stephan, H., Jousseline, E., Questel, R. and Lecomte, A. *Cinesiologie,* 1984, 92-93, p. 97.

2. Fulder, S. "The drug that builds Russians." *New Scientist,* 1215, 576-581, 1987.

3. Dardymov, I.V. "Basic pharmacological properties of eleutherococcus roots." *24th Session of the Comm. to Study Ginseng and Other Medicinal Plants of the Far East,* Vladivostok, 9, 1966, pp. 320.

4. Brekhman, I.I., et al. "Molecular aspects in the mechanism of increasing nonspecific resistivity, caued by an eleutherococcus preparation." *5th Int'l Cong. Pharm.,* San Francisco, 1972, pp. 99-103.

5. Lazarev, N.V. "Antiblastomogenic medical drugs." *Vopr. Onkol.,* 11, 48-54, 1965.

6. Baranov, A.I. "Medicinal uses of ginseng and related plants in the Soviet Union: Recent trends in the Soviet literature." *J. Ethnopharmacology,* 6, 339-353, 1985.

7. Farnsworth, N.R., Kinghorn, A.D. et al. "Siberian ginseng (E. senticosis): current status as an adaptogen." *Economic and Medicinal Plant Research,* 1, 156-215, 1985.

CHAPTER EIGHT

The Concept of a Whole Body Tonic

❧ This chapter will not follow the format of the preceding chapters. It will simply describe one person's reasoning behind the development of a tonic for the whole body, and will attempt to explain why there is a place in the modern world for a liquid tonic.

The concept of a whole body tonic has a "cures what ails you" connotation. In a more conservative approach, these herbs would be combined in powdered form in a capsule, or at the most made into a delightful tea. But our intent is not to be conservative, because a mixture such as the one presented here is absolutely best if made into a whole herb liquid extract—the kind of thing you would take with a tablespoon or by the ounce, every day, just to make sure all the bases were covered. The word panacea comes to mind—so does the phrase "snake oil." But bear with me through a few paragraphs and let's see if we may have been overlooking something of tremendous value in our rush to throw out centuries' worth of herbal lore.

Mankind has always been fascinated by the concept of the panacea, one chemical, plant, magic water, or other food substance that would cure all disease, grant eternal youth, and guarantee continuing virility. Of course, no one has yet found such a miraculous substance, but the search for wonder drugs and the desire to possess perfect health have not abated over the centuries.

At certain times, practitioners of herbal medicine have been guilty of promoting magic elixirs. Panaceas can be found in the folk literature of practically every country in the world. The search for the fountain of youth goes on. In our own country we experienced the great "snake oil" era. Many of the snake oil medicines were little more than straight ethyl alcohol. Others were considerably more genuine in both their claims and their real therapeutic action. Panaceas have existed in several forms, including pills, teas and tinctures, but the most popular in the West has been the liquid extract. European traditions are replete with liquid extracts for the heart, the liver, for digestion and elimination, for nervousness and many other purposes. These are traditionally compounded from several different herbs, and may include nonherbal items such as supplemental iron or other vitamins and minerals. Traveling from one part of Europe to the next, one can find elixirs that are unique to each region and take advantage of local flora, but many are mass-produced and sold throughout the continent. Some of these have even made it to America.

This author has been fascinated by the concept of the liquid tonic for several years. I find myself continually playing with possible combinations of herbs that would make a good product. The idea of a true "panacea" is probably not attainable, but it seems that certain herbs are more likely than others to affect the health of many different body systems. By choosing and combining just the right ones in the just the right way, one could possibly produce a series of synergistic interactions like the way a key acts on the tumblers of a lock, that would then open the way for improved body function.

By carefully selecting plants from around the world, we are capable today of building terrific herbal liquid tonics that don't rely on the "shotgun" approach that has characterized most of the regional elixirs. (The shotgun approach is to put in a little bit of dozens of different plants hoping for therapeutic synergy.) As few as a dozen top-ranked plants (perhaps including a couple of lesser-known herbs, but personal favorites), if properly combined, is about all that is required to produce an effective liquid herbal tonic. The formulation of an herbal elixir is more than a mathematical equation derived from scientific research. It has a personal component that reflects one's own experience and needs. This should be kept in mind while reading the following paragraphs that contain this author's recommendations for just a few herbs that may constitute an effective herbal liquid extract of the elixir variety.

In the current implementation, the immune system would be a primary target. Long before medical science got around to recognizing the importance or even the existence of the immune system, herbal medicine was routinely dealing with the more important aspects of that system. Remember the "blood purifiers," or the "alteratives"? These were nothing less than immune system stimulators, modulators and regulators. And herbal medicine had developed the application of these materials to a very high level. In this area, modern medicine is still very primitive, relying as it does almost exclusively on antimicrobial drugs that weaken the immune system even as they destroy certain strains of germs (and create more resistant strains in the process).

Of the many immunomodulators in the plant kingdom, I think the best are *lapacho, echinacea, astragalus, yerba maté, licorice root,* and all species of *ginseng.* I needn't even depart from the findings of scientific research to state that these herbs have been found to impact just about every aspect of immune system functioning, from the production and stabilization of whole blood cells to the activation of the complement, to the inhibition of allergic reactions, to the regulation of blood platelet activity. The so-called "blood purifiers" of herbal lore also included several that are now known to be antioxidants or free radical scavengers. A few of the herbs already mentioned have this property. Another is *chaparral,* a Southwest American plant utilized by Indians, Mexicans and Whites for centuries to treat and prevent serious immune disorders such as cancer, skin infections and so forth. Working nicely in combination with chaparral and echinacea is *sarsaparilla* or smilax to help maintain the integrity of the body's connective tissues.

Smilax together with ginseng and yerba mate would act to enhance the physical development of muscle tissue. These would help oxygenate cells and help them burn calories. The entire musculoskeletal system would benefit.

Another target of a good herbal liquid tonic should be the cardiovascular system. This is an easy one. *Hawthorn* is without a doubt the world's best cardiotonic plant. Hawthorn combined with ginseng, yerba maté and astragalus would help strengthen the heart muscle, help reduce high blood pressure (without affecting normal blood pressure), would help prevent the absorption of cholesterol and would slowly help remove plaque from the walls of arteries.

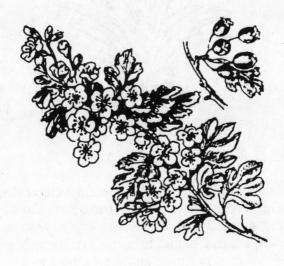

HAWTHORN

Liquid extracts always try to favorably affect the digestive system and often contain a dozen or more plants chosen for this one purpose. That really isn't necessary if the right herbs are chosen in the first place. A simple combination of licorice root, yerba mate, ginseng and *aloe vera* has a remarkably tonic effect on digestion or "constitution" as well as disorders of the gastrointestinal tract, including ulcers, colitis, flatulence and heartburn.

In a related fashion, aloe and licorice root help to maintain the liver, gallbladder, adrenal glands and other organs in good health, repelling disease and increasing effectiveness.

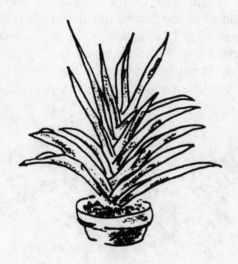

ALOE VERA

Last but certainly not least, I believe a modern elixir should address energy production. Utilizing herbs to help enhance the body's energy production processes has always been a problem. The solution in a liquid extract is to combine the only really good herbs for this effect, yerba maté and ginseng species.

The above formulation embodies the liquid extract idea in its truest sense, but differs from most others in some dramatic ways. First, it contains significant amounts of the South American herb yerba maté. This would give the product a natural energy wallop not shared by other liquid herbal extracts. This natural energy would not interfere with the ability to sleep. On the contrary, it would help regulate sleep cycles and produce a better sleep. It would also allow one to work longer without fatigue, get more done, and feel better about doing it. Indirectly, then, the nervous system benefits, as stress and anxiety are reduced, muscle tension lessens and performance effectiveness increases.

This formulation also differs from most in that it contains superior whole-body tonics from all over the world. These are compounded with the idea of helping to restore balance that is often lost in the day-to-day battles of life, to restore or optimize the delicate balance between mind, body and the emotions that governs daily performance and efficiency. Balance, or homeostasis, is critical to maintaining health and inhibiting the degenerative forces of stress. Imbalance, or loss of homeostasis, leads to sickness, depression, painful inflammation, loss of appetite, constipation, nervousness, sleeplessness, muscle aches, fatigue, etc.

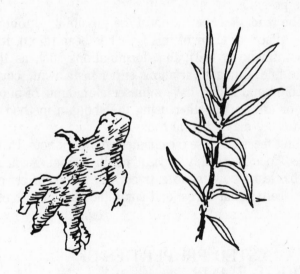

GINGER

A good tonic might also contain a couple of lesser-known plants that are personal favorites. A couple that fit this category for this author that have very nice synergistic action with the other plants in this formulation are *ginger* and *stillingia*. The latter was a popular blood purifier of the 19th century. So far stillingia has not been subjected to a great deal of basic holistic research. Nevertheless, it should be considered a valuable ingredient in any herbal tonic. Ginger root acts as a catalyst to the whole brew, and provides a small amount of zest on its own. The digestive system will accept the entire tonic much more readily with the presence of a little ginger root.

In summary, there is a place in our modern world for herbal liquid elixirs. They may not be panaceas in the true sense of that word, but if compounded properly they can help to maintain the vitality of many of the body's systems and help to rejuvenate a person when he or she is sick or otherwise on the down side of life. These herbs may not bring eternal youth, but they can help make you feel better longer, and retain a youthful appearance, attitude and behavior through many more years than otherwise possible.

If the reader's expectation of the possibility of obtaining in the marketplace an elixir of this type has been raised, it may be a disappointment to learn that formulations such as these are difficult to find. Current variations either taste awful, contain too much alcohol and sugar, have minuscule amounts of pure herbal extracts, or are put together using the shotgun method, and do not contain the major herbal tonics.

I don't mean to close the chapter on a dark note. Readers are encouraged to explore this concept on their own. Acquire a few good herbs, learn how to do extracts (e.g., a *tea* is an extract!). Have fun, learn about herbs, and enjoy the natural side of life.

TEN SUGGESTED PROPERTIES OF AN HERBAL ELIXIR

1. Restores and maintains homeostasis or balance to body systems.

2. Substantially increases production of energy through normal metabolic means.

3. Increases resistance to infectious disease by enhancing the immune system.

4. Decreases stress and anxiety, and increases ability to perform as well as to rest and sleep.

5. Guards against excessive free radical damage by supplying antioxidant activity.

6. Increases body's ability to build new muscle tissue and to lose weight by burning more calories.

7. Regulates digestive processes and prevents indigestion, ulcers, colitis, heartburn and related ailments.

8. Provides substances that strengthen the heart; reduces cholesterol, normalizes blood pressure and prevents undue clotting.

9. Helps keep the liver and related organs and glands in good health.

10. Helps keep bowel movements regular and smooth.

Glossary

Acetylcholine   a chemical neurotransmitter substance secreted at neural synapses of the parasympathetic nervous system and at the neuromuscular junction, in the brain and elsewhere. Facilitates the transmission of a nerve impulse from one neuron or nerve to the next.

Acute   describes a condition that comes on suddenly and lasts for a comparatively short period of time (with appropriate treatment); contrasted with chronic.

Adaptogen   A term coined by Russian scientists to describe the action of Siberian ginseng. Generally, any substance that increases the body's nonspecific resistance to stress or disease; specifically, any substance that acts on the body in a like manner to Siberian ginseng.

Adipose   fatty or fat-containing tissue. White adipose tissue is where the body stores excess calories. Brown adipose tissue burns excess calories so they are not deposited as fat.

Adrenergic   Of or referring to the action of adrenaline (epinephrine) or noradrenaline (norepinephrine); of or referring to the action of the sympathetic nervous system. Opposite of cholinergic.

Aerobic   In the presence of oxygen. Generally refers to metabolism that depends upon oxygen.

Alimentary canal   Another name for the digestive tract, the tube that runs from the mouth to the anus.

Alkaloid   Any of a group of mostly naturally occurring chemicals that contain nigrogen, including caffeine, ephedrine, nicotine, cocaine, morphine and digitalis.

Allergen Any substance that causes an allgeric reaction in the body.

Alterative A substance, typically an herb, that gently detoxifies the bloody and enhances liver, kidney and skin clearance of waste products and toxins.

Alzheimer's disease Formerly called presenile dementia; a condition in which the brain progressively degenerates with age, but before old age.

Anaerobic Living in the absence of oxygen; in contrast to aerobic.

Androgen A general term for any male sex hormone.

Antispasmodics Substances that ameliorate muscle spasms, usually in smooth muscle.

Antioxidant (See Free radical scavenger)

Arteriosclerosis Hardening of the arteries; loss of elasticity of artery wall.

Atherosclerosis A condition characterized by fatty deposits inside medium-to-large arteries that narrow the diameter of the vessel, thereby impairing the flow of blood.

Autonomic nervous system That division of the nervous system that controls involuntary functions, such as heartbeat, blood pressure, and glandular activity. Divided into the sympathetic and parasympathetic systems.

Balance Used in this book to refer to the condition of a body system in which all functions and processes are functioning at optimum levels, i.e., not in a hypo- or a hyper-state of activity.

Bidirectional Refers to the peculiar action of a tonic substance (herb) to restore balance or homeostasis to a body system or a particular function of a body system, no matter which direction current function deviates from normal or optimum; i.e., the ability to either increase or decrease a particular physiological process, depending on the current needs of the body.

Bile Bitter, greenish-yellow fluid produced by the liver and stored in the gallbladder; released into the small intestine to aid in the digestion of fats.

Bitter   A plant that tastes bitter and has the ability to stimulate the secretion of digestive juices throughout the digestive tract.

Body system   A group of organs, glands and other body structures that performs one of several major functions for the body. Examples include the digestive, cardiovascular, reproductive and immune systems.

Cataract   A clouding of the lens of the eye.

Catarrh   Excessive secretion of mucus from the nose and throat as the result of an upper respiratory tract infection.

Cathartic   A strong laxative.

Chilblains   Local swelling, reddening and pain or itching in the fingers, toes, ears or nose that is caused by poor circulation.

Cholagogue   A substance that stimulates the production, storage and release of bile.

Choleretic   A substance that increases the flow of bile from the gallbladder.

Cholinergic   Of or pertaining to the action of acetylcholine, an important neurotransmitter which is generally concerned with anabolic actions, but also critical to proper muscular contraction.

Choliokinetic   A substance that increases the contractive power of the bile duct, resulting in an increased discharge of bile from the gallbladder into the small intestine.

Chronic   Persistent illness; opposed to acute.

Chronotropic   Pertaining to the slowing down of the heartbeat.

Cirrhosis   Chronic liver disease characterized by the destruction of healthy cells and proliferation of fatty or fibrous tissue.

Coldsore   A small sore on or near the lips caused by the herpes simplex virus. May also occur in genital region.

Collagen   Tough, fibrous protein that is a major constituent of connective tissue.

Complement   A series of proteins circulating in the bloodstream that increase the effectiveness of antibodies and phagocytes, and that selectively attack and destroy bacteria.

Cushing's syndrome   A group of symptoms caused by the overproduction of the hormone hydrocortisone and other adrenal hormones: swelling of face and neck, high blood pressure, acne, muscle wasting, obesity, excesive body hair.

Detoxification   The process of eliminating toxic wastes and foreign materials from the bloodstream, lympathatic system, digestive system and other parts of the body.

Duct   Any narrow canal or passageway for secretions or fluids.

Ductless glands   (See Endocrine glands)

Dysmenorrhea   Difficult or painful menstruation.

Edema   Swelling in any part of the body that results from the buildup of fluid in cavities and tissues.

Emetic   Any substance that when swallowed induces vomiting.

Endocrine glands   Glands without ducts that secret hormones directly into the bloodstream. Distinct from exocrine glands.

Endorphin   A type of chemical found in the brain that has tranquilizing and painkilling properties.

Enterohepatic circulation   A special bloodstream circuit that recycles between the stomach and the liver: substances caught up in enterohepatic circulation may pass many times through the liver before being finally filtered out.

Enzyme   Proteinaceous chemicals which act as catalysts to control many biochemical processes within the body and that speed up those actions.

Equilibrium   (See Balance)

Erysipelas   A painful skin infection caused by streptococcal bacteria; marked by redness and swelling on the scalp, face or legs.

Exocrine Glands   Glands that secrete fluids through a duct or tube. Distinct from endocrine glands.

Fatty acids   A common series of organic acids usually formed as breakdown products of fats during digestion.

Feedback mechanisms   The measures the body takes to self-regulate internal processes to help maintain blanace and homeostasis. They involve a system's ability to measure the amount of a reaction and institute appropriate controls, often by glandular secretion. The levels of most circulating hormones are regulated by feedback mechanisms.

Flavonoids   A group of plant substances that affect the body in a variety of different ways, usually in a tonic fashion, to help restore health to blood vessels, cell membranes and other critical parts of the body. Examples: bioflavonoids, quercetin, rutin.

Free radicals Charged particles, or ions, usually of oxygen, that are produced during normal metabolic processes, or that may be ingested in air, food and water, which have the potential of damaging body cells, especially cell membranes and DNA.

Free radical scavengers Substances produced by the body or consumed in many foods which neutralize free radicals; sometimes called anitoxidants or oxygen scavengers.

Gamma globulin A globulin protein in the blood which plays an important role in the immune system. Globulins are a group of proteins sometimes called antibodies, including alpha, beta and gamma.

GAS (General adaptation syndrome) Proposed by Hans Seyle, the GAS describes the body's reactions to stressors and stress and details how the body deals with them, first by adapting, and finally by exhaustion.

GL/GLA Glycyrrhizin and glycyrrhetinic acid; two of the primary active constituents of licorice root; the molecules from which modern anti-ulcer drugs (e.g. carbenoxolone sodium) are formed.

Glaucoma A group of painful eye disorders involving raised pressure in the fluid inside the eye; caused by a narrowing or blockage of the narrow channel that carries fluid away from the eye into the veins.

Glucocorticoid hormones Adrenal cortical hormones that affect numerous important body processes, including the metabolism of carbohydrates.

Ground substance The connective tissue surrounding and connecting the body's cells.

Guaranteed potency herb An herb or herbal extract that has been standardized to contain a fixed amount of a certain ingredient or class of ingredient, which standarized product has been subjected to a substantial amount of research to establish the product's safety and efficacy, which might differ significantly from random samples of raw, unstandardized material.

Hepatic   Pertaining to the liver.

Hepatoprotection   The ability of a substance to protect the liver from the adverse effects of a variety of toxic dietary substances.

Hepatotoxic   Harmful to the liver; many dietary substances contain constituents that damage the liver as it tries to filter them out.

Hepatitis   Inflammation of the liver, most commonly caused by a viral infection.

Homeopathy   A form of medicine based on the idea of treating a disorder with very small amounts of drugs which in a healthy person would produce identical symptoms if administered in large amounts. Inoculation is a comparable idea in orthodox medicine.

Homeostasis   The condition of a body system or process when all aspects are in balance; see Balance.

Hydrocortisone   Cortisol; an important adrenalcortical hormone that regulates the metabolism and action of glucose, fats, and water.

Hypercholesterolemia   The presence of too much cholesterol in the blood; opposite of hypocholesterolemia.

Hyperglycemia   The presence of too much sugar in the blood; opposite of hypoglycemia.

Hyperlipidemia   The presence of too much lipid in the blood; opposite of hypolipidemia.

Hyperpermeability   A pathological condition of the blood vessels in which they become too leaky; leads to the loss of fluids and nutrients from the bloodstream before they reach target organs and tissues.

Hypertension   High blood pressure; opposite of hypotension or low blood pressure.

Hypothalamus   An important structure in the brain that helps regulate pituitary gland secretions and also coordinates the action of the autonomic nervous system.

Infection   Invasion of body tissues by harmful or pathogenic organisms, including viruses, bacteria, fungi and protozoans.

Inflammation   A set of symptoms resulting from the body's reaction to injury or infection. Connective tissues, mucous membranes and blood vessels are most affected. Redness, pain, heat and swelling are characteristic symptoms.

Inotropic Pertaining to the increase of cardiac contractility.

Interstitial space The space between body cells, usually filled with lymph and blood capillaries as well as nutrients traveling from capillaries to cells.

Ischemia Reduced blood supply to a part of the body, resulting in reduced oxygen and nutrient availability to cells.

Ketosis A condition that occurs when fat instead of sugar is used for providing energy; results in building of ketones released when fatty acids are broken down; occurs during starvation, diabetes and other disorders.

Laxative A substance that stimulates the emptying of the bowel; treatment for constipation; may be habituating, or may be toning.

Lupus Any one of a number of chronic diseases that attack the skin; lupus vulgaris is tuberculosis of the skin, marked by facial lesions; lupus erythematosus is an inflammatory disease of the connective tissue, marked by a scaly red rash on the face.

Lymphatic system A network of vessels throughout the body that carry lymph from interstitial spaces to the bloodstream. Lymph glands are located throughout the lymph system, which is the site of many immune system reactions.

Lymphocytes A type of leucocyte or white blood cell responsible for the neutralization of specific allergens and antigens, in contrast to nonspecific resistance provided by phagocytes.

Lymphokines Humoral substances produced by white blood cells that regulate numerous immune system activities.

Mast cell A type of basophil; a histamine-containing component of the immune system that circulates throughout the body and mediates the inflammatory response as well as the allergic reaction.

Neurotransmitter Any one of dozens of natural chemicals that are responsible for transmitting or regulating the transmission of electrochemical potentials from one nerve to another across microscopic gaps called synapses.

Oxygen scavengers (See Free radical scavengers)

Parasympathetic nervous system   Part of the autonomic nervous system mainly involved in anabolic, regenerative processes; contrasted to the sympathetic nervous system.

Phagocytosis   The process by which white blood cells called phagocytes or feeding cells engulf and destroy foreign substances, such as bacteria.

Pituitary gland   Hypophysis; an outgrowth from the underside of the brain that secretes hormones that regulate the function of many other glands.

Platelets   Small, disk-shaped bodies in the blood that adhere to one another to form blood clots.

Platelet aggregation   Refers to the process by which platelets adhere to one another to form blood clots.

Prostaglandins   Highly active fatty acid derivatives that affect dozens of metabolic processes. Taken together, their actions are often bidirectional, or tonic, in nature.

Quercetin   A major flavonoid found in many plants that helps maintain the health of cell membranes, among other things.

Renal insufficiency   The reduced capacity of the kidneys to filter and otherwise function appropriately.

Renin   An enzyme produced by the kidneys whose function it is to raise blood pressure.

RES   Reticuloendothelial system. A network of cells and tissues, found throughout the body, concerned with the formation and destruction blood cells, the storage of fatty materials, the metabolism of iron and pigment, and the course of inflammation and immune responses.

Retina   The light-sensitive cells that line the back of the eye.

Sclerosis   Hardening of tissues or organs because of the growth of fibrous tissue within them or the accretion of material upon them.

Spasm   The sudden involuntary contractin of a muscle.

Standardization, herbal   The process by which certain components of a plant are fixed in a given amount. In practice, it means repeated testing of raw materials to insure the presence of a predetermined amount of one or more chemicals and families of chemicals thought to be responsible for the activity of the plant, or whose concentration is thought to co-vary with the active principles. It may also involve extracting certain fractions of plant material in order to increase the natural concentration, and then, if desired, returning the extracted, concentrated material to a bed of raw herb to maintain some semblance of wholeness.

Stenosis   The abnormal narrowing of a tube or duct in the body, either by accretion of material within the tube, or by thickening of the tube wall.

Stress   A mental and/or physical reaction to overpowering physiological or environmental forces. Such forces cause fear, worry, depression or prolonged excitement, and put huge demands on the body's ability to respond appropriately.

Stressor   Any stimulus that produces a stress reaction.

Sympathetic nervous system   That division of the autonomic nervous system that coordinates the body's different responses to stressors and stress. Prepares the body for emergency action by speeding up the heartbeat, dilating the pupils, relaxing the bladder, etc.

Suppuration   The process of forming and discharging pus.

Synapse   A microscopic gap that separates the end of one neuron from the beginning of the next; the junction between nerves.

System   (See Body system)

Tolerance   The body's ability to endure the effects of pain or of a drug or poison; tolerance to drugs builds up by consumption of progressively larger doses over a prolonged period, and represent one aspect of addiction.

Tonic   Any substance that acts to restore balance, homeostasis or tone to a body system or any aspect of a body system; possessing a bidirectional effect on a body system, tissue or process through which it correct hypo- or hyper-types of deviations from a balanced state.

Toxemia   The presence of bacterial toxins in the blood; sometimes called blood poisoning.

Unidirectional   Describing the action of nontonic substances which tend to push a body system, tissue or process in just one direction, either to decrease or increase activity.

Urea   A chemical formed in the liver from ammonia derived from proteins; found in the blood, urine and lymph.

Index

devil's claw (*Harpagophytum procumbens*), 281
diabetes, 37, 214; herbs that treat
astragalus, 55
bilberry, 136
dandelion, 239
devil's claw, 281
lapacho relieves, 71
Siberian ginseng for, 194
diarrhea, herbs that prevent
linden treats, 190
red raspberry for, 318
turmeric for, 251
digestion, digestive system, 202–
255; herbs that improve
(*see also* indigestion)
aloe vera, 365
balm, 200
chamomile, 187
gentian, 243
ginseng, 365
lapacho, 71
licorice, 365
peppermint, 184
saw palmetto berry, 288
schizandra, 59–62
valerian treats, 149
yerba maté, 365
digestive enzymes, 205, 207
digitalis, hawthorn berry compared
to, 101, 103–104
dihydrotestosterone (DHT), 356–357
Dioscorea spp.: *see* wild yam
diphtheria, echinacea for, 41
diuretic herbs
dandelion, 239
devil's claw, 283
horsetail, 269, 270
lapacho, 72, 81
linden flower, 191
passion flower, 159
pygeum, 342, 344
lapacho, 72
vitex, 334

diverticular disease, 212
wild yam for, 291
dizziness, herbs that prevent
schizandra, 62
ginger, 246
dong quai (*Angelica chinensis, A.
polymorphia, A. acuti-
loba*), 305–309
dopamine synthesis, ginkgo increases, 169
dropsy: *see* diuretic herbs
drug side effects, lapacho relieves,
73
dysentery, herbs that treat
lapacho, 71
miura-puama, 359
red raspberry, 318
dysmenorrhea, 300; herbs that treat
black haw, 311
dong quai, 305
passion flower, 160, 164
wild yam, 291
dyspepsia: *see* indigestion
dysuria (painful urination), 339

echinacea (*Echinacea angustifolium,
purpurea*), 17, 40–46,
292, 364; action on
immune system, 6–7,
12
Eclectic physicians, 41
eczema, 36; licorice relieves, 66,
320, 321
edema: *see* diuretic herbs
elderly, devil's claw recommended
for, 283
elecampane (*Inula helenium*), expectorant herb, 38
Eleutherococcus senticosis, 4,
192–199; *see also*
ginseng
embolism, 95
emetic, large doses of black cohosh,
332

ABOUT THE AUTHOR

Daniel B. Mowrey, Ph.D., is the author of the titles *Fat Management, Next Generation Herbal Medicine, Scientific Validation of Herbal Medicine,* and *Proven Herbal Blends.*